Medical Care of the
NURSING HOME RESIDENT

Also Available from the
American College of Physicians

American College of Physicians Ethics Manual, Third Edition

Clinical Practice Guidelines 1995

Common Diagnostic Tests: Use and Interpretation, Second edition

Common Screening Tests

Computers in Clinical Practice

Diagnostic Strategies for Common Medical Problems

Drug Prescribing in Renal Failure: Dosing Guidelines for Adults, Third edition

Ethical Choices: Case Studies for Medical Practice

Guide for Adult Immunization, Third edition

On Being A Doctor

Who Has Seen A Blood Sugar?: Reflections on Medical Education

MEDICAL *CARE* *OF THE*
NURSING HOME
RESIDENT

What Physicians Need To Know

Edited by

Richard W. Besdine, MD, FACP
Professor of Medicine and Director
Travelers Center on Aging
University of Connecticut Health Center
Farmington, Connecticut

Laurence Z. Rubenstein, MD, MPH, FACP
Professor of Medicine
UCLA School of Medicine
Los Angeles, California
Director, Geriatrics Program
Department of Veterans Affairs
VA Medical Center
Sepulveda, California

Lois Snyder, JD
Ethics and Health Policy Counsel
American College of Physicians
Philadelphia, Pennsylvania

AMERICAN COLLEGE OF PHYSICIANS
PHILADELPHIA, PENNSYLVANIA

A|C|P

Acquisitions Editor: **Mary K. Ruff**
Director of Book and Journal Publishing: **Pamela Fried**
Administrator, Book Publishing: **Diane M. McCabe**
Production Supervisor: **Patricia C. Walter**
Production Editor: **Vicki Hoenigke**
Interior Design: **Patricia C. Walter**
Cover Design: **Colleen Woods-Esposito**
Cover Art: **Michael McNelly**
Index: **Ed Yeager**

Printed in the United States of America.
Composition by ACP Graphic Services.
Printing/binding by Port City Press.
Cover printed by Port City Press.

American College of Physicians
Independence Mall West
Sixth Street at Race
Philadelphia, PA 19106-1572

Library of Congress Cataloging in Publication Data

Medical care of the nursing home resident : what physicians need to know /
   edited by Richard W. Besdine, Laurence Z. Rubenstein, Lois Snyder.
      176p. cm.
   Includes bibliographical references and index.
   ISBN: 0-943126-48-7
   1. Nursing home care.   I. Besdine, Richard W., 1940–
II. Rubenstein, Laurence Z.   III. Snyder, Lois, 1961–
   [DNLM: 1. Geriatrics. 2. Nursing Homes. WT 100 M4885 1996]
RC954.3.M43 1996
362.1' 6—dc20
DNLM/DLC
for Library of Congress
                                        96-12363
                                          CIP

96 97 98 99 00 01 / 9 8 7 6 5 4 3 2 1

CONTRIBUTORS

Cathy A. Alessi, MD
Assistant Professor of Medicine
UCLA School of Medicine
Los Angeles, California
Director, Geriatric Evaluation Services
Department of Veterans Affairs
VA Medical Center
Sepulveda, California

Jerry Avorn, MD
Associate Professor of Medicine
Harvard Medical School
Brigham and Women's Hospital
Boston, Massachusetts

Richard W. Besdine, MD, FACP
Professor of Medicine and Director
Travelers Center on Aging
University of Connecticut Health Center
Farmington, Connecticut

Christine K. Cassel, MD, FACP
Professor and Chair
The Henry L. Schwartz Department of
   Geriatrics and Adult Development
Mt. Sinai Medical Center
New York, New York

Leo Cooney, MD
Director, Continuing Care Unit
Yale–New Haven Hospital
New Haven, Connecticut

Deon Cox Hayley, DO
Assistant Professor of Medicine
University of Chicago
Department of Medicine
Chicago Illinois

Roy V. Erickson, MD
New England Regional Medical Director
Genesis Eldercare
Windsor, Connecticut
Associate Professor of Clinical Medicine
Community Medicine and Health Care
University of Connecticut Health Center
Farmington, Connecticut

James E. Fanale, MD, FACP
Chief of Geriatrics
The Medical Center of Central Massachusetts
Worcester, Massachusetts

Bruce A. Ferrell, MD, FACP
Associate Professor of Medicine
UCLA School of Medicine
Los Angeles, California
Clinical Director
Geriatric Research Education and Clinical Center
VA Medical Center
Sepulveda, California

Jerry H. Gurwitz, MD, FACP
Assistant Professor of Medicine
Harvard Medical School
Brigham and Women's Hospital
Boston, Massachusetts

Karen R. Josephson, MPH
Senior Health Services Researcher
Geriatric Research Education and Clinical Center
VA Medical Center
Sepulveda, California

Paul R. Katz, MD
Associate Professor of Medicine
University of Rochester School of Medicine
Medical Director
Monroe Community Hospital
Rochester, New York

Lawrence Markson, MD
Director of Health Care Research
Geriatrics Division
Boston University School of Medicine
Boston, Massachusetts

John E. Morley, MB, BCh
Professor of Gerontology
St. Louis University School of Medicine
Division of Geriatric Medicine
Director
Geriatric Research Education and Clinical Center
VA Medical Center
St. Louis, Missouri

Dean C. Norman, MD
Chief of Staff
West Los Angeles VA Medical Center
Associate Professor of Medicine
UCLA School of Medicine
Los Angeles, California

Dan Osterweil, MD
Associate Professor of Medicine
UCLA Multicampus Program of
  Geriatric Medicine and Gerontology
Medical Director
Jewish Home for the Aging
Reseda, California

Joseph G. Ouslander, MD
Associate Professor
UCLA Multicampus Program of
  Geriatric Medicine and Gerontology
Associate Director
UCLA Borun Center for Gerontological Research
Medical Director
Jewish Home for the Aging
Reseda, California

Alan S. Robbins, MD
Chief of Staff
Ralph H. Johnson VA Medical Center
Charleston, South Carolina

Laurence Z. Rubenstein, MD, MPH, FACP
Professor of Medicine
UCLA School of Medicine
Los Angeles, California
Director, Geriatrics Program
Department of Veterans Affairs
VA Medical Center
Sepulveda, California

Mark A. Rudberg, MD, MPH
Assistant Professor of Medicine
University of Chicago
Department of Medicine
Chicago, Illinois

John F. Schnelle, PhD
Professor
UCLA Multicampus Program of
  Geriatric Medicine and Gerontology
Director
UCLA Borun Center for Gerontological Research
Director of Research and Quality Assurance
Jewish Home for the Aging
Reseda, California

Andrew Jay Silver, MD
Private Practice
Palm Springs, California

David M. Smith, MD, FACP
Professor of Medicine
Indiana University School of Medicine
Regenstrief Institute
Indianapolis, Indiana

Lois Snyder, JD
Ethics and Health Policy Counsel
American College of Physicians
Philadelphia, Pennsylvania

Thomas T. Yoshikawa, MD, FACP
Chair, Department of Internal Medicine
Charles R. Drew University of Medicine
  and Science
King/Drew Medical Center
Los Angeles, California

CONTENTS

Preface, ix

Acknowledgments, xi

Introduction: Nursing Home Residents Need Physician Care, xiii
Richard W. Besdine, Laurence Z. Rubenstein, Lois Snyder, and *Christine K. Cassel*

PART I   *Getting Started in Nursing Home Care*

1   **Role of the Physician, 3**
James E. Fanale, Lawrence Markson, Leo Cooney, and Paul R. Katz

2   **Physician Evaluation, 15**
Joseph G. Ouslander and Dan Osterweil

PART II   *Common Clinical Conditions in the Nursing Home*

3   **Incontinence, 29**
Joseph G. Ouslander and John F. Schnelle

4   **Fever and Infection, 47**
Thomas T. Yoshikawa and Dean C. Norman

5   **Pressure Ulcers, 61**
David M. Smith

PART III   *Drugs in the Nursing Home*

6   **Drug Use, 77**
Jerry Avorn and Jerry H. Gurwitz

7   **Pain Evaluation and Management, 91**
Bruce A. Ferrell

PART IV   *Special Considerations in the Nursing Home*

8   **Falls and Their Prevention, 103**
Laurence Z. Rubenstein, Karen R. Josephson, and Alan S. Robbins

9   **Nutrition, 117**
John E. Morley and Andrew Jay Silver

10   **Rehabilitation, 131**
Roy V. Erickson

11   **Ethical and Legal Issues, 143**
Deon Cox Hayley, Christine K. Cassel, Lois Snyder, and Mark A. Rudberg

12   **Evaluation and Management of Dementia and Delirium, 155**
Cathy A. Alessi

Index, 169

PREFACE

This book is a project of the Task Force on Aging of the Health and Public Policy Committee of the American College of Physicians. Originally conceived in 1991 when Christine K. Cassel, MD, FACP, was chair, it came to completion under the leadership of the 1994–95 ACP Task Force on Aging chaired by James R. Webster, Jr., MD, FACP. The original Task Force envisioned a series of papers on medical care of the nursing home patient for publication in *Annals of Internal Medicine*. Realizing the potential reach of the papers as a resource for medical education and continuing medical education, it was then decided to compile them into a book.

Twelve papers were commissioned from among the clinical academic leadership of the geriatrics and gerontology community. The series was reviewed by Task Force members and reviewed and endorsed by the American Geriatrics Society. Some papers have been published in *Annals of Internal Medicine*, some in other publications, and others are being published for the first time in this book.

Nursing home residents need your care. We hope this book will help you in providing it.

Richard W. Besdine, MD, FACP, Editor
ACP Task Force on Aging
Laurence Z. Rubenstein, MD, MPH, FACP, Editor
ACP Task Force on Aging
Lois Snyder, JD, Associate Editor
ACP Ethics and Health Policy Counsel

June 1995

ACKNOWLEDGMENTS

The editors acknowledge the efforts of all the members of the Task Force on Aging, 1991–95, who served as reviewers of the chapters of this book:

Christine K. Cassel, MD, FACP, Chair (1991–93)
James R. Webster, Jr, MD, FACP, Chair
(1993–present)
Patricia Barry, MD, FACP
Thomas C. Cesario, MD, FACP
William J. Hall, MD, FACP
Frederick F. Holmes, MD, FACP
Risa Lavizzo-Mourey, MD, MBA, FACP
Francis A. Salerno, MD, FACP
Mark E. Williams, MD, FACP
T. Franklin Williams, MD, FACP
Linda Hiddeman Barondess, American
Geriatrics Society Liaison

We would also like to express gratitude to former ACP staff member Linda Johnson White, Director of Scientific Policy, and to Linda J. Harris and Tom Shotkin for manuscript preparation. Many thanks also go to Pamela Fried, Patricia C. Walter, and the staff of the Publishing Division at the American College of Physicians.

******

Early in the review process, the Task Force recognized that important educational goals would be realized by distributing this book to medical students and residents. To that end, we have received generous support from the Merck Company Foundation to print and distribute the book nationwide to fourth-year medical students and residents in internal medicine and family practice.

The Merck Company Foundation is proud to support this book on the care of persons, including older persons, in nursing homes. Merck is committed to "healthy aging" through the support of education of health professionals and students and through other efforts to improve the care of elderly persons.

Our mutual goal is to provide a resource to help you in providing optimal care to your nursing home patients.

The following chapters have been published elsewhere as journal articles and are presented here in their entirety or with minor revisions, with permission of the respective publishers.

Introduction: *Introduction: Nursing Home Residents Need Physician Care*
Richard W. Besdine, Laurence Z. Rubenstein, Lois Snyder, and Christine K. Cassel
Annals of Internal Medicine. 1994;120(7):616-8

Chapter 1: *Role of the Physician*
James E. Fanale, Lawrence Markson, Leo Cooney, and Paul R. Katz
Journal of the American Geriatrics Society. 1996

Chapter 2: *Physician Evaluation and Management of Nursing Home Residents*
Joseph G. Ouslander and Dan Osterweil
Annals of Internal Medicine. 1994;120(7):584-92

Chapter 3: *Incontinence in the Nursing Home*
Joseph G. Ouslander and John F. Schnelle
Annals of Internal Medicine. 1995;122(6):438-49

Chapter 4: *Approach to Fever and Infection in the Nursing Home*
Thomas T. Yoshikawa and Dean C. Norman
Journal of the American Geriatrics Society. 1996;44(1):74-82

Chapter 5: *Pressure Ulcers in the Nursing Home*
David M. Smith
Annals of Internal Medicine. 1995;123(6):433-42

Chapter 6: *Drug Use in the Nursing Home*
Jerry Avorn and Jerry H. Gurwitz
Annals of Internal Medicine. 1995;123(3):195-204

Chapter 7: *Pain Evaluation and Management in the Nursing Home*
Bruce A. Ferrell
Annals of Internal Medicine. 1995;123(9):681-7

Chapter 8: *Falls in the Nursing Home*
Laurence Z. Rubenstein, Karen R. Josephson, and Alan S. Robbins
Annals of Internal Medicine. 1994;121(6):442-51

Chapter 9: *Nutritional Issues in Nursing Home Care*
John E. Morley and Andrew Jay Silver
Annals of Internal Medicine. 1995;123(11):850-9

Chapter 11: *Ethical and Legal Issues in Nursing Home Care*
Deon Cox Hayley, Christine K. Cassel, Lois Snyder, and Mark A. Rudberg
Archives of Internal Medicine. February 12, 1996;156:249-56

INTRODUCTION

"I am an 84-year-old woman. I have severe arthritis, and about 5 years ago, I broke my hip. As I look around this room, I see the pathetic ones (maybe the lucky ones) who have lost their minds, and the poor souls who should be out but nobody comes to get them, and the sick ones who are in pain. A doctor comes to see me once a month. He spends 3 to 5 seconds with me and then a few more minutes writing in the chart or joking with the nurses (My own doctor doesn't come to convalescent hospitals, so I had to take this one). I pray every night that I may die in my sleep and get this nightmare over with ..." (1).

After reading such a "testimonial," we are relieved that neither we nor anyone we care about lives in a nursing home. Alternatively, if a friend or relative resides in a nursing home, we hope that "hers is different." But more and more Americans can expect to be admitted to a nursing home.

Why should independent, middle-aged adults worry about what goes on in nursing homes? Only 5% of Americans older than 65 years live in nursing homes, and only 10% are admitted in 1 year (2). Some go home, some die, and some remain; that's not so bad. But a more detailed analysis is less comforting. Of persons who were 65 years of age in 1990, 43% will enter a nursing home in their lifetimes; 55% of these will stay at least 1 year, and 21% will stay 5 years or longer (3). The remarkable yet continuing increases in life expectancy, even among the very old (4), strongly suggest that nursing home use will increase because use is strongly associated with age (2), even adjusted for disability. Currently, 1.5 million Americans live in nursing homes; by the year 2030, this number will increase

to 5 million (5,6). In addition, the cost of nursing home care is a sleeping giant. It was $53 billion in 1990 and was the fastest growing component of major health care expense in the national budget (7). It is estimated that the cost in the year 2000 will exceed $140 billion (8); in the year 2030, costs may exceed $700 billion. Because the use and costs of nursing home care are booming, efforts to improve that care are especially important.

Although increased nursing home use by older Americans can confidently be predicted, the real problem is a disturbing shortage of physicians willing to provide care for nursing home residents. Only 1 in 10 primary care physicians spends more than 2 hours per week providing care in nursing homes (9). Although 60% of physicians who visit nursing homes are internists, they spend less time in nursing home care than do family physicians (unpublished data). As with primary care providers, many of the physicians who do visit their patients when they are admitted to nursing homes are themselves older and therefore likely to stop practicing soon; the mismatch between a growing nursing home population and a shrinking pool of physicians willing to attend those patients is yet another maldistribution problem in physician resources. How we train physicians in nursing home care is a moot question until more physicians are recruited to provide care in nursing homes. But the knowledge base is an exciting one, and the challenge to master and apply it to patients in need is itself a recruiting strategy.

Our 84-year-old correspondent suggests that physician practice in the nursing home deserves attention. This book reviews the knowledge base in nursing home care and is directed primarily toward the nongeriatrician. Clinical care and related issues specific to nursing home residents are addressed; careful attention is given to avoid duplication of general information on geriatrics and gerontology now available in many fine texts.

The professional satisfactions of nursing home care are substantial (10). Grateful patients, attentive and motivated staff, advanced pathologic conditions with classic physical findings, and the opportunities to make a difference in a patient's quality of life and sense of self-worth and to master intensive geriatric care are rewards available to physicians who are receptive to learning geriatrics and applying it to nursing home residents. The absence of geriatrics and principles of nursing home care from the medical education of most currently practicing physicians has led to ignorance of the nursing home, negative attitudes toward nursing homes and their residents, and unfamiliarity with the process of nursing home care.

Although the many disincentives for primary care physicians to continue caring for their patients who are admitted to nursing homes must be acknowledged and addressed, none is unique or insurmountable. Travel time and distraction from office- or hospital-based practice, low and slow reimbursement, volumes of paperwork, staff who appear less technically sophisticated than those in hospital or office settings, patients who usually do not get better and go home, and chronic clinical problems that are frustrating and difficult to manage make many good and caring clinicians reluctant to go to the nursing home. And yet those who do care for nursing home residents describe clinical and intellectual satisfactions from meeting human needs that would otherwise be neglected or mishandled. Further, many features of nursing home care are changing with implementation of the Omnibus Budget Reconciliation Act of 1987, which was begun in 1990. This legislation, directed at improving quality of care in nursing homes, mandated 1) a Minimum Data Set to objectively collect clinical information on nursing home residents; 2) standards for training nurses' aides; 3) a reduction in the use of physical and pharmacologic restraints; and 4) a redefinition of the measures used to assess quality. These regulations emphasize improving outcomes of care rather than the previous endless documentation of care; early evaluations indicate that nursing home residents are substantially better off.

There are several additional specific reasons to master and provide nursing home care. Many nursing home residents can and do go to the physician's office for ambulatory care, and nearly all are admitted at some time to a hospital for acute illnesses. It seems sensible for the physician providing office and hospital care to know about and direct care in the nursing home. It is commonly assumed that nursing home residents remain in that setting for life, but many of those admitted return to the community; of Medicaid admissions (best data available) in California, more than one third are discharged to their homes within 6 months (11). The rate for all admissions is estimated to be one half (12). The increasing use of nursing home beds for short-term rehabilitation or other "step-down" care to shorten hospital stay makes such nursing home admissions even more likely; most physicians would probably want to continue caring for their patients during limited nursing home stays. Nursing homes with academic affiliations for teaching and research are becoming more prevalent and increase the intellectual legitimacy of nursing home care. Management of chronic disease and continuity of care over time are the mainstream responsibilities of contemporary medicine, and nursing home residents typify patients who need informed and attentive primary and chronic care. For each nursing home resident, at least two community-dwelling older persons have the same disease and disability burdens but have support systems and care providers (usually unpaid family and friends), allowing them to stay at home. Accordingly, nursing home practice prepares physicians to manage similar, if less intense and less clustered, disorders in the community.

Functional impairment is the final common pathway of most chronic diseases, especially in older persons with multiple advanced disorders (13). Initial identification of lost function, proceeding then to traditional clinical evaluation and finally to therapeutic intervention, is a method well learned in the nursing home. Functional status, best determined by use of standardized brief clinical instruments (14), is a most sensitive clinical indicator with which to follow disease progression or response to therapy in the elderly. The Minimum Data Set, completed by nurses, also assesses functional status well. Recognizing that success is measured by improved function rather than cure is also a major source of physician satisfaction in providing nursing home care. The relevance of emphasizing functional capacity cannot be overstated for older patients, regardless of where they live. Patient satisfaction and preservation or restoration of independence are crucial and dominant themes for older persons. These patients, in or out of the nursing home, are best served by physicians who recognize these priorities and have learned the principles and practice of comprehensive geriatric assessment (15,16).

Critical topics on nursing home care included in this book are 1) the role of the physician in the nursing home; 2) clinical management strategies related to admission evaluation, periodic screening, and efficient continuing care of the nursing home resident; 3) incontinence, including detection, evaluation, behavioral and pharmacologic treatment, and staff training; 4) fever and infection; 5) pressure ulcers, including evaluation, management, and prevention; 6) principles of drug use; 7) pain management; 8) falls and mobility problems; 9) nutritional issues; 10) rehabilitation; 11) ethical and legal issues; and 12) the resident with abnormal mental status.

More than 1.5 million Americans live in nursing homes; they consume a large amount of health care resources, and their number may triple in the next generation. Otherwise good and caring physicians have been insecure and hesitant in delivering care in nursing homes or have been reluctant to visit them at all for many reasons, ranging from convenience to lack of information about or comfort with the common clinical problems encountered. Primary care of older adults increasingly will include the complex clinical issues of care for those who are severely functionally impaired. Specialist geriatricians are not the answer to the care of frail older patients in the community or the nursing home. Generalist physicians now and in the future will be expected to provide primary care to adults of all ages, including those residing in nursing homes.

Richard W. Besdine, MD, FACP
Laurence Z. Rubenstein, MD, MPH, FACP
Lois Snyder, JD
Christine K. Cassel, MD, FACP

REFERENCES

1. Ouslander JG, Osterweil D, Morley JE. Medical Care in the Nursing Home. New York: McGraw-Hill; 1992:1-2.
2. Hing E. Use of nursing homes by the elderly: preliminary data from the 1985 National Nursing Home Survey. In: Advance Data from Vital and Health Statistics. (PHS) 87-1250. Hyattsville, MD: National Center for Health Statistics; 1987.
3. Kemper P, Murtaugh CM. Lifetime use of nursing home care. N Engl J Med. 1991; 324:595-600.
4. Manton KG. Mortality and life expectancy changes among the oldest old. In: Suzman R, Willis DP, Manton KG, eds. The Oldest Old. New York: Oxford University Press; 1992:157-82.
5. Zedlewski SR, Barnes RO, Burt MK, McBride TD, Meyer J. The Needs of the Elderly in the 21st Century. Washington, DC: The Urban Institute; 1989.
6. Doty PJ. The oldest old and the use of institutional long-term care from an international perspective. In: Suzman R, Willis DP, Manton KG, eds. The Oldest Old. New York: Oxford University Press; 1992:251-67.
7. Levit KR, Lazenby HC, Cowan CA, Letsch SW. National health care expenditures: 1990. Health Care Financing Review. 1991;13:29-54.
8. Sonnenfeld ST, Waldo DR, Lemieux JA, McKusick DR. Projections of national health expenditures through the year 2000. Health Care Financing Review. 1991;13:1-27.
9. Katz PR, Karuza J, Parker M, Tarnove L. A national survey of medical directors. Journal of Medical Direction. 1992;2:47-9.
10. Ouslander JG, Osterweil D. Physician evaluation and management of nursing home residents. Ann Intern Med. 1994;120:584-92.
11. Ray WA, Federspiel CF, Baugh DK, Dodds S. Experience of a Medicaid nursing home entry cohort. Health Care Financing Review. 1989;10:51-63.
12. Liu K, Manton KG. The characteristics and utilization pattern of an admission cohort of nursing home patients (II). Gerontologist. 1984; 24:70-7.
13. Besdine RW. The educational utility of comprehensive functional assessment in the elderly. J Am Geriatr Soc. 1983;31:651-6.
14. Applegate WB, Blass JP, Williams TF. Instruments for the functional assessment of older patients. N Engl J Med. 1990;322:1207-14.
15. American College of Physicians. Comprehensive functional assessment for elderly patients. Ann Intern Med. 1988;109:70-2.
16. National Institutes of Health Consensus Development Statement. Geriatric Assessment Methods for Clinical Decisionmaking. J Am Geriatr Soc. 1988; 36:342-7.

PART I

Getting Started
in Nursing Home Care

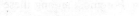

1

Role of the Physician

James E. Fanale, MD, FACP, Lawrence Markson, MD,
Leo Cooney, MD, and Paul R. Katz, MD

Negative attitudes about nursing homes, nursing home residents, and nursing home physicians are prevalent among health professionals and the lay public. These attitudes are rooted in the history of nursing homes. As recently as the early 1900s, nursing homes were warehouses for the indigent and mentally disturbed of all ages, and the care delivered in these settings was notoriously poor and unregulated.

The nursing home began to evolve into its present form in 1935, when the Social Security Act was passed. This legislation provided funds for older persons that could be used for institutional long-term care. Unfortunately, the mechanisms for assuring quality of care were not addressed, with that being left to the individual states, whose efforts were largely ineffectual. It was not until 1965, with the passage of Title 18 (XVIII) and Title 19 (XIX) of the Social Security Act (Medicare/Medicaid), that the federal government began to play an important role in overseeing the quality of nursing home care (1).

Despite increased and seemingly intense scrutiny, a consensus that care in the nursing home remained inferior persisted throughout the 1970s and early 1980s. In response to such concerns and to the limited impact of the Health Care Financing Administration on the quality of health care in the nursing home, the Institute of Medicine undertook an extensive review of nursing home practices in 1983. The final report by the Institute of Medicine highlighted an array of deficiencies and made a series of recommendations for improving nursing home care (2). These recommendations included suggestions to increase the professional level of the nursing staff in nursing homes, enhance the rights of residents, and shift from process-based to outcome-based criteria in the assessment of quality. Most recommendations made by the Institute of Medicine were incorporated into law with the passage of the Nursing Home Reform Amendments of the Omnibus Budget Reconciliation Act of 1987, discussed later in this chapter (3).

Although many physicians care for nursing home patients, such care generally has not been viewed as a prestigious type of practice. This perception has arisen in part from the nursing home's historical reputation for poor quality of care. In addition, rigid regulatory and reimbursement policies can be significant barriers to physician participation in nursing home care. Ironically, many of these policies arose as a response to physicians' reluctance to provide care in the nursing home.

This chapter presents an overview of the nursing home setting and describes proper roles for the physician in this setting. Foremost among these roles is that of primary care provider. Care of the nursing home patient can be a challenging and fulfilling practice that reinforces the most fundamental rewards of medicine.

3

THE NURSING HOME AS A SETTING FOR CARE

Demographic Trends

It has been estimated that for persons who reach the age of 65 years, the risk of nursing home admission before death exceeds 40% (4). Although only 5% of the elderly are institutionalized at any given time, admission to a nursing home increases from 1% for men and women 65 to 74 years of age to 15% for men and 25% for women 85 years of age and older (5). As this "old-old" subset of the older population increases, the number of nursing home residents is expected to exceed two million by the turn of the century. Depending on assumptions made regarding mortality, the number of nursing home residents may balloon to between 3.6 and 5.9 million by the year 2040. In that same year, the subset of nursing home residents who are 85 years or older may include two or three times the number of all residents 65 years of age and older in nursing homes today (5).

Resident Characteristics

The typical nursing home resident is characterized by substantial impairments in some or all of the physical activities of daily living, such as feeding, bathing, ambulating, and bowel and bladder function. The prevalence of mental disorders, especially dementia and depression, is extremely high, exceeding 90% in some studies (6). Table 1.1 compares selected characteristics of nursing home residents with those of community-residing elderly persons.

Since the implementation of the prospective payment system (PPS) in 1983, nursing homes have served an increasingly ill population, as evidenced by a 22% increase in the number of patients discharged from acute care in an "unstable condition" (that is, with shortness of breath, confusion, chest pain, or heart rate or blood pressure abnormality) (7). Of patients discharged to nursing homes, approximately 25% now have one or more such unstable conditions, and approximately half have one or more unresolved medical problems (for example, fever, new incontinence, and new decubiti). Among elderly patients with hip fractures, the number of physical therapy sessions has decreased, as has the maximal distance walked in the hospital and the percentage of patients discharged back to the community after the implementation of PPS (8).

Of 100 consecutive patients admitted to a hospital-based nursing home care unit after the implementation of PPS, 27% required readmission within 30 days (9), a threefold increase compared with pre-PPS rates.

As severity of illness has increased, mortality has risen. Annual death rates in American nursing homes increased from 18.9% in 1982 (pre-PPS) to 21.5% in 1985 (post-PPS); during this same period, hospital death rates decreased from 65% to 61% (10). These figures may reflect an increased mortality rate among long-term residents in nursing homes and a trend toward transferring terminally ill patients to the nursing home to die.

Service Utilization Patterns

Although the current nursing home population is generally "sicker" than previous cohorts, it remains heterogeneous. The duration of stay is less than 3 months for 45% of older persons admitted to the nursing home for conditions such as terminal illness and acute orthopedic or neurologic illnesses (for example, stroke, hip fracture) (11). These conditions generally are amenable to rehabilitation but require longer recovery times than acute-based rehabilitation units typically allow.

Although short stays account for almost half of all admissions, they account for only 5% of all nursing home days. The average duration of stay for all residents is approximately 19 months, and about two thirds of all residents die in the nursing home (11). Approximately 25% of patients discharged from the nursing home return home; of these, about half remain at home 1 year after discharge, and only 7% remain at home 2 years after discharge (12). The cause of death is determined by autopsy in less than 1% of nursing home deaths (13). Infection and cardiac decompensation figure prominently in nursing home–related morbidity and mortality and are among the most common conditions leading to transfer to the acute-care hospital.

With the rapid emergence of subacute-care units, today's nursing homes have assumed a new role in caring for even more seriously ill patients. As the duration of hospital stays continues to decrease, many more patients are now being discharged to nursing homes for acute rehabilitation, intravenous therapy, total parenteral nutrition, and other types of "subacute" care that, until recently, were delivered only in hospitals. Because these patients require a more

TABLE 1.1. Selected characteristics of nursing home residents

Variable	Living in the Nursing Home 1985	Living in the Community 1984
Total 65+		
Number (thousands)	1,318	26,343
%	100.0	100.0
Age		
65–74, %	16.1	61.7
75–84, %	38.6	30.7
85+	45.3	7.6
Sex, %		
Men	25.4	40.8
Women	74.6	59.2
Race, %		
White	93.1	90.4
Black	6.2	8.3
Other	0.7	1.3
Marital status, %		
Widowed	67.8	34.1
Married	12.8	54.7
Never married	13.5	4.4
Divorced or separated	5.9	6.3
With living children, %	63.1	81.3
Requires assistance in, %		
Bathing	91.0	6.0
Dressing	77.6	4.3
Using toilet room	63.2	2.2
Transferring	62.6	2.8
Eating	40.3	1.1
Difficulty with bowel and/or bladder control, %	54.5	NA
Disorientation or memory impairment, %	62.6	NA
Senile dementia or chronic organic brain syndrome, %	46.9	NA

From U.S. Senate Special Committee on Aging and the American Association of Retired Persons, 1991. Aging America. Trends and Projections. Washington, D.C.: USDHHS Pub. No (FCOA) 91-28001.

intensive level of care than do traditional nursing home residents, in managing the care of the nursing home patients, the physician must play both a more active and a more central role than in recent past (14).

Medicare risk contracts are becoming an important mechanism for structuring reimbursements for health care delivered to elders. This parallels similar developments with third-party payers for other patient populations. Because managed care systems pursue the least expensive sites for delivering health services, the nursing home will become an even more important venue for delivering care to patients with subacute and severe chronic illnesses.

Staffing Patterns

The scarcity of well-trained health professionals is an important barrier to providing high-quality care in the nursing home. For example, both total nursing hours and the ratio of professional to nonprofessional nursing staff are commonly used as markers of quality of care. Much of the hands-on care in nursing homes is provided by nursing assistants, only one third of whom have a high school education; although nursing homes typically serve an extremely frail population, registered nurses account for just over 10% of all nursing home employees. On average, there is only 1 registered nurse per 49 residents in the nursing home, as compared with a 1 to 5 ratio in acute-care hospitals. Further, although the federal government has mandated minimum nursing staff requirements, one third of the nation's 19,000 nursing homes fail to meet these standards. Because registered nurses are required to be present in nursing homes only 8 hours per day, it is not surprising that 40% of nursing facilities report

6 minutes or less of registered nurse time per resident per day (15). Retention of staff in nursing homes remains difficult; professional nurses and aides may earn from 35% to 60% less than their counterparts in acute-care hospitals.

Staffing problems are not limited to the nursing profession; physician involvement in nursing homes continues to be limited, due in part to burdensome paperwork, poor reimbursement and regulatory barriers, a lack of role models during formative training years, and the travel time required to visit one or more nursing homes on a regular basis (16). Currently, only 1 in 10 primary care physicians spends more than 2 hours per week in a nursing home facility. Although internists comprise approximately 60% of all nursing home care providers, they are less likely to spend as much time in nursing homes as do their family physician counterparts (17).

The paucity of experienced and knowledgeable physicians in the nursing home has contributed to problems with information transfer between acute- and long-term-care facilities. Much of this difficulty can be traced to a lack of understanding concerning the nature and extent of information required in each setting. Examples include delayed or incomplete discharge summaries and patients sent to hospital emergency rooms without data on vital signs or updated histories; all serve to foster interinstitutional resentment. Ultimately, such practices result in inappropriate placement of patients and diminished quality of care.

THE ATTENDING PHYSICIAN IN THE NURSING HOME

Because the nursing home differs in many respects from other settings, there are several distinct clinical, organizational, and administrative skills that can be useful complements to a physician's core clinical skills (18–20).

Clinical Skills

Foremost, the attending physician in the nursing home should be an expert clinician, using basic diagnostic skills as well as an understanding of specific diseases, syndromes, and problems common in elderly residents (21,22). Examples of such processes include polypharmacy, multiple and interacting illnesses, iatrogenesis, delirium, dementia, incontinence, and malnutrition. Older nursing home residents often manifest illness in ways that are remarkably different from those of their younger counterparts. For example, an older resident with an infection or a metabolic abnormality may simply present with delirium (23). In addition, providing care for older patients requires a more detailed understanding of pharmocotherapeutics, with specific attention to drug interactions.

The approach to managing acute illness in the nursing home often differs from that used in community settings. Through careful use of existing nursing home services, the internist may be able to avoid hospitalization of patients in the treatment of certain acute problems. This, in turn, can reduce one of the more disruptive and wasteful aspects of nursing home care, that is, the frequent transfer of residents between the nursing home and the acute-care hospital. Frail elderly persons are at high risk for iatrogenic complications and functional decline during hospital stays. Further, hospitalization can initiate a cascade of intensive medical interventions that are not always consistent with the patient's preferences or best interests (24). When feasible, management of acute problems in the nursing home setting may be more efficient and cost effective, as well as more comfortable and humane for the resident and family.

The care of an acutely ill elderly patient in the nursing home setting can be one of the more challenging aspects of internal medicine. It requires a strong commitment on the part of the physician and the nursing staff and a close relationship between these professionals. The physician must often depend on nursing staff and other professionals for information about the patient's condition and response to therapy, and diagnosis and treatment must often be carried out without some of the more sophisticated laboratory and diagnostic imaging resources available in the hospital or ambulatory care setting. However, laboratory investigations such as complete blood counts, serum chemistries, urinalysis, and plain radiographs generally are available in the nursing home and can be ordered with rapid response times if necessary. Outside vendors can provide Holter monitors, echocardiograms, and other more elaborate tests in many facilities. In some settings, ventilatory support, wound care, nutritional services (including total parenteral nutrition and enteral hyperalimentation), and intravenous services (including transfusions and chemotherapy) are available.

When managing acute illness in the nursing home, nurses must apply a higher degree of clinical judgment than is required in the hospital setting, where physicians and other specialists are readily available. Physicians must act without the extensive consultative assistance available in the hospital. A physician who visits a facility regularly and develops a rapport with the staff will be better able to organize treatment modalities, such as intravenous antibiotics and fluids, aggressive diuresis, and management of cardiac and respiratory problems. Meeting such challenges and providing coordinated care to acutely ill residents also provides nursing home staff with a sense of pride in accomplishment and improved morale.

The proliferation of subacute-care units demands expert clinical skills on the part of the internist. Patients admitted for short hospitalizations frequently require intravenous medications, rehabilitation, and hyperalimentation. These patients will often need subsequent subacute clinical services, requiring the physician to visit the nursing home more frequently.

Physicians in the nursing home should also be aware of the current guidelines requiring periodic monitoring of chronic illnesses and regular screening for new illnesses and functional decline (25). Physicians should understand that there are relatively few studies that provide a scientific basis for such guidelines; current recommendations are often based on consensus, rather than scientific merit. The value of some practices, such as annual comprehensive physical examinations has been questioned. The physician must apply clinical judgment individually to each case to determine which practices are best.

Team Approach to Care

Nursing home care demands cooperation among all professionals; the physician plays an integral and a key role. Most of the personal care and contact for each resident is provided by nurses' aides, who often become very familiar with the patient. Together with the assistance of nurse, therapists, dietitians, and social workers, the resident's care is managed as a team effort. At the core of this team is the resident's personal physician, who interacts with all of these individuals.

As mandated by the Omnibus Reconciliation Act of 1987 and prescribed by the Institute of Medicine in 1983, the physician should play a pivotal role as care coordinator (2). Managed care companies often require primary care physicians to function as gatekeepers for all of the care that their patients' care. As nursing home expenditures increase, physicians will be asked to participate in certifying the level of care required by their patient and may often be required to act as gatekeepers for nursing home admissions.

Participation in team care often requires the physician to attend team meetings. Recently, subacute-care units began reimbursing physicians for this administrative activity. For other types of team conferences, such as home care planning meetings, the physician may provide prior input and direction to team members in lieu of attending the meeting.

The team approach to care in the nursing home differs in many respects from team models used in the acute-care hospital and in other settings. This is due both to the nature of resident needs as well as differences in the doctor–patient relationship. Residents are usually admitted to nursing homes because of difficulty caring for themselves, rather than because of specific medical conditions. The overall care of these residents is typically managed by a team of individuals that includes a social worker, dietitian, recreational therapist, physical therapist, occupational therapist, and the resident's own aide and nurse. This team should meet regularly to establish goals and a care plan for each resident. Physician participation is essential, because the team must be made aware of underlying conditions, prognoses, limitations to activities, and general safety in carrying out activities. For short-stay residents admitted for rehabilitation or management of an acute problem, participation by the resident's regular attending physician is particularly valuable. Patients with complex medical, social, and ethical issues can also benefit from continued participation by their primary physicians.

The need to relate effectively to the health care team sometimes makes it particularly difficult to care for a relatively small number of patients in the nursing home. A busy physician may be tempted to make occasional visits to the nursing home in the evening or on weekends, during which times other team members may not be available. The presence of the physician in a facility during regular business hours can improve communication between physician and staff and ultimately enhances quality of care.

The relationship between the physician and the nursing home resident is quite distinct from that same relationship in the office or hospital environment. The nature of these differences necessitate a team model in which responsibilities for observing, assessing, and communicating changes differ from those of the acute-care or outpatient settings.

In ambulatory settings the direct, and often long-term, patient–physician relationship is characterized by direct communication. Treatment and advice are rendered to the patient directly by the physician, with occasional involvement in the decision-making process by the patient's spouse or other family members. The patient's social, occupational, and family roles are usually well known to the primary care physician.

The realities of current physician practice patterns often require that a resident change physicians on admission to the nursing home. Without an established patient–physician relationship, knowledge of the resident's social and family roles, treatment preferences, and personality can be severely limited. Even when there is no change in physician, communication between patient and physician is usually less direct in the nursing home. Much of the resident's direct care is provided by nurses and other health professionals. Physicians communicate with the care providers primarily by telephone and therefore rely heavily on the observational skills and clinical judgment of these professionals.

In summary, the physician who cares for the nursing home resident must rely on the skills of the nursing and other professional staff to perform evaluations and interventions with an appropriate level of care. Physicians must develop rapport with team members to be comfortable when dealing with them and delegating responsibility.

Patient Advocate

A team model for care requires a certain amount of negotiation and compromise among team members to forge a consensus as to the appropriate objectives and methods of care. In such negotiations, the physician has a primary ethical obligation to act as an advocate for the patient. In the nursing home, as elsewhere, physicians are ethically obligated to represent the patient's interests in all interactions and communication with other health care team members, with outside parties and with nursing home or hospital administration (26). This point is particularly important in the long-term-care setting, where the physician may be called on to arbitrate a con-

flict or misunderstanding between residents or family and the nursing home.

Nurse Practitioners and Physician Assistants

By employing nurse practitioners and physician assistants, physicians can care for a larger group of nursing home residents than would be otherwise possible. Recent reports have demonstrated the effectiveness of nurse practitioners and physician assistants in improving the quality of care without increasing costs to the health care system (27,28).

Nurse practitioners and physician assistants are providing more nursing home care; they are now allowed to make half of all required medical care visits. In addition, many physician groups use these health professionals to provide emergency nursing home coverage. The prompt and continuing availability of a nurse practitioner or physician assistant often will allow residents to remain in the nursing home during evaluation and treatment of new or recrudescent problems. Visits made by these health professionals are reimbursed by Medicare at 85% of the physician's rate when done under the supervision of the attending physician (29).

Communication

Because the physician is not physically present at the nursing home most of the time, effective communication between physician and nursing home is critical in providing timely, quality care. Communication via the telephone can be a time-consuming process. The use of reporting protocols for events such as falls, injuries, skin tears, and consultant opinions can increase the efficiency of overall communication by requiring direct contact between physician and nurse only for clinically important issues.

In recent years, the increasing use of facsimile machines has begun to revolutionize communication between the nursing home and physician. Laboratory data, physicians' orders, and reports of various kinds can be transmitted between physician and nursing home with fewer interruptions in the daily routine of the staff. In the future, the use of electronic mail (e-mail) messages and forms may be able to make such communications even more efficient.

Effective communication must also be maintained between hospital and nursing home because care in the hospital is provided by a different team of professionals, and sometimes a different physician, from that in the nursing home. To ensure the timely transfer of pertinent information between institutions, physicians should prepare and send complete discharge and transfer summaries when the resident moves either from the hospital to the nursing home, or vice versa. At a minimum, these discharge and transfer summaries should include

1. An accurate list of the patient's current functional status, medical problems, and medications

2. Identification of the next of kin and/or surrogate decision-makers

3. Any available information relating to patient treatment preferences, including written and oral advance directives

Effective information transfer is needed to deliver appropriate care to nursing home residents in both the nursing home and hospital settings.

Quality Improvement

As mentioned earlier, most recommendations from the Institute of Medicine's review of nursing home care were incorporated into law with the passage of the Nursing Home Reform Amendments of the Omnibus Budget Reconciliation Act (OBRA) of 1987 (3). The impact of OBRA on clinical practice in the nursing home is outlined in Box 1.1. All nursing home residents must receive a comprehensive, standardized assessment within 14 days of admission and periodically thereafter upon any important change in condition. The multidisciplinary assessment specified under OBRA emphasizes evaluation of functional capacity and is recorded using standardized documentation known as the Minimum Data Set (MDS). Nursing staff generally are assigned responsibility for completing the MDS, but must rely heavily on information from professionals in a variety of disciplines, including physicians and therapists.

Many of the clinical issues that are highlighted in the MDS fall directly under the purview of the physician (Box 1.2). When a problem is identified that relates to one of these 18 issues, the health care team must then review the appropriate resident assessment protocol (RAP), which outlines a standard diagnostic and therapeutic approach to the specific problem in question. The resident assessment protocols can identify problems that may not have been obvious to physicians and other caregivers. However, these protocols are merely guidelines, and

---

BOX 1.1. OBRA mandates relating to medical practice in the nursing home

1. Nursing facilities must conduct (initially and periodically) a comprehensive, accurate, standardized, reproducible assessment of each residents' functional capacity.
2. Residents have the right to be free from any physical restraints imposed for the purposes of discipline, or convenience, and which are not required to treat the residents medical symptoms.
3. Residents have the right to be free from any psychoactive drug administered for the purpose of discipline or convenience and which are not required to treat the residents' medical symptoms.
4. Residents must be free from unnecessary drugs.
5. Residents have the right to a dignified existence, self- determination, and communication with and access to persons and services inside and outside the facility.
   a. Residents have the right to choose a personal attending physician.
   b. Residents have the right to refuse treatment.
   c. Residents have the right to personal privacy, which includes privacy during medical treatment.
6. Residents must receive in the facility (and the facility must provide) the necessary care and services to attain or maintain the highest practicable physical, mental, and psychosocial well-being in accordance with the comprehensive assessment and plan of care.

Adapted from Elon R, Pawlson LG. The impact of OBRA on medical practice within nursing facilities. J Am Geriatr Soc. 1992; 40:958-63.

BOX 1.2. Clinical issues highlighted in the MSD (Minimum Data Set) resident assessment protocols

1. Delirium
2. Cognitive loss/dementia
3. Visual function
4. Communication
5. ADL functional/rehabilitative potential
6. Urinary incontinence and indwelling catheter
7. Psychosocial well-being
8. Mood state
9. Behavioral problems
10. Activities
11. Falls
12. Nutritional status
13. Feeding tubes
14. Dehydration/fluid maintenance
15. Dental care
16. Pressure ulcer
17. Antipsychotic drug use
18. Physical restraints

Adapted from Elon R, Pawlson LG. The impact of OBRA on medical practice within nursing facilities. J Am Geriatr Soc. 1992; 40:958-63.

physicians are free to employ other approaches that are consistent with sound medical practice.

Many observers have been concerned about the potential overuse of psychoactive agents in the nursing home. New regulations have established systems to identify when high doses of these medications are given for long periods of time without adequate monitoring. The indications for the initial and continued use of these medications now must be identified (3).

Medical practice in the nursing home is guided not only by mandates set forth in federal and state legislation, but also by the manner in which the overseeing of medical care is carried out. Compliance with these regulations may divert time and resources from the bedside to the chart and impede the actual delivery of care. The move from extensive documentation to a more outcome-based quality assurance program is a prime goal toward which many physician groups are working in the long-term-care setting. Active participation by physicians working in the nursing home in these efforts may ultimately decrease the regulatory burden presently faced in nursing homes.

From the physician's point of view, the current regulations may seem to have a perverse, counterproductive intent; from the state's point of view, the contentious nature of current regulations is precisely what is necessary to improve the quality of care in the nursing home. It is unfortunate and perhaps ironic that regulations aimed at improving quality of care may have the unintentional effect of erecting new barriers to such care. Greater understanding and cooperation between providers and regulators may eventually produce methods for monitoring care that identify lapses of quality more efficiently. It may also be possible to use prospective approaches to improving quality (for example, identifying high-risk patients *before* adverse outcomes occur) in conjunction with the retrospective approaches currently in use. In the meantime, physicians who remain sensitive to the potential rift between regulator and provider increase their chances of avoiding conflict and optimizing patient care.

Visits and Reimbursement

In many states, the initial visit by the physician to the nursing home resident must occur within 48 hours of admission. Subsequent visits for all residents must occur every 30 days for the first 3

months and then at least every 60 days thereafter.

During the first visit, it is important for the physician to begin to compile the data necessary to formulate a care plan. Regardless of whether the expected duration of stay is 30 days or several years, each patient should receive a comprehensive assessment that includes 1) evaluation of medical, functional, and nutritional status; 2) review of medications; and 3) discussion of patient treatment preferences, including advance directives and end-of-life planning. This comprehensive assessment may take place over the first several visits.

This initial assessment, as well as the opinions of other members of the health care team, helps the physician to identify and assign relative priorities to the resident's problems. The physician should then establish a complete and comprehensive care plan, with clear goals of therapy, a timetable for accomplishing them, and well-defined parameters for measuring the success of the plan. The plan should be reviewed and amended periodically as new problems develop and existing ones are re-evaluated.

Physician visits are reimbursed based on their level of complexity, as dictated by the resource-based relative value scale. Over the last few years, the American Geriatrics Society and the American Medical Directors Association have negotiated with the Health Care Financing Administration for increased reimbursement in recognition of the increased time involved in caring for nursing home patients. The categories of visits and codes are outlined in Table 1.2.

Medicare will pay for all medically necessary visits. Medicare intermediaries may request verification of medical necessity when more than one visit per month is submitted for reimbursement. Clear documentation of the urgent need for extra visits often will lead to payment; for example, it may be helpful in some cases to include a copy of the progress notes for the emergency visit with the bill.

OTHER ROLES OF THE PHYSICIAN IN THE NURSING HOME

Medical Director

The role of nursing home medical director was created in the early 1970s. More recently, an Institute of Medicine report emphasized the importance of the medical director in the nursing home (2). An

TABLE 1.2. Nursing home visit codes

Code	Description	Comments
99301	NH facility care	E/M new/established patient Detailed history Comprehensive examination Low complexity
99302	NH facility care	E/M new/established patient Detailed history Comprehensive examination Moderate-to-high complexity
99303	NH facility care	E/M new/established patient Comprehensive history Comprehensive examination Moderate-to-high complexity
99311	NH facility care subsequent	E/M new/established patient Problem-focused history Problem examination Low complexity
99312	NH facility care subsequent	E/M new/established patient Expanded history Expanded examination Moderate complexity
99313	NH facility care subsequent	E/M new/established patient Detailed history Detailed examination Moderate-to-high complexity

NH = Nursing home; E/M = evaluation/management.

effective medical director can be instrumental in improving all aspects of care in the nursing home; key responsibilities are shown in Box 1.3. In certain nursing homes, the director may also play an important role in facilitating appropriate research.

The effective medical director provides leadership and functions as the chief of staff, on a hierarchical level with the nursing home administrator and director of nurses. The medical director must be able to communicate effectively with nursing home personnel to develop and implement patient care policies. In addition, the owners and boards of directors of nursing homes often look to the medical director to provide leadership and to work with the medical staff to ensure that patient care is appropriate and timely. To protect the interests of all concerned, it is important for the medical director to have an explicit contract with the nursing home stating the required duties and responsibilities (25,30,31). The American Medical Director's Association currently offers a voluntary certification process for medical directors.

Education

Although physicians have concerns relating to reimbursement, regulation, and documentation, the most powerful barrier to practice in the nursing home is often the physician's lack of experience with, and hence discomfort with, managing the common clinical problems in this setting. On the completion of a residency program, physicians are usually well trained in the management of problems that arise in

BOX 1.3. Responsibilities of the medical director

Organizing comprehensive medical services
Monitoring quality of care
Collaborating with the administrator, the director of nurses, and other department heads regarding policies and procedures
Overseeing the employee health program
Assisting in the development of educational offerings to staff, residents, and families
Representing the nursing home in the community

the hospital and, to a lesser (but recently increasing) extent, in the outpatient setting. Physicians entering practice can usually find more experienced colleagues, as well as a wealth of literature, to help them manage clinical problems in the hospital or ambulatory care setting.

In contrast, physicians typically graduate from residencies with little or no training in nursing home care. New physicians are less likely to encounter mentors, colleagues, and other role models to provide advice on caring for nursing home patients. Despite recent interest in this area, there is still relatively little empirical research to guide medical practice in this setting.

Underlying the scarcity of physicians familiar with nursing home care is the small number of internal medicine residency training programs that currently use the nursing home as a training site. Although the Residency Review Committee strongly encourages the use of nursing homes as training sites, relatively few internal medicine residency training programs have been willing or able to heed this recommendation. The American College of Physicians also has advocated the use of nontraditional training sites as a means to better prepare internists for the challenge of primary care (32). If, as the American College of Physicians advocates, the "internist is the best qualified professional to provide and coordinate long-term care services for the elderly" (33), then the nursing home must become an integral part of postgraduate medical education. Currently, however, only 32% of internal medicine residency training programs offer a nursing home experience, and two thirds of these experiences are optional block rotations (34). Further, internal medicine residents are assigned primary responsibility for patient care in only 12% of programs, whereas 9 of 10 family practice training programs require a longitudinal experience in the nursing home. The type of extended experience that family practice training programs offer is preferable to a block rotation, which encourages brief encounters with large numbers of severely disabled and demented elderly and may reinforce, rather than lessen, negative stereotypical attitudes about caring for the nursing home resident.

It is reasonable to assume that "in a setting where patients have multiple and interacting disabilities, altered presentation of disease and reduced tolerance to stress, the role of a well-trained and interested physician may be critical in providing optimal care" as well as maximizing quality of life (35). Participation of residents has been shown to enhance care and improve patient outcomes in the nursing home (36). Training in a nursing home enhances valuable primary care skills and influences future practice patterns relating to primary care and administrative activities in long-term care settings (37). The use of the nursing home as a site for medical student education also has been well-received (38).

In the future, research in the long-term-care setting should provide more and more scientific knowledge about the natural history, management, and outcomes of clinical problems. Developing this information into a core curriculum for residents in internal medicine and providing practical experience in the nursing home setting should help to train a cadre of competent physicians who are motivated to care for patients in the nursing home setting.

CONCLUSION

Despite past problems, the quality of care in nursing homes has improved dramatically over the past decade. As the nursing home population continues to increase, there will be a growing need for physicians to provide care in this setting. As primary care physicians follow their patients into the nursing home, they must learn to manage these patients efficiently and effectively. They must learn to rely on the clinical skills of the nursing home team, communicating via telephone and facsimile and using physician extenders when possible. They must learn to work within the existing system and to use the skills of the nursing home staff to minimize the burdens of the regulatory process. They must also be willing to act as mentors to more junior physicians who need guidance in the nursing home setting. Physicians who learn to apply these principles will find that providing high-quality care to their patients at what is often their time of greatest need can be tremendously rewarding and satisfying.

REFERENCES

1. The Institute of Medicine. Committee on Nursing Home Regulation. Improving the Quality of Nursing Home Care. Washington, D.C. National Academy Press, 1986.
2. Hawes C. The Institute of Medicine Study: improving the quality of nursing home care. In: Katz PR, Kane RL, Mezy MD, eds. Advances in Long-Term

Care. Vol. 1. New York: Springer Publishing Co. 1991.

3. Elon R. Pawlson LG; The impact of OBRA on medical practice within nursing facilities. J Am Geriatr Soc. 1992;40:958-63.

4. Kemper P, Murtaugh CN. Lifetime use of nursing home care. N Engl J Med. 1991;324:595-600.

5. Schneider EL, Guralnik JM. The aging of America: impact on health care costs. JAMA. 1990;263: 2335-40.

6. Rovner BW, Kafonek S, Filipp L, Lucas KJ, Folstein MF. Prevalence of mental illness in a community nursing home. Am J Psychiatry. 1986;143:1446-9.

7. Koescoff J, Kahn KL, Rogers WH, Reinisch EJ, Sherwood MJ, Rubenstein LV, et al. Prospective payment system impairment at discharge. The "quicker-and-sicker" story revisited. JAMA. 1990; 264:1980-3.

8. Fitzgerald JF, Moore PS, Dittus RS. The care of elderly Patients with hip fracture. Changes since implementation of the prospective payment system. N Engl J Med 1988;319:1392-7.

9. Tresch DD, Duthie EH, Newton M, Bodin B. Coping with diagnosis-related groups: the changing role of the nursing home. Arch Intern Med. 1988;148: 1393.

10. Sager MA, Easterling DV, Kindig DA, Anderson OW. Changes in the location of death after passage of medicare's prospective payment system. N Engl J Med 1989;320:433.

11. Spence DA, Wiener JM. Nursing home length of stay patterns: results from the 1985 National Nursing Home Survey. Gerontologist. 1990;30:16-20.

12. Lewis MA, Kane RL, Cretin S, Clark V. The immediate and subsequent outcomes of nursing care. Am J Public Health. 1985;75:758-62.

13. Katz PR, Seidel G. Nursing home autopsies: survey of physician attitudes and practice patterns. Arch Pathol Lab Med. 1990;114:145-7.

14. American Health care Association. Subacute Care Medical and Rehabilitation Definition and Guide to Business Development. 1994.

15. Mezy M, Knapp M. Nurse staffing in nursing facilities: implications for achieving quality of care. In: Katz PR, Kane RL, Mezy MD, eds. Advances in Long Term Care. Vol 2. New York: Springer-Verlag; 1993.

16. Katz PR, Karuza J, Parker M, Tarnove L. A national Survey of Medical Directors. J Med Direction. 1992;2:81-94.

17. AMA Physician Practice Survey, unpublished.

18. Williams ME. The physician's role in nursing home care: an overview. Geriatrics. 1990;45:47-9.

19. Ouslander JG, Osterweil D. Physician evaluation and management of nursing home residents. Ann Intern Med. 1994;120:584-92.

20. Ouslander JG, Osterweil D, Morley JE. Medical Care in the Nursing Home. New York: McGraw Hill; 1991.

21. Starer P, Libow L. Medical care of the elderly in the nursing home. JGIM 1992;7:350-62.

22. Libow L, Starer P. Care of the nursing home patient. N Eng J Med. 1989;321:93-6.

23. Leukoff S, Evans D, Liptzin B, et al. Delirium: the occurrence and persistence of symptoms among elderly hospitalized patients. Arch Intern Med. 1992;152:334-40.

24. Creditor M. Hazards of hospitalization of the elderly. Ann Intern Med. 1993;118:219-23.

25. Ouslander JG. Medical care in the nursing home. JAMA. 1989;262:2582-90.

26. Powers JS. Helping family and patients decide between home care and nursing care. South Med J. 1989;82:723-6.

27. Kane RL, Garrard J, Skay CL, Radosevich DM, Buchanan JL, McDermott SM, et al. Effects of a geriatric nurse practitioner on process and outcome of nursing home care. Am J Pub Health. 1989;79:1271-7.

28. Garrard J, Kane RL, Radosevich DM, Skay CL, Arnold S, Kepferle L. Impact of geriatric nurse practitioners on nursing home residents' functional status, satisfaction, and discharge outcomes. Med Care. 1990;28:271-83.

29. Medicare and Medicaid: requirements for long-term care facilities–HCFA. Final rule with comment. Federal Register. February 2, 1989;54:5316-73.

30. Fanale JE. The nursing home medical director. J Am Geriatr Soc. 1989;37:369-75.

31. Staats D. The role of the nursing home medical director. Clin Geriatr Med. 1988;4:493-506.

32. American College of Physicians. Geriatric training and the internal medicine residency. Philadelphia: American College of Physicians; 1989.

33. Report of the Institute of Medicine: Academic geriatrics for the year 2000. Committee on Leadership for Academic Geriatric Medicine. J Am Geriatr Soc. 1987;35:773-91.

34. Katz PR, Karuza J, Hall N. Residency education in the nursing home: A national survey of internal medicine and family practice programs. J Gen Intern Med. 1992;7:52-6.

35. Jahnigen DW, Kramer AM, Robbins LJ, Klingbeil H, DeVore P. Academic affiliation with a nursing home: impact on patient outcome. J Am Geriatr Soc. 1985;33:472-8.

36. Wieland D, Rubenstein LZ, Ouslander JG, Martin SE. Organizing an academic nursing home. JAMA. 1986;255:2622-7.

37. Richardson JP, Fredman L, Daly MP. Geriatric education and practice of family practice graduates: an alumni survey. Family Medicine (in press).

38. Grady MJ, Earl JM. Teaching physical diagnosis in the nursing home. Am J Med. 1990;88:519-21.

2

Physician Evaluation

Joseph G. Ouslander, MD, and Dan Osterweil, MD

Physician evaluation of nursing home residents at admission and regularly thereafter is an important part of caring for this rapidly increasing segment of society. The diverse goals of nursing home care, the heterogeneity of nursing home residents, and the varied circumstances under which physicians evaluate them make a single set of recommendations for evaluating all nursing home residents inappropriate. For example, the goals of care and foci of evaluation and management for a nursing home resident admitted for rehabilitation after a hip fracture are very different from those for a resident admitted for terminal care of end-stage cancer or dementia. Similarly, the nature and extent of patient evaluation at admission or at an annual examination are different from those at a routine monthly visit.

The general goals of nursing home care are the following:

1. To provide a safe and supportive environment for chronically ill and dependent persons

2. To maximize individual autonomy, functional capabilities, and quality of life

3. To stabilize and delay, if possible, the progression of chronic illnesses

4. To prevent subacute and acute illnesses and recognize and manage them rapidly when they do occur.

Because nursing home residents are heterogeneous, the goals for caring for specific residents vary. This heterogeneity can be illustrated by categorizing nursing home residents into several types. Examples of subgroups and components of their medical evaluation that need particular emphasis are listed in Table 2.1. Although not all nursing home residents fit neatly into one of these categories, and residents may change from one type to another as their conditions change, this general nosology can help physicians target their evaluations and management for each type of nursing home resident.

As in other comprehensive assessments of geriatric patients in other settings, the timing and purposes for evaluating nursing home residents are important in determining the scope and areas of emphasis for evaluation. Physicians evaluate nursing home residents at the time of admission, at periodic visits every 30 to 90 days, when acute problems occur, and at the time of annual review for residents who stay longer than 1 year. The objectives and elements of evaluation at these different times depend on the clinical status of the resident and goals for care.

Finally, physician evaluation of nursing home residents must be viewed as only one component of a multidisciplinary process that produces an overall care plan for each resident. The goals and context of nursing home care require that a broad range of health professionals participate in care planning and overall management for nursing home residents. In addition, recently implemented federal nursing home regulations mandate comprehensive, multi-

TABLE 2.1. Points of emphasis in the medical evaluation of different types of nursing home residents

Type of Resident	Examples	Points of Emphasis for Medical Evaluation
Short-term (days to 6 months)		
Short-term rehabilitation	Hip fracture; stroke Rehabilitation potential	Functional status
		Status of concomitant medical conditions
		Capabilities of caregivers
		Home environment
Medically unstable	Recovery from infection; poorly controlled diabetes or cardio-vascular or pulmonary disease	Status of medical condition and response to treatment
Terminally ill	End-stage cancer End-stage dementia	Comfort
		Expectations and feelings of family
Long-term (>6 months)*		
Primarily cognitively impaired	Dementia	Functional status
		Behavioral problems
		Affect
Primarily physically impaired	Severe musculoskeletal, neurologic, cardiac, or pulmonary disease	Status of medical condition and response to treatment
		Signs of drug side effects
		Functional status
Both cognitively and physically impaired	Dementia in combination with musculoskeletal, neurologic, cardiac, or pulmonary disease	All of the above under long-term

* Monitoring, screening, and preventive practices were also important in this group (see Appendix Tables 2.1 and 2.2).

faceted assessment with interdisciplinary communication and participation. Specific components of the physician evaluation are presented below. However, the relevant federal rules and the role of the interdisciplinary team are reviewed first.

The specific recommendations made in this article are based on literature review and experience, not on a meta-analysis of research. In fact, no research on the most cost-effective strategies to evaluate and care for subgroups of nursing home residents exists. We hope the recommendations described stimulate discussion and research on these issues. These recommendations may be difficult to achieve given the nature of the nursing home environment, the need to spend more time in the nursing home, and inadequate Medicare reimbursement for physician care in nursing homes. Despite recent increases in the relative value of nursing home visit codes achieved by the American Medical Directors Association and the American Geriatric Society, creative and efficient strategies and close cooperation among the interdisciplinary team and physician

extenders (where available) are needed to fulfill our recommendations.

FEDERAL RULES AND THE ROLE OF THE INTERDISCIPLINARY TEAM

The Omnibus Budget Reconciliation Act (OBRA) of 1987 contained new federal rules for nursing home care. After considerable public comment, debate, and revision, the new rules became effective in 1991 (2). Although these rules address a broad range of general and administrative aspects of nursing home care, the process and quality of clinical care are heavily emphasized (3). With this act, the goal of care is achieving the highest practicable level of functioning (as opposed to custodial care). The act also requires that when a resident's condition deteriorates or complications develop, documentation must show why such situations were "medically unavoidable." Although many physicians, nurses, and other health professionals believe OBRA 1987 represents unnecessary governmental intrusion into the clinical care of nursing home residents, the rules were developed in response to an Institute of Medicine report (4). When read carefully, the rules provide a sound basic paradigm for improving the process and outcomes of nursing home care. Federal and state nursing home inspectors have interpretive guidelines for these new regulations and will focus increasingly on compliance with OBRA 1987 in the next several years.

One of the central elements of OBRA 1987 is the mandate for a comprehensive, reproducible assessment of all nursing home residents within 14 days of admission, including the "Minimum Data Set," a standard 4-page form composed of 16 sections (5). Selected areas of the Minimum Data Set must be updated quarterly, and the entire assessment must be updated whenever an important change in patient condition occurs (Table 2.2).

On a national level, the Minimum Data Set will be used to compile standardized data on nursing home residents, as a tool for quality assurance, and eventually as a component of a prospective reimbursement system. For the individual nursing home, the Minimum Data Set provides health professionals a tool to identify clinical problems and to develop a comprehensive care plan for each resident. Selected items from the Minimum Data Set, called "triggers," are designed to alert the interdisciplinary team that a particular problem or set of problems should be evaluated further. A standard set of assessment protocols (the Resident Assessment Protocols) address 18 common problems in

TABLE 2.2. Areas covered by the minimum data set and resident assessment protocols*

Sections of the Minimum Data Set	Problems Addressed by Resident Assessment Protocols	Discipline(s) Responsible for Completion[†]
Demographic and background information (includes advanced directives)		Medical record staff, nursing
Cognitive patterns[‡]	Delirium	Nursing
	Cognitive loss or dementia	Social work
Communication/hearing patterns	Communication	Nursing, audiology, and speech therapy
Vision patterns	Visual function	Nursing, optometry
Physical functioning[‡]	Activities of daily living, functional rehabilitation potential, falls	Nursing Occupational therapy Physical therapy
Continence[‡]	Urinary incontinence/indwelling catheter	Nursing
Psychosocial well-being	Psychosocial well-being (feelings about self and social relationships)	Nursing Social work, psychology
Mood and behavior[‡]	Mood state (depression, anxiety)	Nursing
	Behavior problems (wandering, verbal abuse, physical aggression)	Social work Psychology
Activity pursuit patterns	Activity (inactivity, lack of participation)	Activities
Disease diagnoses[‡]		Nursing
Health conditions		Nursing
Oral/nutritional status[‡]	Nutritional status	Nursing
	Feeding tubes	Dietary
	Dehydration/fluid maintenance	
Oral/dental status	Dental care	Dental
Skin condition	Pressure ulcers	Nursing
Medication use[‡]	Psychotropic drug use	Nursing, psychology, psychiatry
Special treatments and procedures (dialysis, intravenous medication, restraints)	Physical restraints	Nursing

* The Minimum Data Set must be completed within 14 days of admission. Selected items on the Minimum Data Set are intended to trigger use of one or more Resident Assessment Protocols to assess specific problems in residents (see text).
† The physician should be involved in the assessment of all problems identified on the Minimum Data Set that trigger use of a Resident Assessment Protocol (see text).
‡ Area must be updated quarterly.

nursing home residents (6) (Table 2.2). The Resident Assessment Protocols were developed by experts in geriatric medicine, gerontologic nurses, and other gerontologists through a contract with the Health Care Financing Administration. The Resident Assessment Protocols provide recommendations on critical elements of the history, physical examination, and diagnostic testing useful in identifying potentially treatable conditions that may underlie the clinical problem. Most nursing homes have not adequately developed the interdisciplinary cooperation and communication required to make full use of the Minimum Data Set and Resident Assessment Protocols, and the reliability and validity of the data recorded on the Minimum Data Set by typical nursing home staff need further study. In fact, based on our experience and on discussions with other nursing home professionals across the country, the Minimum Data Set is often viewed as just another component of the onerous paperwork required of nursing home staff. Yet, these tools can help physicians and members of the interdisciplinary team to identify important problems in their nursing home residents and to incorporate evaluations from multiple disciplines into the overall care plan. Table 2.2 lists the disciplines generally responsible for completing specific sections of the Minimum Data Set and the Resident Assessment Protocols. This is usually accomplished at care plan meetings, in which the interdisciplinary team establishes a comprehensive care plan for each resident and updates it quarterly. Because physicians generally do not attend these quarterly meetings, medical aspects of the Minimum Data Set, Resident Assessment Protocols, and care plan must be discussed regularly on routine rounds with the nurses, social service providers, rehabilitation therapists, and other members of the interdisciplinary team. When available, nurse practitioners and physician assistants may play an important role in communicating with the interdisciplinary team and implementing the care plan.

ADMISSION EVALUATION

Physicians evaluate nursing home residents within three admission contexts: direct admission from home, admission from an acute-care hospital after an acute illness that requires nursing home care, and readmission of a nursing home resident after hospitalization for an acute illness. Often, the primary physician changes during these transitions. Thus, adequate and timely transfer of information critical to patient care among nursing homes, hospitals, and physicians' offices is important. Explicit policies and procedures should be developed to address information exchange, and simplified, comprehensive, and standardized documents should be used during these transfers.

Box 2.1 lists the key elements of the physician evaluation during nursing home admission. Some elements require greater emphasis than others, depending on the circumstances of the admission.

BOX 2.1 Key components of the physician evaluation at nursing home admission*

History
    Reason(s) for seeking admission
    Status of active medical problems
    Past medical history
        Chronic medical conditions
        Surgical procedures
    Preventive care
        Vaccinations
        Dental, optometric, podiatric care
    Medications
    Review of symptoms
Physical examination
    In addition to traditional system approach
        include
        Orthostatic changes in blood pressure
        Nutritional status
        Screening for hearing problems[†]
        Visual capabilities
        Mobility (direct observation of ability to
           walk or transfer)[†]
        Cognitive function[†]
        Affective status[†]
Functional status
    Ability to perform:
        Instrumental activities of daily living[†]
        Basic activities of daily living[†]
Socioeconomic status
    Nature of family relationships
    Relevant financial information (private pay,
        Medicaid, Medicare, other)
Advance directives
    Designation of proxy decision maker
    Intensity of care desired

* Nursing home admission may be directly from home, from an acute care hospital, or readmission after hospitalization for an acute condition. Different areas of the evaluation may deserve special emphasis, depending on the context of the admission (see text).
† Standardized tests may be helpful (see text).

In addition, an interdisciplinary team can conduct several of the recommended assessments because they are requirements of the Minimum Data Set (*see* Table 2.2). Standardized assessment instruments besides the Minimum Data Set are available to assist in selected areas of the evaluation, including hearing (7,8), mobility (9,10), cognitive function (11,12), affective status (13–15), and overall function (16,17). To screen for hearing impairment, hand-held audioscopes are available that provide frequency sounds at several decibel levels. Detecting hearing loss is an important part of the evaluation and may lead to improved quality of life even among frail nursing home residents (18). Standardized assessments of mobility involve observing the resident's sitting balance, ability to stand and transfer, stability while standing, and balance and safety while walking. Such assessments are helpful to predict the risk for falls among frail older patients (19) and to identify potentially reversible factors and comorbid conditions that may cause subsequent falls (20,21). The Mini-Mental State examination, a 30-point scale that tests orientation, attention, short-term memory, and selected components of higher cognitive function, is the most commonly used standardized screening test of cognitive function. It is reasonably sensitive and specific for detecting dementia (11,12), is a more objective assessment than is included in the Minimum Data Set, and is sensitive to change. Level of education, primary language, and cultural considerations are important factors to consider when interpreting the results of screening tests for cognitive impairment. Screening questions and scales are available to help detect depression (13,14), but their reliability and validity for use in cognitively impaired persons have been questioned (22,23). Given the high prevalence of untreated depression and its association with death in nursing home residents (24–27) and the frequent coexistence of dementia and depression in this setting (28), identification of depression is an important component of the evaluation process. The Minimum Data Set provides a detailed assessment of basic activities of daily living (such as dressing, grooming, using the toilet, eating) that is similar to the well-established Katz Activities of Daily Living index (29). For some nursing home residents, particularly those receiving rehabilitation to return to their homes, an assessment of instrumental activities of daily living (such as housekeeping, using the telephone, cooking, and managing finances and medications) may determine their potential for discharge (30).

Relatively few nursing home residents are admitted directly from home. When they are, their need for nursing home care may be based on a broad range of medical, physical, cognitive, affective, and socioeconomic factors. Epidemiologic data suggest that for every nursing home resident, two or three similarly dependent persons live in the community and that most of their care is provided by relatives (31). Thus, admission of a person to a nursing home from home often is precipitated by a weakening or failure of the support system that kept that person in the community or by the development of behavioral disturbances (such as wandering, night-time agitation, physical or verbal aggression, or incontinence) that family caregivers cannot manage. In addition, many of these persons are treated with several medications, with the potential for adverse effects. Thus, an assessment of socioeconomic status, prescription and nonprescription medications, and behavioral problems should be included in the initial evaluation of persons admitted from home.

Most often, admission to a nursing home occurs after hospitalization for an acute condition. In this case, the acute medical problem is usually the focus of care. But if this is the first nursing home admission, focusing only on the acute problem often leaves many important areas inadequately evaluated. Such areas include concomitant chronic medical conditions, physical and cognitive function, affective status, and socioeconomic status. Thus, when admitting a nursing home resident, whether directly from home or from an acute care hospital, the physician should assess several areas (Box 2.1).

Acute hospitalization of nursing home residents is common, and infections, fractures, and cardiopulmonary and gastrointestinal conditions are the most frequent causes (32–34). The readmission evaluation should summarize the status of the acute condition(s) that precipitated hospitalization and update areas outlined in Box 2.1 that may have changed (for example, overall functional status, mobility, continence, or cognitive function) or been addressed during hospitalization (diagnostic tests related to cognitive function or nutritional status or decisions about intensity of care, for example). Nurse practitioners and physician assistants can be especially helpful in completing these readmission summaries.

CONTINUING CARE

Periodic Visits

Physicians are generally required by federal or state requirements to re-evaluate nursing home residents every 30 to 60 days. When visits for intercurrent subacute problems are used to meet this requirement, important aspects of the resident's overall condition may be unevaluated for several months. Thus, physicians (or nurse practitioners or physician assistants who can make every other required visit after the first one) should use a standardized format for progress notes to ensure that all relevant areas are addressed (Box 2.2). Software is available to generate notes on a laptop computer and to structure the documentation to include the elements listed in Box 2.2 (35).

In addition to the periodic evaluation, selected practices are recommended to monitor specific aspects of chronic disease or therapy (1,36) (Appendix Table 2.1). Although no data support the efficacy of such practices for preventing morbidity or death, the frailty of nursing home residents, the high prevalence of multiple chronic conditions, and nonspecific evidence of many acute and subacute conditions that could result from complications of therapies warrant a systematic approach to patient monitoring. The monitoring practices we recommend can be accomplished by standing orders, with the results reviewed at periodic visits. Criteria can be set for physician notification of abnormal results (37), and nurse practitioners and physician assistants, when available, can help implement these recommendations.

Acute and Subacute Problems

Many physicians are fortunate to work with nurse practitioners or physician assistants who can evaluate acute and subacute problems at the nursing home. Protocols are available to assist nurse practitioners and physician assistants in these evaluations (1,38), and both can be reimbursed for their services by Medicare. Involving nurse practitioners and physician assistants gives the nursing staff better access to medical input when problems arise; improves the information physicians receive, which in turn facilitates better decision making; and can prevent some emergency room visits and acute care hospitalizations (39–41).

BOX 2.2. Format and key data for medical progress notes on nursing home residents*

Subjective
  New complaints
  Symptoms related to active medical conditions
Objective
  General appearance
  Weight
  Vital signs
  Physical findings relevant to new complaints and active medical conditions
  Reports from nursing staff (functional and behavioral status)
  Progress in rehabilitative therapy (if relevant)
  Reports of other interdisciplinary team members
  Laboratory data
  Consultant reports
Assessment
  Presumptive diagnoses of new complaints or changes in status
  Stability of active medical conditions
  Response to interventions, especially psychotropic medications and rehabilitative therapy
Plans
  Changes in medications or diet
  Nursing interventions (monitoring of vital signs, skin care)
  Assessments by other disciplines (rehabilitation therapists, consultants)
  Laboratory studies
  Discharge planning (if relevant)

* Adapted from Ouslander and colleagues (1).

Most physicians do not, however, have a nurse practitioner or physician assistant who can evaluate nursing home residents in person when problems occur. As a result, physicians usually do the initial evaluation of acute changes in a nursing home resident's status over the telephone. We developed a policy and procedure on "When to Call the Doctor" that delineates specific problems that require immediate or nonimmediate physician notification (1,37). This policy helps nursing staff to identify clinically important acute and subacute conditions or laboratory values that require physician evaluation and assists nurses and physicians by eliminating unnecessary telephone calls. When a nurse does call a physician, she or he should have the chart available, have taken the resident's vital signs, and have described the resident's new condition in detail. Physicians on call (who may not be familiar with the resident) should ask, at a minimum, the following questions: What are the resident's vital

APPENDIX TABLE 2.1. Examples of periodic monitoring practices in selected nursing home residents*

Practice	Recommended Frequency	Comments
All residents		
Vital signs, including weight	Monthly	More often if unstable or subacutely ill
Diabetics		
Fasting and postprandial glucose	Monthly	More often if unstable; finger-stick tests may also be useful if staff can do them reliably
Glycosylated hemoglobin	Every 3 to 4 months	
Residents receiving diuretics or who have with renal insufficiency (creatinine >2 mg/dL or BUN >35 mg/dL)		
Electrolytes, BUN, creatinine	Every 2 to 3 months	Nursing home residents are more vulnerable to dehydration, azotemia, hyponatremia, and hypokalemia
Residents receiving nonsteroidal anti-inflammatory drugs		
Hemoglobin/hematocrit, stool for occult blood BUN, creatinine	Every 1 to 2 months	Bleeding is frequently asymptomatic
Anemic residents who are receiving iron replacement or who have hemoglobin level <10 g/dL		
Hemoglobin/hematocrit	Monthly until stable, then every 2 to 3 months	Iron replacement should generally be discontinued once hemoglobin value stabilizes
Blood level of drug for residents on specific drugs		
Digoxin Dilantin Quinidine Procainamide Theophylline Nortriptyline	Every 3 to 6 months	More frequently if drug treatment has just been initiated, dosage adjusted, or toxicity suspected

* Adapted from Ouslander and colleagues (1). Date for the efficacy and timing of these practices are limited (see text). Thus, these recommendations should not be considered guidelines based on scientific merit but rather opinions based on literature review and clinical experience. BUN = blood urea nitrogen.

signs? What medications is the resident receiving? Has the resident's mental status changed? Is the resident eating and drinking fluids? Does the resident have a "No CPR" order or a "No Hospitalization" order? The answers to these questions are critical to understanding the acuity of the situation and the need for hospitalization. Medical directors and nursing directors should develop a policy and procedure regarding nurse physician communication. A medical fact sheet, which includes a succinct summary of the resident's medical, functional, and psychosocial status on one page, can be used by nurses to give physicians a more comprehensive description of a resident's overall medical and functional status (1,42). When laboratory tests are ordered or other orders are requested, communication by facsimile may be an efficient strategy in some settings. Facsimile orders to nursing homes are recognized as legitimate by the Health Care Financing Administration (43).

Annual Review

Although the value of the routine annual history and physical examination for nursing home residents has been questioned (44,45), long-term nursing home residents should have a comprehensive annual review performed by a physician to summarize relevant findings from 1) the Minimum Data Set (which must be updated annually); 2) the physician's evaluation of the resident's medical status; and 3) the results of selected screening procedures. Substitution of a history and physical examination done during hospitalization for an intercurrent acute illness for the required annual examination will inadequately address many issues, such as underlying chronic conditions and cognitive and functional status, that should be reviewed at least annually.

Few data exist on which to base recommendations for screening practices that might be included in the annual review of long-term nursing home residents. We recommend selected screening practices (Appendix Table 2.2), recognizing that these recommendations differ somewhat from those offered by the U.S. Preventive Services Task Force (46) and that they are based on our review of the literature and opinion, not on data from clinical trials. The areas included in functional status should be assessed by members of the interdisciplinary team during the required annual updating of the Minimum Data Set *(see* Table 2.2) and summarized briefly in the physician's annual review. Selected laboratory tests (listed in Appendix Table 2.2) may be useful to identify potentially treatable conditions in nursing home residents (47–50). Screening for tuberculosis with a PPD (purified protein derivative) should be done on admission and annually if the result is initially negative because of the high risk for conversion and spread of infection in the nursing home (51–54). A repeated test should be done in 10 to 14 days if the admission PPD test result is negative to rule out the booster phenomenon (a positive test result developed in response to the PPD, which generally does not represent true conversion or reactivation of tuberculosis) (55,56). A chest roentgenogram and an electrocardiogram (57) are often useful as baseline examinations for comparison during subsequent illnesses, but annual examinations are probably not cost-effective (49). Screening for cervical cancer with a Papanicolaou test is probably unnecessary after age 65 years if the resident has had at least two negative results (58, 59).

Screening for breast cancer with an annual mammogram and for prostate cancer with a prostate-specific antigen test is controversial. The guiding principle should be to do these tests only if the results would change the patient's care plan. In this context, a mammogram would make sense for some long-term nursing home residents because curative treatment is available (60). However, because most breast carcinomas grow slowly, the value of detecting and treating an early cancer in an 85-year-old woman with a short life expectancy is debatable (61). Discovery of early-stage prostate cancer through prostate-specific antigen screening in a man older than 75 years who has substantial comorbid conditions would probably not prompt initiation of curative therapy, because life expectancy and the natural history of the disease suggest that these men will die of another illness (62–67). In addition, the number of false-positive results in these patients could lead to substantial morbidity and expense from further evaluation (such as prostate ultrasonography and biopsy). The recommendations outlined above are different from those published for younger persons (68,69) and for older noninstitutionalized adults (46,70), for whom some data support the recommendation. Until better data are available, decisions to use these screening tests for nursing home residents must be based on specific patient needs.

Box 2.3 outlines a format for annual physician evaluation of long-term nursing home residents. Rather than simply dictating a standard history and physical examination and medically oriented problem list, physicians should use the annual review to summarize succinctly data gathered from their medical evaluation, the Minimum Data Set completed by the interdisciplinary team, and the results of selected screening procedures. Establishing overall goals for the resident's medical care and documenting information relevant to advance directives are essential components of this review. This type of annual review is useful for the interdisciplinary team, provides critical documentation should the resident be hospitalized or transferred to another physician or health care facility, and helps set realistic expectations of the resident, family, and nursing home staff for subsequent medical care. Medicare reimburses the cost of one comprehensive nursing home evaluation each year, and nurse practitioners and physician assistants can help complete this annual evaluation.

APPENDIX TABLE 2.2. Examples of screening practices in the nursing home*

Practice	Recommended Approximate Frequency	Comments
Comprehensive history and physical examination	Yearly	Should include careful assessment of mental status, skin condition, rectal examinatioin, breast examination, and pelvic examination in selected women
Weight	Monthly	Substantial weight loss (3 to 5 pounds) should prompt a search for treatable medical, psychiatric, and functional problems
Functional status Gait/mobility Cognitive function Basic activities of daily living	Yearly[†]	Should be done by interdisciplinary team as components of Minimum Data Set (see Table 2.2) Physician should review to identify changes that may be amenable to intervention
Affective and behavioral status		Standardized tests are available for these assessments in addition to the Minimum Data Set (see text)
Vision testing	Yearly	Assess acuity and identify correctable problems
Hearing testing	Yearly	Identify correctable problems (cerumen impaction; hearing loss that might be improved by an assistive device)
Dental	Yearly	Assess status of any remaining teeth and fit of dentures; identify any disease
Podiatric	Yearly	More frequently in diabetic patients and residents with peripheral vascular disease
Tuberculosis	At admission and yearly	All residents and staff should be tested; control skin tests and booster testing are generally recommended for nursing home residents
Laboratory tests Stool for occult blood Complete blood count Fasting glucose Electrolytes Renal function tests Albumin, calcium, phosphorus Thyroid function tests	Yearly in selected residents	These tests appear to have reasonable yield in the nursing home population
Chest radiograph	On admission if recent radiograph not available	May be helpful as baseline
Electrocardiogram	On admission if recent tracing not available	May be helpful as baseline
Mammography	Yearly	May benefit some women; those at high risk and those who would receive curative therapy if cancer discovered

* Adapted from Ouslander and colleagues (1). Data for the efficacy and timing of these practices are limited (see text). Thus, these recommendations should not be considered guidelines based on scientific merit but rather opinions based on literature review and clinical experience.

† Functional status assessment is an ongoing process in the nursing home. These domains are assessed quarterly using the Minimum Data Set (see Table 2.2).

BOX 2.3. Suggested format for annual physician review of long-term nursing home residents

1. Active medical problem list
2. Medical history
   a. Description of acute medical conditions that have occurred in the past year
   b. Comment on results of laboratory tests done to monitor active medical problems
   c. Summarize symptoms relevant to active medical problems
   d. List current medications
3. Symptom review
   a. Review symptoms common in nursing home residents
4. Physical examination
   a. Note any new physical findings
5. Functional status
   a. Briefly summarize current status, hightlighting changes in
      1) Ability to perform basic activities of daily living
      2) Mobility
      3) Continence
      4) Cognitive function
      5) Affective status (including behavioral disturbances)
   b. Assess rehabilitation potential (if relevant)
6. Social status
   a. Review any family involvement, family concerns, or problems
7. Health maintenance
   a. Review the results of screening evaluations, including
      1) Audiologic
      2) Ophthalmologic/optometric
      3) Dental
      4) Podiatric
      5) Tuberculosis testing
8. Screening laboratory tests (not done to monitor active medical conditions)
   a. Brief summary of results
9. Advanced directive
   a. Existence of directive
   b. Identification of proxy
   c. Whether the resident can still make or participate in decisions about his or her health care
   d. Intensity of care (no CPR, etc)
10. Plans
    a. Summarize overall goals for care
    b. List specific plans related to findings from the entire review

Acknowledgments. The authors thank members of the American College of Physicians Subcommittee on Aging and the *Annals of Internal Medicine* reviewers who provided many suggestions to improve this chapter. They also thank Laura Hodson for help in preparing the manuscript.

REFERENCES

1. Ouslander JG, Osterweil D, Morley JE. Medical Care in the Nursing Home. New York: McGraw-Hill; 1991.
2. The Federal Register. 56(187):48865-921.
3. Elon R, Pawlson LG. The impact of OBRA on medical practice within nursing facilities. J Am Geriatr Soc. 1992;40:958-63.
4. The Institute of Medicine. Improving the Quality of Care in Nursing Homes. Washington, DC: National Academy Press; 1986.
5. Morris JN, Hawes C, Fries BE, Phillips CD, Mor V, Katz S, et al. Designing the national resident assessment instrument for nursing homes. Gerontologist. 1990;30:293-307.
6. Health Care Financing Administration. Resident assessment protocols for long term care facilities. Baltimore, MD; 1991.
7. Uhlman RF, Rees TS, Psaty BM, Duckert LG. Validity and reliability of auditory screening tests in demented and non-demented older adults. J Gen Intern Med. 1989;4:90-6.
8. Mulrow CD, Lichtenstein MJ. Screening for hearing impairment in the elderly: rationale and strategy. J Gen Intern Med. 1991;6:249-58.
9. Tinetti ME. Performance-oriented assessment of mobility problems in elderly patients. J Am Geriatr Soc. 1986;34:119-26.
10. Tinetti ME, Ginter SF. Identifying mobility dysfunctions in elderly patients. Standard neuromuscular examination or direct assessment? JAMA. 1988;259:1190-3.
11. Siu AL. Screening for dementia and investigating its causes. Ann Intern Med. 1991;115:122-32.
12. Tombaugh TN, McIntyre NJ. The mini mental state examination: a comprehensive review. J Am Geriatr Soc. 1992;40:922-35.
13. Yesavage JA, Brink TL, Rose TL, Lum O, Huang V, Adey M, et al. Development and validation of a geriatric depression screening scale: a preliminary report. J Psychiatr Res. 1983;17:37-49.
14. Alexopoulos GS, Abrams RC, Young RC, Shamoian CA. Use of the Cornell scale in nondemented patients. J Am Geriatr Soc. 1988;36: 230-6.
15. Burke WJ, Nitcher RL, Roccaforte WH, Wengel SP. A prospective evaluation of the Geriatric Depression Scale in an outpatient geriatric assessment center. J Am Geriatr Soc. 1992;40:1227-30.
16. Applegate WB, Blass JP, Williams TF. Instruments for the functional assessment of older patients. N Engl J Med. 1990;322:1207-14.
17. Lachs MS, Feinstein AR, Cooney LM Jr, Drickamer MA, Marottoli RA, Pannill FC, et al. A simple procedure for general screening for functional disability in elderly patients. Ann Intern Med. 1990;112: 699-706.
18. Mulrow CD, Aguilar C, Endicott JE, Tuley MR, Velex R, Charlip WS, et al. Quality-of-life changes and hearing impairment. A randomized trial. Ann Intern Med. 1990;113:188-94.

19. Tinetti ME, Speechley M, Ginter SF. Risk factors for falls among elderly persons living in the community. N Engl J Med. 1988;319: 1701-7.
20. Tinetti ME, Speechley M. Prevention of falls among the elderly. N Engl J Med. 1989;320:1055-9.
21. Rubenstein LZ, Robbins AS, Josephson KR, Schulman BL, Osterweil D. The value of assessing falls in an elderly population. A randomized clinical trial. Ann Intern Med. 1990;113:308-16.
22. Burke WJ, Houston MJ, Boust SJ, Roccaforte WH. Use of the Geriatric Depression Scale in dementia of the Alzheimer type. J Am Geriatr Soc. 1989;37: 856-60.
23. Kafonek S, Ettinger WH, Roca R, Kittner S, Taylor N, German PS. Instruments for screening for depression and dementia in a long- term care facility. J Am Geriatr Soc. 1989;37:29-34.
24. Parmelee PA, Katz IR, Lawton MP. Depression among institutionalized aged: assessment and prevalence estimation. J Gerontol. 1989;44:M22-9.
25. Parmelee PA, Katz IR, Lawton MP. Incidence of depression in long-term care settings. J Geronol. 1992;47:M189-96.
26. Parmelee PA, Katz IR, Lawton MP. Depression and mortality among institutionalized aged. J Gerontol. 1992;47:P3-10.
27. Rovner BW, German PS, Brant LJ, Clark R, Burton L, Folstein MF. Depression and mortality in nursing homes. JAMA. 1991;265:993-6.
28. Rovner BW, German PS, Broadhead J, Morriss RK, Brant LJ, Blaustein J, et al. The prevalence and management of dementia and other psychiatric disorders in nursing homes. Int Psychogeriatr. 1990;2:13-24.
29. Katz S, Ford AB, Moskowitz RW, Jackson BA, Jaffee MW. Studies of illness in the aged. The index of ADL: a standardized measure of biological and psychosocial function. JAMA. 1963;185:914-9.
30. Lawton MP, Brody EM. Assessment of older people: self-maintaining and instrumental activities of daily living. Gerontologist. 1969; 9:179-86.
31. Kane RA, Kane RL. Long-Term Care: Principles, Programs, and Policies. New York: Springer; 1987.
32. Irvine PW, Van Buren N, Crossley K. Causes for hospitalization of nursing home residents: the role of infection. J Am Geriatr Soc. 1984;32:103-7.
33. Gordon WZ, Kane RL, Rothenberg R. Acute hospitalization in a home for the aged. J Am Geriatr Soc. 1985;33:519-23.
34. Kayser-Jones JS, Wiener CL, Barbaccia JC. Factors contributing to the hospitalization of nursing home residents. Gerontologist. 1989; 29:502-10.
35. Med4th Systems, Ltd. Care 4th. Milwaukee, Wisconsin, 1993.
36. American Society of Consultant Pharmacists. Drug Regimen Review: A Process Guide for Pharmacists. Arlington, VA: American Society of Consultant Pharmacists; 1992.
37. Ouslander J, Turner C, Delgado D, Reid D, Sannes G, Osterweil D. Communication between primary physicians and staff on long-term care facilities [Letter]. J Am Geriatr Soc. 1990;38:490-2.
38. Martin SE, Turner CL, Mendelsohn SE, et al. Assessment and initial management of acute medical problems in a nursing home. In Bosker G, ed. Principles and Practice of Acute Geriatric Medicine. 2d ed. St. Louis: Mosby-Year Book; 1990.
39. Wieland D, Rubenstein LZ, Ouslander JG, Martin SE. Organizing an academic nursing home. Impacts on institutionalized elderly. JAMA. 1986;255:2622-7.
40. Kane RL, Garrard J, Skay CL, Radosevich DM, Buchanan JL, McDermott SM, et al. Effects of a geriatric nurse practitioner on process and outcome of nursing home care. Am J Public Health. 1989;79:1271-7.
41. Garrard J, Kane RL, Radosevich DM, Skay CL, Arnold S, Kepferle L, et al. Impact of geriatric nurse practitioners on nursing home residents' functional status, satisfaction, and discharge outcomes. Med Care. 1990;28:271-83.
42. Ouslander JG. Medical care in the nursing home. JAMA. 1989;262: 2582-90.
43. Tangalos EG, Freeman PI, Garness SL, Kosiak CP. Nursing home fax machines [Letter]. JAMA. 1990;264:693-4.
44. Gambert SR, Duthie EH, Wiltzius F. The value of the yearly medical evaluation in a nursing home. J Chronic Dis. 1982;35:65-8.
45. Irvine PW, Carlson K, Adcock M, Slag M. The value of annual medical examinations in the nursing home. J Am Geriatr Soc. 1984;32:540-5.
46. Sox HC Jr, Woolf SH. Evidence-based practice guidelines from the US Preventive Services Task Force [Editorial]. JAMA. 1993;269: 2678.
47. Domoto K, Ben R, Wei JY, Pass TM, Komaroff AL. Yield of routine annual laboratory screening in the institutionalized elderly. Am J Public Health. 1985;75:243-5.
48. Wolf-Klein GP, Holt T, Silverstone FA, Foley CJ, Spatz M. Efficacy of routine annual studies in the care of elderly patients. J Am Geriatr Soc. 1985; 33:325-9.
49. Levinstein MR, Ouslander JG, Rubenstein LZ, Forsythe SB. Yield of routine annual laboratory tests in a skilled nursing home population. JAMA. 1987; 258:1909-15.
50. Joseph C, Lyles Y. Routine laboratory assessment of nursing home patients. J Am Geriatr Soc. 1992; 40:98-100.
51. Cooper JK. Decision analysis for tuberculosis prevention treatment in nursing homes. J Am Geriatr Soc. 1986;34:814-7.
52. Stead WW, Lofgren JP, Warren E, Thomas C. Tuberculosis as an endemic and nosocomial infection among the elderly in nursing homes. N Engl J Med. 1985;312:1483-7.
53. Stead WW, To T. The significance of the tuberculin skin test in elderly person. Ann Intern Med. 1987;107:837-42.
54. Stead WW, To T, Harrison RW, Abraham JH 3d. Benefit-risk considerations in preventive treatment for tuberculosis in elderly persons. Ann Intern Med. 1987;107:843-5.

55. Finucane TE. The American Geriatrics Society statement on two- step PPD testing for nursing home patients on admission. J Am Geriatr Soc. 1988;36:77-8.
56. Yoshikawa TT. Tuberculosis in aging adults. J Am Geriatr Soc. 1992;40:178-87.
57. Ziemba SE, Hubbell FA, Fine MJ, Burns MJ. Resting electrocardiograms as baseline tests: impact on the management of elderly patients. Am J Med. 1991;91:576-83.
58. Fahs MC, Mandelblatt J, Schechter C, Muller C. Cost effectiveness of cervical cancer screening for the elderly. Ann Intern Med. 1992; 117:520-7.
59. American Geriatrics Society Clinical Practice Committee. Position Statement on Screening for Cervical Carcinoma in the Elderly. New York: American Geriatrics Society, 1993.
60. Balducci L, Schapira DV, Cox CE, Greenberg HM, Hyman GH. Breast cancer of the older woman: an annotated review. J Am Geriatr Soc. 1991;39:1113-23.
61. American Geriatrics Society Clinical Practice Committee. Position Statement on Screening for Breast Cancer in Elderly Women. New York: American Geriatrics Society; 1993.
62. Catalona WJ, Smith DS, Ratliff TL, Dodds KM, Coplen DE, Yuan JJ, et al. Measurement of prostate-specific antigen in serum as a screening test for prostate cancer. N Engl J Med. 1991;324:1156-61.
63. Brawer MK, Chetner MP, Beatie J, Buchner DM, Vessella Rl, Lange PH. Screening for prostatic carcinoma with prostate specific antigen. J Urol. 1992;147:841-5.
64. Johansson JE, Adami HO, Andersson SO, Bergstrom R, Holmberg L, Krusemo UB. High 10-year survival rate in patients with early, untreated prostatic cancer. JAMA. 1992;267:2191-6.
65. Moon TD. Prostate cancer. J Am Geriatr Soc. 1992;40:622-7.
66. Garnick MB. Prostate cancer: screening, diagnosis, and management. Ann Intern Med. 1993;118:804-18.
67. Kramer BS, Brown ML, Prorok PC, Potosky AL, Gohagan JK. Prostate cancer screening: what we know and what we need to know. Ann Intern Med. 1993;119:914-23.
68. Oboler SK, LaForce FM. The periodic physical examination in asymptomatic adults. Ann Intern Med. 1989;110:214-26.
69. Cebul RD, Beck JR. Biochemical profiles. Applications in ambulatory screening and preadmission testing of adults. Ann Intern Med. 1987;106:403-13.
70. Woolf SH, Kamerow DB, Lawrence RS, Medalie JH, Estes EH. The periodic health examination of older adults: the recommendations of the U.S. Preventive Services Task Force. Part II. Screening tests. J Am Geriatr Soc. 1990;38:933-42.

PART II

Common Clinical Conditions
in the Nursing Home

3

Incontinence

Joseph G. Ouslander, MD, and John F. Schnelle, PhD

Incontinence is one of the most common conditions encountered in the nursing home population. Recently implemented rules and regulations for nursing home care (Omnibus Budget Reconciliation Act [OBRA] 1987) (1) require that incontinent nursing home residents have a basic diagnostic assessment and that residents managed by an indwelling bladder catheter have an appropriate indication for this device documented in their medical record. The federally mandated Minimum Data Set (MDS) (2) includes a separate section for the documentation of continence status that is completed by nursing home staff within 14 days of admission and updated on a quarterly basis. Incontinence documented on the MDS should "trigger" the use of the Resident Assessment Protocol for incontinence (3). Some of this assessment can be done by a trained nurse practitioner, physician's assistant, or clinical nurse specialist with input from members of the nursing home interdisciplinary team. The assessment does, however, require the involvement of the primary physician. We provide an overview of the assessment and treatment of incontinence in the nursing home setting.

PREVALENCE AND MORBIDITY

Urinary incontinence affects approximately half of nursing home residents (4,5). The prevalence varies among individual facilities depending on the case mix; rates may range from 40% to 70% or even higher in facilities with a functionally impaired resident population. In contrast to urinary incontinence among ambulatory community-dwelling geriatric patients, urinary incontinence among nursing home residents is more severe and more commonly associated with fecal incontinence. Incontinent nursing home residents generally have multiple episodes of urinary incontinence throughout the day and night, and approximately half are also incontinent of stool more than once per week (5,6).

Urinary incontinence in the nursing home is associated with substantial morbidity and cost. It can predispose patients to skin irritation, make pressure ulcers difficult to heal (7), and result in symptomatic urinary tract infection when urinary retention with overflow urinary incontinence remains undiagnosed or when urinary incontinence is inappropriately managed by long-term use of an indwelling catheter (8,9). It may also lead to falls among residents with nocturia and urge urinary incontinence and impaired balance or gait (10). The adverse psychological effects of urinary incontinence among nursing home residents have been difficult to document systematically (11), but incontinent residents who do not have severe dementia are often embarrassed and frustrated by their urinary incontinence. Nursing home staff generally consider urinary incontinence to be one of the most onerous and difficult conditions for which they care, and they perceive that they spend a disproportionate amount of time on the care of incontinent residents. The economic costs of urinary incontinence in the nursing home have been estimated to be close to $5 billion annually, including the costs of staff time, laundry, and supplies (12).

TYPES AND CAUSES OF URINARY INCONTINENCE

The pathogenesis of urinary incontinence among nursing home residents is often multifactorial, involving urologic and gynecologic conditions, neurologic disorders, behavioral and psychological factors, and functional impairments. Thus, the approach to assessment and treatment must be comprehensive and consider all of these potential factors. The most important factors to consider are those that are reversible. Potentially reversible conditions that can contribute to urinary incontinence in nursing home residents are listed in Table 3.1. These factors can be recalled by the acronym DRIP (delirium; restricted mobility, retention;

TABLE 3.1. Potentially reversible conditions that can cause or contribute to urinary incontinence in nursing home residents

Conditions	Management
Impaired ability or willingness to reach a toilet	
Delirium	Diagnosis and treatment of underlying causes of acute confusional state
Illness, injury, or restraint that interferes with mobility	Regular toileting assistance
	Use of toilet substitutes
	Environmental alterations (e.g., bedside commode)
Depression	Appropriate pharmacologic or nonpharmacologic treatment, or both
Irritation or inflammation in or around the lower urinary tract	
Urinary tract infection (symptomatic with frequency, urgency, sudden onset or worsening of incontinence, unexplained fever, or functional decline)	Antimicrobial therapy*
Atrophic vaginitis or urethritis	Oral or topical estrogen†
Stool impaction	Disimpaction
	Appropriate use of stool softeners and laxatives if necessary
	Adequate mobility and fluid intake
Increased urine production	
Metabolic (hyperglycemia, hypercalcemia)	Better control of diabetes mellitus
	Therapy for hypercalcemia depends on underlying cause
Excess fluid intake	Reduction in intake of diuretic fluids (e.g., caffeinated beverages)
Volume overload	
Venous insufficiency with edema	Support stockings
	Leg evaluation
	Sodium restriction
	Diuretic therapy
Congestive heart failure	Medical therapy
Drug side effects	
Rapid-acting diuretics causing frequency and urgency	Discontinuation of therapy with the medication if possible
Anticholinergics, narcotics, calcium channel blockers, α-adrenergic agonists (in men) causing urinary retention	Dosage reduction or modification (e.g., flexible scheduling of rapid-acting diuretics)
α-Adrenergic antagonists causing urethral relaxation and stress incontinence	
Psychotropic drugs with sedative or extrapyramidal effects causing sedation and immobility that interfere with toileting	

* For nursing home residents with bacteriuria (with or without pyuria) who have chronic, stable symptoms of incontinence and no other symptoms of urinary tract infection, antimicrobial therapy is not indicated.
† See text for specific recommendations.

infection, inflammation, impaction; polyuria, pharmaceuticals). Although identification and management of these reversible factors may not cure the urinary incontinence, its severity may be reduced and thereby be made more manageable by other interventions. In addition, identification and management of these conditions may have important benefits for the resident's overall functioning and quality of life.

A classification of the basic types of persistent urinary incontinence is shown in Table 3.2. Three important features of this classification should be noted. First, from a neurologic perspective, this classification is greatly simplified and does not include all of the pathophysiologic types of urinary incontinence. For example, patients with suprasacral spinal cord lesions, such as those that can occur in multiple sclerosis, may have detrusor hyperreflexia with external sphincter dyssynergy that can result in incontinence and incomplete bladder emptying

(detrusor-sphincter dyssynergy). Second, many incontinent nursing home residents have mixtures of these types of incontinence. The predominant abnormality of lower urinary tract functioning found among nursing home residents is detrusor hyperactivity (involuntary bladder contractions found on cystometry; also called detrusor instability, unstable bladder, and detrusor hyperreflexia [the latter occurs in the presence of a neurologic disorder]). Although most often associated with urge urinary incontinence, detrusor hyperactivity is commonly seen with sphincter weakness and stress urinary incontinence among women and with obstruction in men with benign or malignant enlargement of the prostate. Interestingly, detrusor hyperactivity is also seen in continent elderly people (men more frequently than women) (13,14); thus, its precise role in the pathogenesis of incontinence in the nursing home population is incompletely understood. In nursing home residents,

TABLE 3.2. Types and causes of urinary incontinence

Type	Symptoms	Common Causes
Stress	Involuntary loss of urine (usually small amounts) occurring with increases in intra-abdominal pressure (such as those caused by coughing, sneezing, and laughing)	Weakness and laxity of pelvic-floor musculature resulting in hypermobility of the bladder base and proximal urethra Bladder outlet or urethral sphincter weakness (intrinsic sphincter deficiency) related to previous surgery or trauma
Urge	Leakage of urine (usually larger, but often varying, volumes) because of inability to delay voiding after sensation of bladder fullness is perceived	Detrusor hyperactivity isolated or associated with one or more of the following: Local genitourinary condition such as cystitis, urethritis, tumors, stones, diverticula, outflow obstruction; impaired bladder contractility (detrusor hyperactivity with impaired contractility) Central nervous system disorders such as stroke, dementia, parkinsonism, spinal cord injury, and disease
Overflow	Leakage of urine (usually small amounts) resulting from mechanical forces on an overdistended bladder	Anatomical obstruction by prostate or large cystocele Acontractile bladder associated with diabetes mellitus or spinal cord injury
Functional*	Urinary leakage associated with inability to use the toilet because of impairment of cognitive or physical functioning, psychological unwillingness, or environmental barriers	Severe dementia Immobility Physical restraints Inaccessible toilets Unavailability of regular toileting assistance Depression

* Functional incontinence should be a diagnosis of exclusion. Most nursing home residents have functional factors that may contribute to incontinence but may also have reversible and specifically treatable conditions underlying the incontinence.

detrusor hyperactivity is commonly associated with impaired bladder contractility that results in incomplete bladder emptying (called detrusor hyperactivity with impaired contractility) (15,16). Nursing home residents with this disorder may have symptoms that mimic stress, overflow, or urge incontinence. Third, and most importantly, functional urinary incontinence should be a diagnosis of exclusion because most nursing home residents have impairments of cognitive or physical functioning that may interfere with their ability to use a toilet. These residents may also have other potentially treatable conditions that contribute to their urinary incontinence. Thus, a search for reversible factors and other types of urinary incontinence should be done before a nursing home resident's urinary incontinence is labeled as "functional."

ASSESSMENT

Nursing home residents are heterogeneous, and a realistic and appropriate goal for one type of resident may be unrealistic and inappropriate for another (17,18). The approach to urinary incontinence brings this concept into sharp focus. A resident having active rehabilitation after a hip fracture or a stroke may, after a thorough incontinence assessment, benefit from a specific bladder-retraining protocol or pharmacologic therapy for detrusor hyperactivity; incontinence undergarments and indwelling catheters are probably inappropriate for this type of resident. On the other hand, a resident with end-stage dementia and severe agitation may be most appropriately managed by an incontinence undergarment after reversible causes of their urinary incontinence have been excluded. Thus, an important aspect of incontinence care is to determine, through the interdisciplinary care-planning process, if a particular resident has the potential to respond to specific interventions for the urinary incontinence. Because even severely impaired residents may respond well to a prompted voiding program (see below), a bias in favor of thorough assessment and a therapeutic trial is appropriate.

Basic assessment of bladder and bowel function as indicated on the MDS is required for all newly admitted nursing home residents. A bladder and bowel record is helpful in documenting the continence status of new residents and can also be used as part of periodic reassessments. A legible record,

such as the one shown in Figure 3.1, should be used (19). The specific symbols used are not important, but the record should provide a simple way of documenting wetness, dryness, appropriate toileting, and bowel status and a space for comments. Records such as the one shown in Figure 3.1 can be reduced so that several records fit on one page. This type of record is also helpful in monitoring responses to therapeutic interventions. Because many newly admitted residents come from acute-care hospitals, they frequently arrive at the nursing home with an indwelling bladder catheter. In this situation, it is essential to determine why the catheter was placed (for example, to monitor urinary output or for urinary retention or management of urinary incontinence) and to consider the resident for a bladder-retraining program. The catheter should be removed unless there is an appropriate indication for retaining it.

Basic Evaluation

After these initial assessments and documentation, incontinent nursing home residents should have a basic evaluation that includes a history, physical examination, urinalysis, and determination of postvoid residual urine volume. Much of this evaluation can be done by nursing home staff and a "physician extender" (nurse practitioner, physician's assistant, or clinical nurse specialist). This basic evaluation has three objectives:

1. To identify potentially reversible factors (Table 3.1)
2. To identify potentially serious underlying conditions or conditions that may require further urologic, gynecologic, or urodynamic evaluation (Table 3.3)
3. To determine the type of incontinence (urge, stress, overflow, or mixed) and an appropriate management plan.

Both the Resident Assessment Protocol for incontinence and the Agency for Health Care Policy and Research (AHCPR) clinical practice guideline on urinary incontinence (20) contain specific recommendations for the assessment of incontinence in nursing home residents. The information summarized below is consistent with these recommendations, but readers should become familiar with the Resident Assessment Protocol and the AHCPR guidelines as well.

HISTORY

Medical records should be reviewed to identify medications, medical conditions, and genitourinary history that may be relevant to the resident's incontinence. A precise history and report of symptoms may be difficult to obtain from many nursing home residents because incontinence is closely associated with dementia in this population. Residents who can reliably report symptoms should be questioned about irritative and other symptoms that suggest urge incontinence (frequency, urgency, nocturia [more than two episodes]); symptoms of stress incontinence (leakage simultaneous with coughing, sneezing, laughing, bending); voiding difficulty (hesitancy, poor or intermittent stream, straining to finish voiding); and other associated symptoms such as dysuria or pain. Pain related to voiding is unusual and should be carefully evaluated.

Nursing home staff can be helpful in identifying many of these symptoms among residents who cannot reliably report them, as well as in assessing the timing and nature of fluid intake and monitoring voiding activity using a record such as the one shown in Figure 3.1.

INCONTINENCE MONITORING RECORD

INSTRUCTIONS: EACH TIME THE PATIENT IS CHECKED:
1. Mark one of the circles in the BLADDER section at the hour closest to the time the patient was checked.
2. Make an X in the BOWEL section if the patient has had an incontinent or normal bowel movement.

| ◗ = Incontinent, small amount | O = Dry | ✗ = Incontinent BOWEL |
| ◗ = Incontinent, large amount | △ = Voided Correctly | ✗ = Normal BOWEL |

PATIENT'S NAME: _____ ROOM NO. _____ DATE _____

| TIME | BLADDER | | | | BOWEL | | | |
	INCONTINENT OF URINE	DRY	VOIDED CORRECTLY	INCONTINENT ✗	NORMAL ✗	INITIALS	COMMENTS
12 am	● ●	O	△ cc ___				
1	● ●	O	△ cc ___				
2	● ●	O	△ cc ___				
3	● ●	O	△ cc ___				
4	● ●	O	△ cc ___				
5	● ●	O	△ cc ___				
6	● ●	O	△ cc ___				
7	● ●	O	△ cc ___				
8	● ●	O	△ cc ___				
9	● ●	O	△ cc ___				
10	● ●	O	△ cc ___				
11	● ●	O	△ cc ___				
12 pm	● ●	O	△ cc ___				
1	● ●	O	△ cc ___				
2	● ●	O	△ cc ___				
3	● ●	O	△ cc ___				
4	● ●	O	△ cc ___				
5	● ●	O	△ cc ___				
6	● ●	O	△ cc ___				
7	● ●	O	△ cc ___				
8	● ●	O	△ cc ___				
9	● ●	O	△ cc ___				
10	● ●	O	△ cc ___				
11	● ●	O	△ cc ___				

FIGURE 3.1. Example of a record that is helpful in assessing incontinent nursing home residents and in following their response to intervention.

PHYSICAL EXAMINATION

Because impairments of cognitive and physical function are commonly associated with incontinence among nursing home residents, the physical examination should include an assessment of these areas specifically related to the resident's ability to respond to a prompt to urinate, use the toilet, and manage their clothing and hygiene. Physical and occupational therapists can be helpful in completing this assessment.

The general physical examination should exclude volume overload (for example, venous insufficiency or congestive heart failure) and previously undiagnosed neurologic conditions that might contribute to the incontinence (such as signs of parkinsonism or spinal cord compression). Rectal examination is done to assess resting and active sphincter tone, to exclude fecal impaction, and, in men, to assess the prostate. The size of the prostate on physical examination can neither establish nor exclude the presence of urethral obstruction.

The pelvic examination should assess perineal and vulvar skin condition, exclude pelvic masses and marked pelvic prolapse (such as uterine descensus or a cystocele that protrudes through the vaginal introitus), and evaluate the vaginal epithelium for signs of inflammation (erythema, friability, or bleeding) that suggest atrophic vaginitis. A cough test to detect stress incontinence can also be done during the pelvic examination, but it is best done while the patient is standing and has at least 200 mL of urine in the bladder (3).

URINALYSIS

The urinalysis is primarily done to exclude significant bacteriuria in residents who have symptoms (other than incontinence) suggesting a urinary tract infection (dysuria, recent onset or worsening of incontinence, or unexplained fever or functional decline) and to exclude sterile hematuria, which may indicate bladder or upper urinary tract disorders.

Clean urine may be difficult to obtain from incontinent, cognitively impaired, immobile nursing home residents. However, it is possible to noninvasively obtain from both men and women a clean-catch urine that accurately matches culture results from a catheterized specimen. For women, the technique involves carefully cleaning the perineum with a sterile preparation kit and then having the patients void into a disinfected collection device (a toileting insert or "hat" or a fracture bedpan) (21). For men, a clean condom catheter can be applied after the penis is cleaned with a sterile preparation such as iodine-povidone (Betadine) (22).

Although rapid-urine screening methods are generally considered inaccurate in the nursing home population, they can be used to exclude bacteriuria with reasonable accuracy. The combination of negative dipstick test results for both nitrite and leukocyte esterase counts and a negative enzyme-based screen for bacteriuria (Uriscreen, Ventrex Laboratories, Portland, Maine) has a negative predictive value of more than 95% for significant bacteriuria among incontinent nursing home residents (23). Whether such screening tests are practical depends on the availability of personnel who can reliably collect the urine and do the tests and on the costs relative to sending a specimen to the laboratory for urinalysis.

ESTIMATE OF POSTVOID RESIDUAL VOLUME

Significant degrees of urinary retention can occur without symptoms or signs of obstruction or bladder contractility problems. In addition, physical examination (suprapubic palpation, bimanual examination) is neither sensitive nor specific in detecting significant residual volume. The postvoid residual is usually determined by catheterization, but a portable ultrasound device is now available (Bladder Volume Instrument; Bard Urological, Covington, Georgia) that can noninvasively measure residual urine volume with reasonably good accuracy in incontinent nursing home residents (24). It is important to note that postvoid residual volumes can substantially vary within individual patients. The timing of the determination in relation to a void, the degree to which the void was natural for the patient, the nature of instructions given to the patient, the amount of straining, and body position can all influence the postvoid volume obtained. Thus, when moderately elevated urine volumes are detected (for example, 150 to 300 mL), repeated determinations may be appropriate. In these situations, ultrasonography may be especially valuable in avoiding the need for repeated catheterizations. Repeated residual volumes of more than 200 mL should prompt consideration of whether the resident should be referred for further evaluation (Table 3.3).

TABLE 3.3. Conditions that may require further urologic, gynecologic, or urodynamic evaluation

Condition	Comments
History	
Recurrent symptomatic urinary tract infections in addition to incontinence	A structural abnormality or pathologic condition in the urinary tract predisposing the patient to symptomatic infection should be excluded
Physical examination	
Marked pelvic prolapse protruding through the vaginal introitus	Surgical repair or pessary management should be considered to prevent discomfort and tissue erosion to treat the incontinence
Suspicion of prostate cancer	Although surgical intervention to cure the cancer would not be appropriate for most nursing home residents, diagnosis of the cancer may be important in managing the incontinence and other complications
Urinalysis	
Hematuria (sterile)	Urologic evaluation should be considered to identify pathologic conditions of the urinary tract
Determination of postvoid residual volume	
Residual volumes >200 mL	Although no precise cutoff point can be recommended, residual volumes >200 mL are abnormal and should prompt consideration of further evaluation of the urinary tract to identify complications (such as hydronephrosis or renal function impairment) and to determine the cause of the retention (such as obstruction, impaired bladder contractility, or both)

Further Evaluation

Selected incontinent nursing home residents may benefit from further urologic, gynecologic, or urodynamic evaluation. Examples of conditions that may require further evaluation are outlined in Table 3.3. In determining the need for further evaluation, the most important consideration is whether the results will change the management of the resident's incontinence. Thus, for example, a nursing home resident with urinary retention who is not a candidate for surgical intervention is unlikely to benefit from a urodynamic evaluation to diagnose the cause of the retention; such a patient should be managed by intermittent or long-term catheterization. On the other hand, urodynamic evaluation is essential for a resident for whom surgery is being considered (for example, a woman with symptoms and signs of severe stress incontinence or a man with symptoms and signs suggesting obstruction).

Complex urodynamic tests (including cystometry with simultaneous measurement of bladder and abdominal pressure; voiding pressure-flow study; measurement of urethral pressure at rest, during voiding, and with straining; sphincter electromyography; and videourodynamic studies) have been shown to be safe and feasible in the nursing home population (16). This type of testing is essential for the accurate diagnosis of obstruction, detrusor hyperactivity with impaired contractility, and the type of stress incontinence (that is, primarily caused by urethral hypermobility or by intrinsic sphincter deficiency). Because the testing procedures are relatively expensive, involve some discomfort, and require specialized equipment and trained personnel, they should only be done in incontinent nursing home residents for whom the results are necessary to determine an appropriate treatment plan.

Some simple urodynamic tests, including a pad test for stress incontinence and "bedside" cystometry, do not require specialized equipment (17,25,26). The Resident Assessment Protocol recommends a stress test for nursing home residents whose incontinence persists after the basic evaluation and management of reversible conditions (3). The stress test is done by having the patient cough forcefully several times, preferably in the standing position, when their bladder is relatively full (but not when the patient has a strong urge to void). The test result is positive if there is immediate leakage similar to the volume and circumstance of the resident's usual incontinence. If the test result is negative and the total bladder volume (voided volume plus residual volume) is less than 200 mL, the test should be repeated. If the postvoid residual determination has been done by catheterization, the bladder can be filled with sterile water (by gravity) to a volume of 200 mL for the stress test. Simple cystometry can also be done immediately after catheterization (25) by filling the bladder in 50-mL aliquots through a 50-mL catheter-tip syringe without the piston, while asking the resident to hold as much as possible. Involuntary bladder contractions are shown by continuous upward movement of the fluid column in the syringe in the absence of abdominal straining (which can sometimes be detected by palpating the abdomen) or by leakage of the water around the catheter. When involuntary contractions do not occur, the volume at which the resident has a strong urge to void (cystometric bladder capacity) can be determined. Although this test can be helpful in identifying involuntary bladder contractions (27), the results may be difficult to interpret in cognitively impaired nursing home residents. Straining may be difficult to detect and may be misinterpreted as an involuntary contraction, and low-pressure involuntary contractions (such as those seen in many patients having detrusor hyperactivity with impaired contractility) are easily missed.

In our studies, we have not found stress tests and simple cystometry helpful in identifying the substantial proportion of incontinent residents (25% to 40%) who respond well to daytime prompted voiding (28). Other investigators have also shown that urodynamic diagnosis does not predict responsiveness to bladder training in community-dwelling older women (29). We therefore suggest that if behavioral interventions such as prompted voiding and bladder training are to be used as the initial therapy, urodynamic testing is not necessary before a therapeutic trial. Urodynamic testing to help differentiate stress from urge and mixed (both stress and urge) incontinence should be considered for residents who do not respond well to the behavioral intervention and for whom more specific therapy (such as pharmacologic treatment) is planned.

APPROACHES TO THERAPY

Reversible Factors

The first step in treating incontinence is to attempt to reverse the potentially reversible factors (Table

3.1). Conditions that may interfere with the resident's ability or willingness to get to a toilet or use a toilet substitute should be addressed. New or worsening incontinence may, for example, be a manifestation of delirium, a condition with myriad potential underlying causes and substantial morbidity and mortality if it remains unidentified and untreated. Immobility caused by musculoskeletal pain (such as hip fracture or exacerbation of arthritis) may precipitate incontinence. In these situations, regular toileting assistance and the optimal use of toilet substitutes (such as fracture bedpans) and other environmental interventions should be used. Physical restraints may also contribute to incontinence and, consistent with OBRA rules (1), should be avoided whenever possible. Unrecognized and untreated depression is another major cause of morbid conditions in the nursing home population and can interfere with a nursing home resident's motivation to be continent. Underlying depression should be considered if a patient repeatedly refuses to cooperate with toileting assistance.

Data do not support treating asymptomatic bacteriuria in incontinent nursing home residents because eradicating bacteriuria does not appear to alter morbidity, mortality, or the severity of chronic incontinence in this population (30–32). The presence of pyuria in this population (defined as more than 10 leukocytes per high-power field on routine microscopic examination of centrifuged urine) does not necessarily indicate the presence of symptomatic infection that requires treatment (32,33). However, manifestations of a symptomatic urinary tract infection in this population may be subtle and include the onset or worsening of incontinence, unexplained low-grade fever, anorexia, and functional decline. Thus, clinicians should not treat asymptomatic bacteriuria on the one hand but have a high index of suspicion for symptomatic infection in the presence of such nonspecific symptoms on the other. Atrophic vaginitis, manifested by inflamed or friable epithelium on pelvic examination, may cause irritative symptoms, including urge incontinence, and should be treated by either a vaginal estrogen cream (1 to 2 g applied 3 to 5 nights per week) or oral conjugated estrogen (0.3 to 0.625 mg/d). No data support any specific treatment protocol (34). The goal is not necessarily to cure the incontinence but to reduce the frequency of incontinent episodes and possibly make the resident more responsive to other forms of treatment. If a clear

response is shown, estrogen therapy can either be continued or discontinued and reinitiated if symptoms and signs recur. Prolonged, unopposed estrogen therapy (that is, lasting longer than 1 to 2 years) in a woman with a uterus should prompt consideration of adding a progestational agent (35).

Fecal impaction is an important reversible cause of urinary (and fecal) incontinence. The mechanisms by which impaction contributes to urinary incontinence has never been fully explained. Impactions can generally be prevented by a bowel regimen similar to the one presented in the section below on fecal incontinence. Factors contributing to polyuria or nocturia should be addressed. Although controlling diabetes in some nursing home residents is difficult, the osmotic diuresis induced by glucosuria can certainly exacerbate urinary incontinence, and better glucose control should be attempted. Edema that is mobilized in the supine position, especially in the evening and night hours, can cause bothersome polyuria and nocturia. This may be hazardous for residents who are prone to falls. It is therefore reasonable in some situations to initially manage the urinary incontinence by adding (or increasing the dose of) a rapid-acting diuretic in the morning to reduce the edema, which will make the resident urinate more often when they have better access to a commode.

Drugs that may be contributing to urinary incontinence (Table 3.1) should be stopped whenever possible, especially if urinary retention is present. If it is not possible to discontinue therapy, reducing the dose or modifying the dosage schedule may help manage the urinary incontinence.

Behavioral Interventions

Most nursing homes have bladder training protocols that consist of simple scheduled toileting every 2 hours (6). Although this is practical for staff and may help some residents, it is probably not the most efficient procedure and should be combined with other techniques whenever feasible. Behavioral interventions can be divided into two basic types: patient-dependent and caregiver-dependent. Patient-dependent procedures include pelvic muscle (Kegel) exercises, bladder training, biofeedback, and other similar behavioral therapies. All have some demonstrated efficacy among community-dwelling incontinent patients (36–38). None of these procedures, or other adjunctive therapies such as electrical stimulation (39), has been adequately studied among nursing home residents. The goal of patient-dependent interventions is to restore a normal pattern of voiding and continence, and it is presumed that the resident will be capable of independent toileting once bladder functioning is improved. Because of the high prevalence of dementia among incontinent nursing home residents, the learning and practice required for these techniques to be successful are obstacles to their widespread use in this population. Bladder retraining is a patient-dependent behavioral intervention that is relevant in the nursing home. This intervention is applicable in the common situation in which an incontinent resident has been admitted (or readmitted) to the nursing home from an acute-care hospital with an indwelling bladder catheter that was inserted for either urinary retention or accurate monitoring of urine output. (Under these circumstances, the bladder retraining may serve as a "void-

ing trial," as suggested by the Resident Assessment Protocol [3].) An example of a bladder-retraining protocol is shown in Box 3.1. The precise protocol depends on the resident's bladder function. If the catheter was placed to measure urine output or to manage urinary incontinence during a hospitalization, the bladder is probably irritable and has a small capacity; in this instance, progressively increasing the intervals between voiding can be attempted. In highly functional residents, pelvic-muscle exercises and other behavioral techniques may be helpful in this process. If the catheter was inserted for urinary retention, the bladder muscle may be decompensated; in this situation, regular attempts to void should be combined with routine estimation of residual urine volume and postvoid intermittent catheterizations as needed. During this phase, ultrasound determination of postvoid residual volume can be helpful in avoiding repeated catheterizations. It may take weeks for the bladder to begin func-

---

BOX 3.1. Bladder retraining protocol for use after the removal of an indwelling catheter*

Goal: to restore a normal pattern of voiding and continence after the removal of an indwelling catheter
Monitor the resident's urine output every 8 hours for 1 or 2 days
Remove the indwelling catheter (clamping the catheter before removal is not necessary)†
Initiate a toileting schedule
    Begin by taking the resident to the toilet
        Every 2 hours during the day and evening
        Before getting into bed
        Every 4 hours at night
    Instruct the resident on techniques to trigger voiding (such as running water, stroking inner thigh, and suprapubic tapping) and to help completely empty bladder (such as bending forward, suprapubic pressure, and double voiding)
If the resident cannot void by the time the expected bladder volume is 800 mL (on the basis of monitoring in step 1) or if the postvoid residual is >400 mL, reinsert the catheter and consider a urodynamic evaluation or the use of a permanent catheter
If the postvoid residuals are 100 to 400 mL, continue to monitor until they are consistently less than approximately 200 mL‡
Monitor the resident's voiding and continence pattern with a record (see Figure 3.1) that allows the recording of the following:
    Frequency, timing, and amount of incontinence episodes
    Fluid-intake pattern
    Postvoid or intermittent catheter volume
If the resident is voiding frequently (that is, more often than every 2 hours), encourage the resident to delay voiding as long as possible and instruct him or her (if possible) to use pelvic-muscle exercises and techniques to help empty bladder completely
If the resident continues to have incontinence:
    Rule out reversible causes (see Table 3.1)
    Consider urodynamic evaluation to determine cause and appropriate treatment

* Indwelling catheters should be removed from all residents who do not have an indication for their short- or long-term use (see Box 3.3). For those who have had significant retention (volume >400 mL), the catheter should be kept in for several days to decompress the bladder.
† Clamping routines have never been shown to be helpful and are not appropriate for residents who have had overdistended bladders.
‡ A precise value cannot be recommended on the basis of available data. Residual volumes <200 mL generally do not cause upper urinary tract complications.

tioning again. If postvoid residual volumes remain elevated and the resident remains incontinent, a urologic evaluation should be considered. Note that in either situation, clamping the catheter before removal is not necessary; it has never been shown to be beneficial and may be harmful to residents who already have a decompensated bladder after an episode of urinary retention.

Caregiver-dependent techniques, including habit-training and prompted voiding, have been shown to be effective for some incontinent nursing home residents (40–46). These interventions can be used with demented and physically impaired residents who are not candidates for patient-dependent procedures. Habit-training involves establishing a pattern for assisting residents with voiding and toileting according to their own pattern. This technique may be difficult to implement because it requires that multiple nursing home staff keep track of individual toileting schedules (45), and it is not clear what types of residents respond to this intervention. In prompted voiding, residents are asked (prompted) on a 2-hour schedule if they will try to use the toilet. See Box 3.2 for an example of a prompted voiding protocol. As opposed to bladder retraining (Box 3.1), the goal is not necessarily to restore a normal pattern of voiding and continence but rather to prevent wetness. Prompted voiding has been shown to be highly effective in reducing incontinence frequency during the day and evening hours when motivated staff implement it properly. Because it appears to be effective in nursing home

BOX 3.2. Prompted voiding protocol

Goal: To reduce the frequency of wetness in selected residents from 7 a.m. to 7 p.m.
Assessment period (3 to 5 days)
    Contact the residents every 2 hours from 7 a.m. to 7 p.m.
    Focus their attention on voiding by asking them whether they are wet or dry
    Check them for wetness, make notation on bladder record, and give feedback on whether they were correct
        or incorrect
    Whether wet or dry, ask residents if they would like to use the toilet (or urinal)
        If they say yes:
            Assist them
            Record the results on the bladder record
            Give them positive reinforcement by talking with them for extra minute or two
        If they say no:
            Inform them that you will be back in 2 hours and request that they try to delay voiding until then
            If they have not attempted to void in the last 4 hours, request once or twice before leaving that they use
                the toilet
    Measure voiding volumes as often as possible by the following:
        Placing a measuring "hat" in the commode
        Preweighing and then reweighing incontinence pads or garments
Targeting
    Prompted voiding is more effective in some residents than others
    The best candidates for continuing an effective prompted voiding program are residents who show the
        following characteristics during the assessment period:
        Usually correct about their wet or dry status
        Void in the toilet, commode, or urinal (as opposed to being incontinent in a pad or garment) more than half
            the time
        Have a maximum voided volume of 200 mL or more
        Lower voiding frequencies
        Substantial reduction in incontinence frequency as shown in bladder records
    Residents who do not show any of these characteristics should be considered for one of the following:
        Further evaluation to determine the specific type of incontinence
        Palliative management by containment devices and a checking and changing protocol
Prompted voiding (ongoing protocol)
    Contact the resident every 2 hours from 7 a.m. to 7 p.m.
    Use same procedures as those for the assessment period
    For nighttime management, use either a modified prompted voiding schedule or a containment device
    If a resident who has been responding well has an increase in incontinence frequency despite adequate staff
        implementation of the protocol, they should be evaluated for reversible factors (*see* Table 3.1)

residents with different types of lower urinary tract dysfunction and has almost no side effects, it is a reasonable initial approach to managing most incontinent nursing home residents after reversible factors have been identified and treated. Data collected in nearly 30 nursing homes suggest that 25% to 40% of incontinent residents respond well, with a reduction in their daytime incontinence frequency from three to four episodes per day to one or fewer (28, 40–42, 46–50). Nursing home staff can use simple behavioral and other observations from a 3- to 5-day trial of prompted voiding to target those most likely to respond well (Box 3.2) (28,47,50). An intense quality-assurance program, based on principles of statistical quality control or other management techniques, is necessary for the ongoing effectiveness of prompted voiding or any other caregiver-dependent intervention in nursing homes (48–51).

The best results from prompted voiding have been documented from 7 a.m. to 7 p.m. Prompted voiding has not been systematically studied between 7 p.m. and 7 a.m., even though evidence suggests that incontinence is at least as severe during this nighttime period (52). The frequency of incontinence during night hours is similar to that observed during daytime periods, but the volume of the incontinence episodes at night is significantly higher. Although volume overload (congestive heart failure, venous insufficiency with edema) and benign prostatic hyperplasia may contribute to nighttime incontinence, the mechanism or mechanisms underlying increased urine production at night in this population are not well understood. Hormonal abnormalities such as altered secretion of antidiuretic hormone or atrial natriuretic peptide may be responsible, but further research is needed in this area. Nursing rounds during the night to change incontinent residents frequently disrupt sleep (53,54). Prompted voiding schedules have not yet been designed to improve night-time incontinence management without disrupting resident's sleep. It is therefore not clear whether the potential benefits of regular toileting throughout night-time hours are outweighed by disruption of the resident's sleep. In addition, staffing patterns at night may preclude an effective prompted voiding program, even in targeted residents. Thus, until further data are available, nursing homes should modify the prompted voiding procedures for night-time hours or should use incontinence undergarments.

Drug Therapy

Because of the close association between functional disability and urinary incontinence among nursing home residents, drug therapy must generally be used as an adjunct to some form of toileting program. Drug therapy in this population is directed at one of two abnormalities of lower urinary tract functioning, or a combination of both. Detrusor hyperactivity (involuntary bladder contractions on urodynamic testing), the most common urodynamic abnormality found in incontinent nursing home residents, is generally associated with urge urinary incontinence (16,26,55). Drugs with anticholinergic effects, including propantheline (15 to 30 mg three to four times per day), oxybutynin (2.5 to 5 mg two to four times per day), and imipramine (10 to 25 mg three times per day) have been most commonly used as bladder relaxants. Several studies suggest that frail and functionally impaired incontinent patients do not respond well to bladder relaxant medications (56–60). A recent placebo-controlled trial in which oxybutynin was added to prompted voiding suggests that a modest subgroup (approximately 25%) of incontinent nursing home residents with detrusor hyperactivity may benefit from this drug when it is added to a prompted-voiding protocol (61). If one of these medications is given in a therapeutic trial, careful observation is needed for anticholinergic side effects such as dry mouth, constipation and fecal impaction, blurry vision, urinary retention, and worsening cognitive function. Imipramine can also cause postural hypotension. Women with urge incontinence associated with atrophic vaginitis should be treated with estrogen as described above. New types of bladder-relaxant drugs and long-acting preparations (for example, slow-release capsules and skin patches) are being developed but are not currently available.

For sphincter weakness with stress urinary incontinence in women, drug treatment involves a combination of estrogen and an α-agonist. Estrogen can be given by vaginal cream, 1 g at bedtime, or orally, 0.625 mg conjugated estrogen daily. Few data support the effectiveness of estrogen, especially when given alone, for treating stress incontinence (20,34). Either pseudoephedrine, 30 to 60 mg three times per day, or phenylpropanolamine, 75 mg twice per day, can be used as the α-agonist. Phenylpropanolamine has been shown to be as effective as pelvic-muscle exercises among noninstitutionalized older women with stress incontinence (62). Drug treatment for stress urinary incontinence should be combined with a toileting program (to keep the bladder volume as low as possible) and pelvic-muscle exercises (for residents who can cooperate). Women who have prominent pelvic prolapse or who fail a 3- to 6-month trial of drug or behavioral therapy, or both, should be considered for surgical intervention.

For women with mixed urge and stress urinary incontinence, a combination of the above approaches can be used. Imipramine, in doses of 10 to 25 mg three times per day, may be tried as a combination anticholinergic–α-agonist. Imipramine can worsen cardiac conduction abnormalities and, in addition to its anticholinergic side effects, can cause significant postural hypotension in ambulatory nursing home residents. Thus, this drug should be used cautiously in the nursing home population.

Drug treatment for overflow urinary incontinence has not been adequately studied in incontinent geriatric patients. Cholinergic agonists such as bethanechol have not been consistently effective when given orally on a long-term basis in patients with urinary retention caused by poor bladder contractility (63). Nursing home residents having bladder retraining after an episode of urinary retention (Box 3.1) may benefit from a therapeutic trial of bethanechol if urinary retention persists. Other drugs, such as metaclopramide, have also been used for this purpose. Both bethanechol and metaclopramide can have significant side effects in frail geriatric patients and must be used cautiously. α-Antagonists (such as prazosin and terazosin) have been somewhat successful in men with obstructive symptoms (hesitancy, straining, frequency, urgency, and nocturia) that are associated with benign prostatic hyperplasia (64–66). Because these drugs can cause postural hypotension and result in falls and related injuries in frail older men, it is recommended that therapy be initiated with a small bedtime dose and that postural vital signs be monitored as the dose is increased.

Surgery

Surgical intervention for urinary incontinence is a consideration for a small but important subgroup of incontinent nursing home residents. Because uri-

nary incontinence is not a life-threatening problem, elective surgery should be pursued only if the incontinence is bothersome enough to a resident who is a candidate for such treatment.

There are two types of surgery for urinary incontinence. First, women with stress urinary incontinence associated with significant pelvic prolapse and urethral hypermobility may benefit from bladder-neck suspension and repair of the pelvic prolapse. Although studies have not been done in the nursing home population, the short-term (1 to 5 years) success of this type of surgery for properly selected older women is approximately 75% for significant reduction or elimination of wetness (20). Artificial urinary sphincters have been used for younger patients with stress incontinence associated with intrinsic urethral deficiency. This requires a relatively major surgical procedure and is probably not appropriate for nursing home residents. Periurethral injections of collagen have recently been approved for patients with intrinsic urethral deficiency. Although studies have not yet included very frail patients, periurethral injection has reportedly been effective in younger patients (67).

The other type of surgical intervention for urinary incontinence is the removal of anatomical obstruction, most commonly an enlarged prostate in men or a urethral stricture. Detailed discussion of the evaluation and surgical treatment of lower urinary tract obstruction is beyond the scope of this article, but nursing home residents who are candidates for surgery and who are suspected of having obstruction should be referred for complex urodynamic evaluation. Newer, less invasive techniques are now available for the surgical relief of obstruction in men and may be especially appropriate for consideration in frail, older nursing home residents.

Pads and Undergarments

Highly absorbent launderable and disposable pads and undergarments are the most common method of managing urinary incontinence in the nursing home. This method of management is appropriate for the subgroup of incontinent nursing home residents who remain incontinent despite more specific treatments. Pads and garments may also be helpful at night for residents who are managed by prompted voiding or other interventions during the day and evening. Many factors should be considered when selecting the optimal pad or undergarment for an individual resident, including comfort and fit, absorbency relative to the degree of leakage, availability of laundry services (for reusable products), skin sensitivity, and cost. No adequate well-controlled studies are available on which to base the choice of one specific type of product over another (68). Pads and undergarments should not be used as the sole solution to urinary incontinence in the nursing home, or in a manner that fosters further dependency. When pads or garments are used, residents should still be regularly checked and given the opportunity to use the toilet or be changed if necessary to avoid skin irritation and breakdown.

Catheters and Catheter Care

Three basic types of catheters and catheterization procedures are used to manage urinary incontinence in nursing homes: external catheters, intermittent straight catheterization, and long-term indwelling catheterization. External catheters consist of some type of condom connected to a drainage system. Improvements in design and observance of proper procedure and skin care when applying the catheter will decrease the risk for skin irritation and the frequency with which the catheter falls off. Few studies have been done on complications associated with the use of these devices, but existing data suggest that male nursing home residents with external catheters are at increased risk for developing symptomatic urinary tract infections (69). External catheters should therefore only be used to manage intractable incontinence in male residents who do not have urinary retention and who are extremely physically dependent. As with incontinence undergarments and padding, these devices should not be used for convenience because they may foster dependency. The safety and effectiveness of external catheters for women have not been documented in nursing homes.

Intermittent catheterization is used to manage urinary retention and overflow incontinence. The procedure involves straight catheterization two to four times daily to keep the bladder volume below approximately 400 mL. Studies done primarily in younger paraplegic patients have shown that this technique is practical and, compared with long-term catheterization, reduces the risk for symptomatic infection (70). Intermittent self-catheterization has also been shown to be feasible

for elderly female outpatients who are functional, willing, and able to catheterize themselves (71). However, the results of studies done in young paraplegic patients and elderly female outpatients cannot automatically be extrapolated to the nursing home population. The technique may be useful for certain nursing home residents (72), but the practicality and safety of this procedure in nursing homes have not been well documented. Elderly nursing home residents, especially men, may be difficult to catheterize, and the anatomical abnormalities commonly found in the lower urinary tract of nursing home residents may increase the risk for infection because of repeated straight catheterizations. In addition, using this technique in an institutional setting (which may have an abundance of organisms relatively resistant to many commonly used antimicrobial agents) may yield an unacceptable risk for nosocomial infections. The use of sterile catheter trays for the multiple catheterizations is expensive. Thus, it may be difficult to implement such a program in a typical nursing home.

Long-term indwelling catheterization has been overused in the nursing home (73) and increases the incidence of several other complications, including chronic bacteriuria, symptomatic urinary tract infection, bladder stones, periurethral abscesses, and even bladder cancer (8,9,74–78). Elderly nursing home residents managed by this technique, especially men, are at relatively high risk for developing symptomatic urinary tract infection (9). Given these risks, it seems appropriate to recommend that long-term indwelling catheterization be limited to certain specific situations, and, when indwelling catheterization is used, sound principles of catheter care should be observed so that complications are minimized (Box 3.3). Recently implemented federal regulations require that an appropriate indication be documented for nursing home residents with long-term indwelling catheterization (1) (Box 3.3); similar recommendations were made some 35 years ago (79). Although few data are available on the most effective routine care regimens for long-term indwelling catheterization, the closed system should be broken as infrequently as possible, and the catheter should be changed every 4 to 8 weeks (in addition to when symptomatic infection occurs [Box 3.3]) to help prevent the build-up of encrustations, which can lead to catheter blockage and infection (80,81).

BOX 3.3. Long-term indwelling catheterization

Appropriate indications
 Urinary retention characterized by the following:
  Causes persistent overflow incontinence, symptomatic infections, or renal dysfunction
  Cannot be corrected surgically or medically
  Cannot be managed practically with intermittent catheterization
 Skin wounds, pressure sores, or irritations that are being contaminated by incontinent urine
 Care of terminally ill or severely impaired persons for whom bed and clothing changes are uncomfortable
  or disruptive
 Preference of patient or caregiver when patient has not responded to more specific treatments
Ongoing care
 Maintain sterile, closed, gravity drainage system and avoid breaking the closed system
 Use clean techniques in emptying and changing the drainage system; wash hands between patients in
  institutional settings
 Secure the catheter to the upper thigh or lower abdomen to avoid perineal contamination and urethral irritation
  caused by movement of the catheter
 Avoid frequent and vigorous cleaning of the catheter entry site; washing with soapy water once a day is sufficient
 Do not routinely irrigate
 If bypassing occurs in the absence of obstruction, consider the possibility of a bladder spasm, which can be
  treated with a bladder relaxant
 Change the catheter every 4 to 8 weeks to avoid the build-up of encrustations
 If catheter obstruction occurs frequently, increase the patient's fluid intake and acidify the urine if possible
  (diluted acetic acid irrigations may be helpful)
 Do not routinely use prophylactic or suppressive urinary antiseptic or antimicrobial agents
 Do not perform routine surveillance cultures to guide management of individual patients because all patients
  with long-term catheters have bacteriuria (which is often polymicrobial) and the organisms change frequently
 Do not treat infection unless symptoms develop; symptoms may be nonspecific, and other possible sources of
  infection should be carefully excluded before symptoms are attributed to the urinary tract
 If a symptomatic infection develops, the catheter should be changed before a specimen is collected for culture
  (specimens obtained from the old catheter may be misleading because of colonization of the catheter lumen)
 If symptomatic urinary tract infections frequently develop, a genitourinary evaluation should be considered to
  rule out pathologic conditions such as stones, periurethral or prostatic abscesses, and chronic pyelonephritis

FECAL INCONTINENCE

Fecal incontinence is less common than urinary incontinence, but a large proportion (50% to 75%) of nursing home residents with frequent urinary incontinence also have episodes of fecal incontinence (5,6). Defecation, like urination, is a physiologic process that involves smooth and striated muscles, central and peripheral innervation, coordination of reflex responses, mental awareness, and physical ability to get to a toilet. Disruption of any of these factors can lead to fecal incontinence.

The most common causes of fecal incontinence are problems with constipation and laxative use, hyperosmotic enteral feedings, neurologic disorders, colorectal disorders, and functional dependence (82,83). Iatrogenic causes (such as laxatives, hyperosmotic feedings, and some antacids) and dietary factors (such as lactose intolerance) should be excluded. Hypothyroidism and hyperthyroidism can also cause bowel symptoms and should be considered. Constipation is common in the elderly and,

when chronic, can lead to fecal impaction and incontinence. The hard stool (or scybalum) of fecal impaction irritates the rectum and results in the production of mucus and fluid. This fluid leaks around the mass of impacted stool and precipitates incontinence. Appropriate management of constipation will help prevent fecal impaction and resultant fecal incontinence. The management of constipation in nursing home residents involves several approaches, including adequate intake of fluid and fiber; the appropriate use of stool softeners; and regular toileting with the use of glycerin suppositories if necessary. Some residents have acquired laxative dependence and require the intermittent use of more potent osmotic or irritant laxatives or suppositories.

Fecal incontinence caused by neurologic disorders is sometimes amenable to biofeedback therapy, although most elderly nursing home residents with dementia cannot cooperate or learn the techniques. Prompted voiding improves bowel and urinary continence in some nursing home residents. For those residents with end-stage dementia, a strategy of alternating constipating agents (if necessary) and laxatives on a routine schedule is generally effective in controlling defecation and preventing fecal incontinence. Such strategies are generally referred to as bowel-training programs. The basic components of most bowel-training programs include the regular use of stool softeners or fiber and adequate fluid intake to prevent fecal impaction; regular toileting after breakfast (to take advantage of the gastrocolic reflex); and the intermittent use (commonly three to four times per week) of either an oral laxative such as milk of magnesia or sorbitol, or a suppository (glycerin or bisacodyl) to stimulate a bowel movement. Periodic enemas may be necessary for residents who do not respond to these measures.

REFERENCES

1. Federal Register. 1991;56:48865-921.
2. Morris JN, Hawes C, Fries BE, Phillips CD, Mor V, Katz S, et al. Designing the national resident assessment instrument for nursing homes. Gerontologist. 1990;30:293-307.
3. Morris JN, Hawes C, Murphy K, Nonemaker S, Phillips C, Fries BE, et al. Resident Assessment Instrument Training Manual and Resource Guide. Natick, Massachusetts: Eliot Press; 1991.
4. Mohide EA. The prevalence and scope of urinary incontinence. Clin Geriatr Med. 1986;2:639-55.
5. Ouslander JG, Kane RL, Abrass IB. Urinary incontinence in elderly nursing home patients. JAMA. 1982;248:1194-8.
6. Ouslander JG, Fowler E. Incontinence in Veterans Administration nursing homes. J Am Geriatr Soc. 1985;33:33-40.
7. United States Agency for Health Care Policy and Research. Pressure Ulcers in Adults: Prediction and Prevention. Rockville, Maryland: U.S. Department of Health and Human Services, Pubic Health Services, Agency for Health Care Policy and Research; 1992.
8. Warren JW, Damron D, Tenney JH, Hoopes JM, Deforge B, Muncie HL Jr. Fever, bacteremia and death as complications of bacteriuria in women with long-term urethral catheters. J Infect Dis. 1987;155:1151-8.
9. Ouslander JG, Greengold BA, Chen S. Complications of chronic indwelling urinary catheters among male nursing home patients: a prospective study. J Urol. 1988;138:1191-5.
10. Stewart RB, Moore MT, May FE, Marks RG, Hale WE. Nocturia: a risk factor for falls in the elderly. J Am Geriatr Soc. 1992;40:1217-20.
11. Ouslander JG, Morishita L, Blaustein J, Orzeck S, Dunn S, Sayre J. Clinical, functional, and psychosocial characteristics of an incontinent nursing home population. J Gerontol. 1987;42:631-7.
12. Hu TW. The cost impact of urinary incontinence on health-care services. In: AHCPR Clinical Practice Guideline on Urinary Incontinence in Adults. Rockville, Maryland: U.S. Department of Health and Human Services, Public Health Service, Agency for Health Care Policy and Research; 1994.
13. Diokno AC, Brown MB, Brock BM, Herzog AR, Normolle DP. Clinical and cystometric characteristics of continent and incontinent noninstitutionalized elderly. J Urol. 1988;140:567-71.
14. Elbadawi A, Yalla SV, Resnick NM. Structural basis of voiding dysfunction. I. Methods of a prospective ultrastructural/urodynamic study and an overview of the findings. J Urol. 1993;150:1650-6.
15. Resnick NM, Yalla SV. Detrusor hyperactivity with impaired contractile function. An unrecognized but common cause of incontinence in elderly patients. JAMA. 1987;257:3076-81.
16. Resnick NM, Yalla SV, Laurino E. The pathophysiology of urinary incontinence among institutionalized elderly persons. N Engl J Med. 1989;320:1-7.
17. Ouslander JG, Osterweil D, Morley JE. Medical Care in the Nursing Home. New York: McGraw-Hill; 1991.
18. Ouslander JG, Osterweil D. Physician evaluation and management of the nursing home resident. Ann Intern Med. 1994;121:584-92.
19. Ouslander JG, Urman HN, Urman GC. Development and testing of an incontinence monitoring record. J Am Geriatr Soc. 1986;34:83-90.
20. United States Agency for Health Care Policy and Research. Urinary Incontinence in Adults: Clinical Practice Guideline. Rockville, Maryland: Rockville, Maryland: U.S. Department of Health and Human Services, Public Health Service, Agency for Health Care Policy and Research; 1992.
21. Ouslander JG, Schapira M, Schnelle JF. Urine specimen collection from incontinent female nursing home residents. J Am Geriatr Soc. 1995; [In press].
22. Ouslander JG, Greengold BA, Silverblatt FJ, Garcia JP. An accurate method to obtain urine for culture in men with external catheters. Arch Intern Med. 1987;147:286-8.
23. Schapira M, Ouslander J, Nigam J, Tuico E, Schnelle J. Accuracy of rapid screening methods for bacteriuria among incontinent nursing home residents [Abstract]. J Am Geriatr Soc. 1994;11:SA4.
24. Ouslander J, Schnelle J, Simmons S, Tuico E, Bates-Jensen B. Use of a portable ultrasound to measure residual urine among nursing home residents. J Am Geriatr Soc. 1994; 1189-92.
25. Ouslander JG, Leach GE, Staskin DR. Simplified tests of lower urinary tract function in the evaluation of geriatric urinary incontinence. J Am Geriatr Soc. 1989;37:706-14.
26. Ouslander JG, Leach G, Staskin D, Abelson S, Blaustein J, Morishita L, et al. Prospective evaluation of an assessment strategy for geriatric urinary incontinence. J Am Geriatr Soc. 1989;37:715-4.
27. Ouslander JG, Leach G, Abelson S, Staskin D, Blaustein J, Raz S. Simple versus multichannel cys-

tometry in the evaluation of bladder function in an incontinent geriatric population. J Urol. 1988;140:1482-6.

28. Ouslander J, Schnelle J, Nigam J, Uman G, Fingold S, Tuico E. Predictors of responsiveness to prompted voiding among incontinent nursing home residents [Abstract]. J Am Geriatr Soc. 1994;11:SA25.

29. McClish DK, Fantl JA, Wyman JF, Pisani G, Bump RC. Bladder training in older women with urinary incontinence: relationship between outcome and changes in urodynamic observations. Obstet Gynecol. 1991;77:281-6.

30. Nicolle LE, Bjornson J, Harding GK, MacDonell JA. Bacteriuria in elderly institutionalized men. N Engl J Med. 1983;309:1420-5.

31. Nicolle LE, Henderson E, Bjornson J, McIntyre M, Harding GK, MacDonell JA. The association of bacteriuria with resident characteristics and survival in elderly institutionalized men. Ann Intern Med. 1987;106:682-6.

32. Ouslander J, Schapira M, Nigam J, Tuico E, Schnelle J. Effects of eradicating bacteriuria on the frequency of urinary incontinence among nursing home residents [Abstract]. J Am Geriatr Soc. 1993;SA11:A44.

33. Schapira M, Ouslander J, Nigam J, Tuico E, Schnelle J. Pyuria among incontinent nursing home residents [Abstract]. J Am Geriatr Soc. 1994;11:SA24.

34. Fantl JA, Cardozo L, McClish DK. Estrogen therapy in the management of urinary incontinence in postmenopausal women: a meta-analysis. First report of the Hormones and Urogenital Therapy Committee. Obstet Gynecol. 1994;83:12-8.

35. American College of Physicians. Guidelines for counseling postmenopausal women about preventive hormone therapy. Ann Intern Med. 1992;117:1038-41.

36. Fantl JA, Wyman JF, McClish DK, Harkins SW, Elswick RK, Taylor JR, et al. Efficacy of bladder training in older women with urinary incontinence. JAMA. 1991;265:609-13.

37. Wells TJ. Pelvic (floor) muscle exercises. J Am Geriatr Soc. 1990;38:333-7.

38. Burns PA, Pranikoff K, Nochajski TH, Hadley EC, Levy KJ, Ory MG. A comparison of effectiveness of biofeedback and pelvic muscle exercise treatment of stress incontinence in older community-dwelling women. J Gerontol. 1993;48:M167-74.

39. Lamhut P, Jackson TW, Wall LL. The treatment of urinary incontinence with electrical stimulation in nursing home patients: a pilot study. J Am Geriatr Soc. 1992;40:48-52.

40. Schnelle JF, Traughber B, Sowell VA, Newman DR, Petrilli CO, Ory M. Treatment of urinary incontinence in nursing home patients. A behavior management approach for nursing home staff. J Am Geriatr Soc. 1989;37:1051-7.

41. Schnelle JF, Newman DR, Fogarty T. Management of patient continence in long-term care facilities. Gerontologist. 1990;30:373-6.

42. Schnelle JF. Treatment of urinary incontinence in nursing home patients by prompted voiding. J Am Geriatr Soc. 1990;38:356-60.

43. Hu TW, Igou JF, Kaltreider DL, Yu LC, Rohner TJ, Dennis PJ, et al. A clinical trial of a behavioral therapy to reduce urinary incontinence in nursing homes. Outcome and implications. JAMA. 1989;261:2656-62.

44. Engel BT, Burgio LD, McCormick KA, Hawkins AM, Scheve AA, Leahy E. Behavioral treatment of incontinence in the long-term care setting. J Am Geriatr Soc. 1990;38:361-3.

45. Colling J, Ouslander J, Hadley BJ, Eisch J, Campbell E. The effects of patterned urge-response toileting (PURT) on urinary incontinence among nursing home residents. J Am Geriatr Soc. 1992;39:135-41.

46. Schnelle JF, Traughber B, Norgan DB, Embry JE, Binion AF, Coleman A. Management of geriatric incontinence in nursing homes. J Appl Behav Anal. 1983;16:235-41.

47. Schnelle JF, Ouslander JG, Simmons SF. Predicting nursing home resident responsiveness to a urinary incontinence treatment protocol. International Urogynecology. 1993;J4:89-94.

48. Schnelle JF, Newman DR, Fogarty T. Statistical quality-control in nursing homes: assessment and management of chronic urinary incontinence. Health Serv Res. 1990;25:627-37.

49. Schnelle JF, Newman D, White M, Abbey M, Wallston KA, Fogarty T, et al. Maintaining continence in nursing home residents through the application of industrial quality control. Gerontologist. 1992;33:114-21.

50. Schnelle JF. Managing Urinary Incontinence in the Elderly. New York: Springer Publishing; 1991.

51. Schnelle JF, Ouslander JG, Osterweil D, Blumenthal S. Total quality management: administrative and clinical application in nursing homes. J Am Geriatr Soc. 1993;41:1259-66.

52. Ouslander JG, Schnelle J, Simmons SF, Bates-Jensen B, Zeitlin M. The dark side of incontinence: incontinence at night in nursing homes. J Am Geriatr Soc. 1993;41:371-6.

53. Schnelle JF, Ouslander JG, Simmons SF, Alessi CA, Gravel MD. Nighttime sleep and bed mobility among incontinent nursing home residents. J Am Geriatr Soc. 1993;41:903-9.

54. Schnelle JF, Ouslander JG, Simmons SF, Alessi CA, Gravel M. The nighttime environment, incontinence care, and sleep disruption in nursing homes. J Am Geriatr Soc. 1993;41:910-4.

55. Pannill FC 3d, Williams TF, Davis R. Evaluation and treatment of urinary incontinence in long term care. J Am Geriatr Soc. 1988;36:902-10.

56. Castleden CM, Duffin HM, Asher MJ, Yeomason CW. Factors influencing outcome in elderly patients with urinary incontinence and detrusor instability. Age Ageing. 1985;14:303-7.

57. Zorzitto ML, Jewett MA, Fernie GR, Holliday PJ, Bartlett S. Effectiveness of propantheline bromide in the treatment of geriatric patients with detrusor

instability. Neurourology and Urodynamics. 1986;5: 133-40.

58. Zorzitto ML, Holliday PJ, Jewett MA, Herschorn S, Fernie GR. Oxybutynin chloride for geriatric urinary dysfunction: a double-blind placebo-controlled study. Age Ageing. 1989;18:195-200.

59. Tobin GW, Brocklehurst JC. The management of urinary incontinence in local authority residential homes for the elderly. Age Ageing. 1986;15:292-8.

60. Wiseman PA, Malone-Lee J, Rai GS. Terodiline with bladder retraining for treating detrusor instability in elderly people. BMJ. 1991;302:994-6.

61. Ouslander J, Schnelle J, Uman G, Nigam J, Fingold S, Tuico E. Does oxybutynin enhance the effectiveness of prompted voiding for incontinence among nursing home residents? J Am Geriatr Soc. 1995; 43:610-7.

62. Wells TJ, Brink CA, Diokno AC, Wolfe R, Gillis GL. Pelvic muscle exercise for stress urinary incontinence in elderly women. J Am Geriatr Soc. 1991;39:785-91.

63. Finkbeiner AE. Is bethanechol chloride clinically effective in promoting bladder emptying? A literature review. J Urol. 1985;134:443-9.

64. Caine M. The present role of alpha-adrenergic blockers in the treatment of benign prostatic hypertrophy. J Urology. 1986;136:1-4.

65. Kirby RS, Coppinger SW, Corcoran MO, Chapple CR, Flannigan M, Milroy EJ. Prazosin in the treatment of prostatic obstruction. A placebo-controlled study. Br J Urol. 1987;60:136-42.

66. Lepor H, Meretyk S, Knapp-Maloney G. The safety, efficacy, and compliance of terazosin therapy for benign prostatic hyperplasia. J Urol. 1992;147: 1554-7.

67. Cole HM. Diagnostic and therapeutic technology assessment. Use of Teflon preparations for urinary incontinence and vesicoureteral reflux. JAMA. 1993;269:2975-80.

68. Brink CA. Absorbent pads, garments, and management strategies. J Am Geriatr Soc. 1990;38:368-73.

69. Ouslander JG, Greengold B, Chen S. External catheter use and urinary tract infections among incontinent male nursing home patients. J Am Geriatr Soc. 1987;35:1063-70.

70. Lapides J, Diokno AC. Clean, intermittent self-catheterization. In: Raz S, ed. Female Urology. Philadelphia: W.B. Saunders; 1983.

71. Bennett CJ, Diokno AC. Clean intermittent self-catheterization in the elderly. Urology. 1984;24:43-5.

72. Terpenning MS, Allada R, Kauffman CA. Intermittent urethral catheterization in the elderly. J Am Geriatr Soc. 1989;37:411-6.

73. Warren JW, Steinberg L, Hebel RJ, Tenney JH. The prevalence of urethral catheterization in Maryland nursing homes. Arch Intern Med. 1989;149:1535-7.

74. Warren JW, Muncie HL, Berquist EJ, Hoopes JM. Sequelae and management of urinary infection in the patient requiring chronic catheterization. J Urol. 1981;125:1-7.

75. Warren JW, Muncie HL Jr, Hall-Craggs M. Acute pyelonephritis associated with bacteriuria during long-term catheterization: a prospective clinico-pathological study. J Infect Dis. 1988;158:1341-6.

76. Kunin CM, Chin QF, Chambers S. Morbidity and mortality associated with indwelling urinary catheters in elderly patients in a nursing home confounding due to the presence of associated diseases. J Am Geriatr Soc. 1987;35:1001-6.

77. Ribeiro BJ, Smith SR. Evaluation of urinary catheterization and incontinence in a general nursing home population. J Am Geriatr Soc. 1985;33:479-82.

78. Marron KR, Fillit H, Peskowitz M, Silverstone FA. The nonuse of urethral catheterization in the management of urinary incontinence in the teaching nursing home. J Am Geriatr Soc. 1983;31:278-81.

79. Beeson PB. The case against the catheter [Editorial]. Am J Med. 1958;24:1-3.

80. Muncie HL Jr, Warren JW. Reasons for replacement of long-term urethral catheters: implications for randomized trials. J Urol. 1990;143:507-9.

81. Kunin CM, Chin QF, Chambers S. Indwelling urinary catheters in the elderly. Relation of catheter life to formation of encrustations in patients with and without blocked catheters. Am J Med. 1987;82:405-11.

82. Goldstein MK, Brown EM, Holt P, Gallagher D, Winograd CH. Fecal incontinence in an elderly man. Stanford university geriatrics case conference. J Am Geriatr Soc. 1989;37:991-1002.

83. Madoff RD, Williams JG, Caushaj PF. Fecal incontinence. N Engl J Med. 1992;326:1002-7.

———— 4 ————

Fever and Infection

Thomas T. Yoshikawa, MD, FACP, and Dean C. Norman, MD

EPIDEMIOLOGY OF INFECTIONS IN NURSING HOMES

Scope of Problem

The number of infections that occur annually in long-term care facilities such as a nursing home approaches that reported for acute-care hospitals. It is estimated that approximately 1.5 million infections occur each year in nursing homes (1). Reported prevalence rates from one dozen studies range from 5.4 to 32.7 infections per 100 residents per month, and incidence rates range from 10.7 to 20.1 infections per 100 residents per month (2).

However, precise data on the number and types of infections in nursing homes are not easily obtainable. In addition, it is difficult to compare surveillance data among different studies of infections in long-term-care settings. Numerous factors are responsible for the imprecision and heterogeneity of information on nursing home–acquired infections (3, 4). These factors include type of long-term-care facility (skilled nursing facility, Veterans Affairs); reporting methods (prevalence; incidence; numbers of infections per month, 100 days, 1000 days, or per year); study design (retrospective, prospective, chart reviews, clinical examination, duration of surveillance—for example, 1 day, 1 month, 1 year); and definition of infection (criteria for infection, use of laboratory confirmation).

The importance of infections in the long-term-care setting is underscored by the fact that estab-

lished or suspected infections are often the most frequent reason for the transfer of residents from a nursing home to an acute-care facility (5,6).

Types of Infection

The three most frequently encountered sites (types) of infections in nursing home patients are the respiratory tract (pneumonia, bronchitis), urinary tract (cystitis, pyelonephritis), and skin or soft tissue (infected pressure ulcer, cellulitis). Investigations of residents who reside in long-term-care facilities and develop sepsis show that these three sites of infections account for 70% to 80% of all proven cases of bacteremia (7–11). Table 4.1 summarizes clinical data on bacteremia cases reported in long-term-care facilities (7–10). The urinary tract is the primary site of infection in 55% to 60% of all bacteremic nursing home residents. In contrast, studies of nursing home–acquired infections in which bacteremia was not present showed the lower respiratory tract (pneumonia and bronchitis) to be the dominant site of infection (12–16). Other less common sites of infections in this population include the gastrointestinal tract (gastroenteritis) and the eyes (conjunctivitis). Bacteria are most frequently isolated from serious infections in nursing home residents. However, viral infections such as influenza and respiratory syncytial virus can occasionally cause serious morbidity in this population. Infection with mycobacteria also occurs in nursing home residents (see the section Tuberculosis).

47

TABLE 4.1. Bacteremia cases in long-term care facilities

Author (Ref.)	Episodes	Incidence*	Mortality	Mean Age	Male	Infection† P	U	S	O*	Gram-neg Bacilli	Gram-pos Cocci	Poly-microbial
	n		%	*y*	←———————————— % ————————————→							
Setia et al. (7)	100	0.3	35	79	36	10	56	14	20	67	24	9
Rudman et al. (8)	42	0.3	21	69	100	7	56	7	22	60	36	15
Muder et al. (9)	163	0.2–0.36‡	22	69	NS§	11	55	9	25	NS‖	NS‖	22
Marrie (10)	13¶	NS	29	80	8	8	54	0	38	60	32	8

* per 1000 patient days.

† P = pneumonia; U = urinary tract infection; S = skin/soft tissue infection; O = other sites or unknown.

‡ From beginning (1984) to end (1989) of study period.

§ Not stated but most likely predominantly male (veteran population).

‖ Not stated. However, of 267 isolates of 163 episodes, 59% were gram-negative bacilli and 35% were gram-positive cocci.

¶ Number of patients (episodes not stated).

The mortality rate from nursing home–acquired infections ranges from 12% to 35% and increases with the severity of chronic underlying disorders and in the presence of bacteremia, pulmonary involvement, and more virulent pathogens, especially gram-negative bacilli (7–10,14,15).

CLINICAL MANIFESTATIONS OF INFECTION

Altered Clinical Features

Although the majority of older patients exhibit typical features of various infections, the symptoms and signs of illness—including infectious diseases—in some elderly patients may be altered, that is, atypical, nonspecific, masked, or confounded by coexisting chronic conditions and age-related changes, or they may even be absent (17). Such findings are especially common in frail, debilitated and very old nursing home residents (18). In addition, cognitive impairments may prevent nursing home residents from being aware of clinical changes or from communicating about their symptoms.

Fever

Fever is the cardinal manifestation of infection (17, 18). Although the criterion for fever (for example, a rectal or oral temperature of at least 100 °F or 101 °F) varies among clinicians and investigators, an acute febrile response in an elderly person is highly diagnostic for the presence of a serious infectious disease and is most often due to a bacterial infection (19). In elderly patients, no data correlate

the magnitude of fever with severity of infection. However, the higher the body temperature, the more likely it is that an infectious disease process is present (19). No definitive studies have been done assessing noninfectious causes of acute onset of fever or prolonged fever of undetermined origin in nursing home residents. Despite the common finding of fever in association with infection, a substantial proportion of older patients (that is, 25%) do not exhibit fever in the presence of such serious infectious diseases as pneumonia, tuberculosis, infective endocarditis, and sepsis (20–23). Diminished febrile responses to infections in nursing home patients have also been shown (24). However, some of the infected "afebrile" nursing home residents did manifest an appropriate temperature response, (that is, body temperature increased at least 2.4 °F above baseline body temperature but failed to reach a predetermined accepted criterion for fever of 101°F); in such cases, the residents had lower baseline ("normal") core body temperatures (less than 98.6 °F). Thus, change in body temperature is as important as the absolute temperature value for the diagnosis of an infection in frail, elderly nursing home residents (25): An increase in body temperature of at least 2.4 °F indicates a "febrile" response. In this regard, it might be a useful practice to document baseline body temperatures for all nursing home residents, although the clinical utility of this has yet to be proven in a prospective study. Likewise, the optimal frequency of measuring body temperature in nursing home residents has not been determined in terms of clinical usefulness and cost effectiveness (that is, with regard to the limited number of nursing personnel). Nevertheless, recording measurements at least once daily at same time of day (for example, late afternoon) may facilitate early detection of infections.

Other Manifestations of Infection

Elderly patients who harbor an infection often manifest other symptoms and signs with or without a fever (Box 4.1). Although precise frequency data are not available, acute confusion or delirium is a common presenting clinical finding of older patients who have infections (26). In nursing home residents in whom confusion, delirium, or any change in baseline mental status occurs, infection as well as drug reactions, hypoperfusion to the brain (for example, secondary to stroke, heart failure, dehydration, cardiac arrhythmia), and metabolic disorders (for example, electrolyte imbalance, hypoglycemia) should be considered in the differential diagnosis.

GENERAL APPROACH TO SUSPECTED INFECTION

Diagnostic Approach

If infection is suspected in a nursing home resident (that is, based on clinical clues or specific symptoms and signs), knowledge or awareness of the most common sites of infection in such patients is very helpful in directing the examination and diagnostic evaluation. Because approximately 75% of all nursing home–acquired infections occur in the respiratory tract, urinary tract, and skin, an evaluation for pneumonia (or bronchitis), urinary tract infection, and infected pressure ulcers (or cellulitis) should be pursued initially unless clinical manifestations are present indicating another potential infectious disease (for example, diarrhea secondary to bacterial or viral gastroenteritis) (11).

An initial assessment done by the nurse should include a careful recording of body temperature (rectal temperature is preferred if the resident is unable to cooperate fully for an oral measurement), as well as any change in body temperature from the usual (normal) baseline value. The resident's blood pressure should be measured, and any decrease in blood pressure from baseline or any postural changes in blood pressure should be recorded. The respiratory rate of the resident should be noted; tachypnea may be an early sign of sepsis or lower

BOX 4.1. Clinical clues to infections

Fever ≥100 °F
Change in body temperature from baseline of ≥2.4 °F
Acute confusion or delirium
Unexplained change in behavior pattern
Unexplained change in functional status
Loss of appetite or unexplained weight loss or both
Weakness
Lethargy
Urinary incontinence
Falls
Tachypnea
Orthostatic hypotension

respiratory infection. The resident's current and previous body weights are useful in providing insight with regard to potential volume depletion, nutritional status, and chronicity of illness (18).

If the resident has a fever, the nurse should contact the responsible physician. Residents who are deemed clinically ill or unstable (for example, hypotensive, toxic, tachypneic) should be transferred immediately to the hospital, where the initial examination and diagnostic evaluation can take place. In addition, because many physicians have a busy clinical practice, they are often unable to examine the resident in the nursing home, and many nursing facilities are unable to do routine tests such as radiography and blood tests. Under these circumstances, too, the nursing home resident who is suspected of having an infection will have to be transferred to a hospital where a physician can examine the resident and preliminary studies can be done. Otherwise, the initial examination and laboratory tests should be performed in the nursing home.

A careful general physical examination should be done, whether the resident remains in the home or is transferred to an acute-care facility. Particular attention needs to be focused on the examination of mental status, oral cavity, conjunctiva, skin, chest, heart, abdomen, genitalia, perirectal area, and central nervous system. If the initial clinical evaluation does not suggest a specific site or type of infection, preliminary laboratory studies should include a chest radiograph, urinalysis with culture, and a complete blood count with a differential leukocyte count *regardless* of the total leukocyte count (a left shift of the leukocyte count—even with leukopenia—is a reliable indicator of bacterial infection) (26). If these preliminary studies are not revealing and the resident remains clinically ill, the resident should be transferred to an acute-care facility for further diagnostic evaluation. Blood cultures are indicated if the resident is ill enough to be hospitalized or the resident has shaking chills.

Hospitalization

If the resident is clinically unstable or if a severe or moderately severe infection is present, the resident should be hospitalized. Conversely, residents who are mildly ill with a serious infection may be considered for management in the nursing home provided that a physician, nursing personnel, emergency equipment, laboratory, and radiographic tests are readily available on a 24-hour basis. The issue of advanced directives always must be considered. In cases in which it has been decided that a terminally ill resident should not receive acute intervention, hospitalization would ordinarily not be an appropriate option. In such residents or other residents who are not candidates for hospitalization, management must be individualized. For some, diagnostic procedures should be minimized and empiric antimicrobial therapy (based on most likely source of infection from clinical assessment) should be initiated in the nursing home. Long-acting antibiotics (for example, cefonicid, ceftriaxone) may be administered intramuscularly, or oral agents may be prescribed if intravenous administration is not feasible in the long-term-care facility.

Supportive Management

Whether the infection is treated with antibiotics in the hospital or nursing home, an initial period of bed rest is recommended. However, depending on the severity of illness, the resident's functional capabilities, and the response to treatment, prolonged bed rest should be discouraged to minimize aspiration pneumonia, deconditioning, thrombophlebitis, and pressure ulcers. Adequate fluid intake should be monitored because dehydration secondary to inadequate fluid intake and increased loss of water from fever and elevated metabolic rate may occur rapidly. Similarly, adequate nutrition must be maintained during the catabolic state of infection.

Antipyretic agents should be discouraged for modest fevers (under 101 °F or 38.3 °C) unless the increase in temperature is causing other adverse consequences (for example, tachycardia in a resident with serious cardiac disease). Although not

proved in humans, fever is considered to be a host defense mechanism against infection and is generally associated with improved mortality and morbidity (25).

IMPORTANT INFECTIOUS DISEASES

Pneumonia

The mortality rate for nursing home–acquired pneumonia may reach 40% (28). In addition, other complications such as bacteremia, empyema, and meningitis are more likely to develop in elderly patients with pneumonia (29).

The clinical manifestations of pneumonia in institutionalized elderly persons may be atypical or subtle. Fever, chills, cough, sputum production, rales, and rhonchi are often absent, and may be replaced by symptoms of confusion, anorexia, and nausea (28).

It is highly likely that most cases of bacterial pneumonia in older patients result from aspiration of organisms colonizing the oropharynx (29). Studies indicate that both hospitalized and institutionalized elderly patients are at high risk for oropharyngeal colonization with facultative or aerobic gram-negative bacilli (30). However, the data on the microbiology of nursing home–acquired pneumonia are limited because 1) nursing home residents frequently cannot cooperate in providing reliable sputum, 2) expectorated sputa are likely to be contaminated by the oropharyngeal flora, and 3) invasive diagnostic procedures (for example, transtracheal aspiration) are not recommended routinely for this population (31). Nevertheless, available data indicate that *Streptococcus pneumoniae* and facultative or aerobic gram-negative bacilli are the two most frequently isolated pathogens from residents with nursing home—acquired pneumonia (32–35). In addition, *Haemophilus influenzae, Staphylococcus aureus,* and anaerobic bacteria have been implicated as respiratory pathogens in this population (32–35). Although *Legionella* species have been implicated in elderly patients with community-acquired pneumonia (36), this pathogen has not been reported to occur often in nursing home residents.

Based on such limited data, antimicrobial therapy should be directed against *S. pneumoniae,* gram-negative bacilli, *H. influenzae, S. aureus,* and anaerobes in residents in whom empiric therapy is necessary or in whom a specific causative pathogen cannot be identified. Monotherapy is preferred, although combined drug regimens are equally effective. Antibiotic regimens that have been suggested for empiric therapy include second-generation cephalosporins (for example, cefuroxime, cefoxitin), third-generation cephalosporins (for example, ceftriaxone, cefoperazone), ticarcillin-clavulanic acid, ampicillin-sulbactam, penicillin plus aztreonam, or a quinolone (31,37). The decision of which antibiotic to select will depend on the clinician's experience with certain drugs, on the antibiotic-resistance patterns of organisms in the nursing home, and on the resident's tolerance to the drugs. Penicillin-allergic patients may be given trimethoprim-sulfamethoxazole, clindamycin, erythromycin, aztreonam, metronidazole, or a quinolone, in various combinations. Parenteral antibiotics should be administered for at least 7 days. Depending on the presumed or proven cause of the pneumonia, the clinical response to the parenteral antibiotic(s), and the patient's ability to comply with oral administration, parenteral antibiotics may substituted with oral antibiotics and treatment completed, for a total of 2 weeks of therapy. Oral drugs that can be considered include cefuroxime axetil, amoxicillin-clavulanic acid, trimethoprim-sulfamethoxazole, clindamycin, metronidazole, and a quinolone. Supportive care should be as described earlier (see Supportive Management). In addition, supplemental oxygen should be prescribed, and expectoration of accumulated sputum should be encouraged.

Urinary Tract Infection

The functional status and physical impairment(s) of the elderly person, as well as genitourinary manipulation, anatomy, and function predict how likely bacteriuria and urinary tract infection are present. Risk factors occur more frequently in older persons residing in nursing homes and other chronic-care facilities.

Most bacteriuric older persons, including nursing home residents, experience bacteriuria without associated genitourinary or systemic complaints or functional changes (38–40). Studies on noncatheterized elderly institutionalized women with asymptomatic bacteriuria showed that the majority of the infections (67%) were localized to the kidney (41). In addition, autopsy data on long-term catheterized nursing home residents showed a high prevalence of acute and chronic renal inflammation as well as of chronic pyelonephritis (42,43). Thus, although bacteriuria in the majority of both noncatheterized and catheterized nursing home residents is asymptomatic, subclinical infection and inflammation occur and often persist in the renal parenchyma.

When symptoms do develop from bacteriuria (that is, urinary tract infection), the resident may typically complain of fever, dysuria, urinary frequency, nocturia, and urgency. Alternatively, the resident may manifest urinary tract infection as acute confusion, urinary incontinence, functional capacity deterioration, anorexia, nausea, or hypotension. Catheterized residents who have active urinary tract infection will generally not express genitourinary symptoms; fever, cognitive impairment, functional changes, changes in appetite, tachypnea, tachycardia, and orthostatic or nonorthostatic hypotension are more likely to be the presenting manifestations.

The microbial causes of bacteriuria and urinary tract infection in noncatheterized, chronically institutionalized elderly persons are primarily enteric gram-negative bacilli, that is, *Escherichia coli, Proteus* species, *Klebsiella* species, and *Enterobacter* species, as well as occasional isolates of *Pseudomonas aeruginosa* and *Enterococcus* species (41,44). It appears that elderly men experience a significantly higher frequency of polymicrobial bacteriuria than elderly women (41,44). In elderly patients with chronic bladder catheters, polymicrobial bacteriuria is found in the majority of urine specimens, with two to four bacterial species being a common finding (45, 46). In addition to enteric pathogens, *Enterococcus* species may be recovered from 25% of urine samples of chronically catheterized patients (46).

Nursing home residents who have asymptomatic bacteriuria, with or without a chronic bladder catheter and even in the presence of pyuria, generally do not warrant antimicrobial therapy (47). In prospective, randomized studies comparing antimicrobial therapy with no therapy for asymptomatic bacteriuria in institutionalized, noncatheterized elderly men and women, no differences in mortality and genitourinary or infectious morbidity between the participants who received treatment and those who did not were noted (44,48). However, if urinary obstruction coexists with asymptomatic bacteriuria, active antimicrobial therapy is indicated (38,47) Nevertheless, although there is a high prevalence of bacteriuria in this population, the development of fever, clinical changes, or functional deterioration should not necessarily be attributed to a urinary tract infection, and other infectious diseases should be excluded (for example, pneumonia, infected pressure ulcers).

Symptomatic infections should be promptly treated after a Gram stain of the urine and appropriate cultures are obtained. The Gram stain of urine is useful in determining whether bacteriuria is present (although the sensitivity of the test is only 80% with presence of 310^5 organisms/mL urine) and if the organisms are gram-negative bacilli or gram-positive coccus or both. Because 55% of all cases of bacteremia in nursing home patients (Table 4.1) originate from a urinary tract infection, undue delays in therapy can result in sepsis and deaths. All clinically unstable residents or residents who appear moderately to severely ill should be hospitalized and treated with parenteral antibiotics and supportive measures (see the section Supportive Management on page 50). Blood cultures should be obtained from such patients before chemotherapy. Patients with chronic catheters should have their old catheters changed before urine specimens are collected for culture because of the chronic colonization of organisms that occurs with such catheters (49).

For noncatheterized bacteriuric residents who require parenteral therapy, empiric antimicrobial regimens could include a second- or third-generation cephalosporin, aztreonam, ticarcillin-clavulanic acid, ampicillin-sulbactam, or a quinolone. For severely ill residents in whom *Pseudomonas aeruginosa* is a likely pathogen, treatment with an aminoglycoside should be considered (38). If residents are able to receive treatment in the nursing home but require parenteral agents, such antibiotics as cefonicid (second-generation cephalosporin), ceftriaxone (third-generation cephalosporin) or amikacin (aminoglycoside) may be administered intramuscularly on an every-12-hour or every-24-hour dosage schedule for gram-negative bacilli uropathogens. In noncatheterized residents with urinary tract infection who are able to receive treatment with oral agents, trimethoprim-sulfamethoxazole, amoxicillin-clavulanic acid, second-generation cephalosporins (for example, cefuroxime), or a quinolone (for example, norfloxacin, ciprofloxacin) are potentially useful antibi-

otics. Catheterized residents with urinary tract infections should receive a parenteral or oral regimen that is effective against both gram-negative bacilli and enterococci—for example, ampicillin plus aztreonam, quinolone, third-generation cephalosporin, or aminoglycoside; ampicillin-sulbactam; or amoxicillin-clavulanic acid—until culture data are available to guide adjustment in therapy. Duration of antibiotic therapy will generally be 7 to 14 days. Chronically catheterized residents may be treated for 7 to 10 days unless sepsis or other complications occur (in which case the duration of treatment should be 14 days). In noncatheterized residents with uncomplicated urinary tract infection (no sepsis, recurrences, underlying genitourinary abnormalities, immunocompromising conditions, or stones), antibiotics may be prescribed for 7 to 10 days for women and 14 days for men (50). For noncatheterized residents, a repeat urine culture should be done 1 week after completion of therapy to prove that the bacteriuria has been eradicated. Catheterized residents only require clinical response as the end point of therapy; urine cultures obtained after therapy are not useful because the catheter will soon become colonized (50).

Skin Infections

CELLULITIS

Cellulitis of the lower extremities occurs with greater frequency in elderly patients, probably because of peripheral vascular disease, chronic venous insufficiency, edema, and trauma (51). The most common microbial causes (excluding cellulitis secondary to pressure ulcers and diabetic ulcers) are *S. aureus* and beta-hemolytic streptococci (52). Management should be guided by the clinical status of the patient. Oral therapy may be instituted with dicloxacillin, cloxacillin, amoxicillin-clavulanic acid, or a first-generation cephalosporin. Penicillin-allergic residents should be treated with oral clindamycin. If parenteral therapy is necessary, such agents as cefazolin (first-generation cephalosporin), cefuroxime or nafcillin-oxacillin may be administered intramuscularly. If sepsis is a complication of cellulitis, the nursing home resident should be hospitalized and treated with parenteral antibiotics such as oxacillin, nafcillin, or first-generation cephalosporin.

Infected Pressure Ulcers

Pressure ulcers occur commonly in nursing home residents, with a prevalence of approximately 20% to 25% and an incidence at the end of 1 and 2 years of 13% and 22%, respectively (53). Infection is a frequent complication of pressure ulcers (10% to 65%, depending on the severity and chronicity of the lesion) and may develop into contiguous osteomyelitis or sepsis or both (54,55). The microbial flora of infected pressure ulcers depends on the severity and duration of the lesion. Superficial ulcers without necrotic tissue are most often colonized or infected with facultative aerobic bacteria, including streptococci, staphylococci, and gram-negative bacilli; deeper ulcers associated with tissue necrosis more frequently reveal obligate anaerobes as well as facultative gram-negative bacilli (56).

Management of infected pressure ulcers includes standard therapy and preventive measures for pressure ulcers (not discussed in this chapter). The extent of infection should be assessed for tissue damage and the potential for osteomyelitis. If clinical suspicion is high for osteomyelitis, plain radiographs should be obtained. Surface swab cultures have little diagnostic value. Needle aspiration through uninfected intact skin of the infected lesion (an injection of 1 mL of nonbacteriostatic saline) provides findings of the microbiology of the infection nearly equal in accuracy to those of tissue biopsy (56). If osteomyelitis is suspected, bone biopsy for culture is recommended (56).

Local wound care, including debridement as needed, followed by saline-soaked, wet-to-dry dressings, is the most effective method to reduce the microbial counts in the lesion. Topical antibiotics and disinfectants are not recommended. Systemic antibiotics, however, are recommended in the presence of cellulitis, sepsis, or osteomyelitis (56). Early or superficial infected lesions are most likely to respond to antibiotics directed toward facultative aerobes, that is, second- or third-generation cephalosporins. Ulcers that are believed likely to harbor anaerobes should be treated with a therapeutic regimen that includes cefoxitin, cefotetan, clindamycin, or metronidazole.

SCABIES

Scabies is a mite infestation caused by *Sarcoptes scabies*, which occasionally can occur as a widescale problem in nursing homes. The infestation causes a severely pruritic, crusted papular or nodular skin lesion, typically found on the hands, wrists, elbows, anterior axillary folds, buttocks, genitals, and periumbilical area (57). Diagnosis is confirmed by placing skin scrapings of the lesion in mineral oil on a glass slide with a coverslip. Under light microscopy, a positive test result is the presence of a mite (in some stage of development), eggs or typical fecal pellets (scybala). Treatment is most effective with 1% lindane solution (Kwell) or 5% permethrin cream (Elimite); the latter is believed to be more effective in eliminating the organism and controlling scabies epidemics (58). These agents should be applied topically to all skin surfaces from the neck down, including the gluteal cleft, toe webs, and beneath fingernails. Then, 8 to 12 hours later, the medication should be removed by showering or bathing. Some clinicians recommend repeating the treatment after 1 week. All persons who have had physical contact with a resident with scabies should also be treated.

Methicillin-Resistant *Staphylococcus aureus* Infection

Methicillin-resistant *S. aureus* colonization and infection are increasingly common in nursing homes. Approximately 10% to 25% of all nursing home residents may be harboring this infection (59). Carriage rate of methicillin-resistant *S. aureus* increases in patients who are bedridden, have poor functional status, require feeding tubes and urinary catheters, and have wounds. Despite a high carriage rate of methicillin-resistant *S. aureus* in nursing home patients, the *infection* itself is relatively infrequent (occurs in only 3% to 4% of residents) (60,61). Furthermore, transmission of methicillin-resistant *S. aureus* from roommate to roommate occurs infrequently. Thus, active antibiotic treatment for methicillin-resistant *S. aureus* colonization is not indicated. In addition, recolonization occurs relatively soon after discontinuation of the antibiotics, and resistance to the antibiotic very often develops (59).

Residents with methicillin-resistant *S. aureus infection* are best treated with vancomycin. Unfortunately, because vancomycin may be administered intravenously only (and not intramuscularly), infected patients require hospitalization unless the nursing home is staffed to provide intravenous medications. Isolation procedures for residents with methicillin-resistant *S. aureus* colonization or infection remain somewhat controversial. Contact isolation, with careful handwashing techniques and use of gloves when touching residents or handling clinical specimens, is appropriate for the management of residents with small wounds or urinary tract infection with methicillin-resistant *S. aureus*. Residents who are colonized with this bacteria may remain in the same room with those noncolonized residents who are at minimal risk for developing this infection (high-risk residents include those who are immunosuppressed or who have gastric feeding tubes, intravenous catheters, or wounds), or they may be isolated with other methicillin-resistant *S. aureus*–colonized residents (59).

Tuberculosis

Currently, persons 65 years of age and older account for approximately 26% of all cases of tuberculosis in the United States and for 60% of deaths due to this infection (62). Even though 80% to 90% of cases of tuberculosis in older adults occur in the community setting, the incidence rate for tuberculosis in nursing home residents is three to four times higher than that in elderly community dwellers (63,64).

All older persons entering a long-term care facility should receive a two-step tuberculin skin test (64). A two-step process involves repeating the skin test within 1 to 2 weeks in residents who respond with induration of less than 10 mm (that is, a negative test result). A positive test result on second application (called the booster effect) is a skin test response of 10 mm or more induration and an induration of ≥6 mm that of the initial skin test response. Control dermal antigens (mumps, *Candida*, tetanus toxoid) may be applied concurrently (or at a later time) to exclude cutaneous anergy. In residents with positive tuberculin skin test results (induration of ≥10 mm to an intermediate-strength purified protein–derivative antigen), a chest x-ray should be obtained to assess for new or old pulmonary involvement with *Mycobacterium tuberculosis*. An abnormal chest radiograph that is consistent with tuberculosis (active or inactive) requires evaluation with sputum examination for the presence of mycobacteria. Pulmonary or occult miliary tuberculosis should be suspected in a nursing home resident who has prolonged unexplained fever, weight loss, respiratory symptoms, or cognitive impairment; a two-step tuberculin skin test with dermal controls, chest radiography, a complete blood count, and liver function tests should be done in these residents. Some residents may require bronchoscopy and bronchial biopsy.

Recently, the Centers for Disease Control and Prevention and the American Thoracic Society established new treatment guidelines regarding tuberculosis and tuberculosis infection (65). Unless there is evidence that a patient is at low risk for drug-resistant tuberculosis, most patients with suspected or proven (active) tuberculosis receive treatment with a four-drug regimen of isoniazid, rifampin, pyrazinamide, and ethambutol or streptomycin until culture and susceptibility data are available (65). However, drug-resistant *M. tuberculosis* is infrequently isolated from elderly patients with tuberculosis (62). Treatment should generally begin with isoniazid (300 mg/d) and rifampin (600 mg/d) for 9 months. If sputum smear and culture are negative in persons with active tuberculosis and if there is low possibility of drug resistance, therapy may be shortened from 9 to 4 months (65). Box 4.2 shows those risk factors that are indicators for isoniazid chemoprophylaxis for nursing home residents (that is, those ≥35 years of age). Clinicians should be aware of (as well as follow) the guidelines that were established by the Centers for Disease Control and Prevention for the prevention and control of tuberculosis in long-term-care facilities for elderly persons (66).

Clostridium difficile Colonization and Colitis

Increasingly, *Clostridium difficile* colonization and infection have been found in nursing home residents as the use of antibiotics increases in long-term-care settings (67, 68). After the disruption of normal bowel flora by systemic antibiotics, colonization with *C. difficile* occurs. In some patients, toxin will be released by the organism, causing mucosal damage and inflammation (69). Infection with *C. difficile* may cause diarrhea or colitis or both. However, many persons who are colonized with *C. difficile* are not infected with the organism (68).

The diagnosis of *C. difficile* diarrhea or colitis can be made by the toxin assay. The toxin assay is highly sensitive and specific (70). However, results of the assay may be positive in some asymptomatic *C.*

BOX 4.2. Indications for tuberculous chemoprophylaxis in nursing home patients*

With ≥5 mm PPD reactivity
- Close contact with active tuberculosis case
- Known or suspected HIV infection
- Abnormal chest radiograph with fibrosis consistent with old healed tuberculosis

With ≥10 mm PPD reactivity
- Intravenous drug use with no HIV infection
- Silicosis
- Gastrectomy or jejunoileal bypass
- Weight loss ≥10% ideal body weight
- Chonic renal failure
- Diabetes mellitus
- Immunosuppression
- Hematologic malignancies (leukemia, lymphoma)

With ≥15 mm PPD reactivity
- Skin test conversion within 2 years

Treatment
- Isoniazid, 300 mg/d or 900 mg twice weekly (observed) for 6 to 12 months

* At least 35 years and older. PPD = Purified protein derivative; HIV = human immunodeficiency virus.

difficile carriers or, in persons with frank antibiotic-associated colitis, they may occasionally be negative. In these persons with negative toxin assays, diagnosis of *C. difficile* diarrhea or colitis may be made by sigmoidoscopy and the finding of classic mucosal changes. Therapy is not indicated for asymptomatic carriers; however, efforts should be made to discontinue all antibiotics. Symptomatic residents should initially receive treatment with oral metronidazole (250 mg four times daily) for 10 days. If the patient fails to respond to metronidazole therapy, oral vancomycin (125 mg four times daily) should be prescribed. If parenteral therapy is required, intravenous metronidazole can provide effective treatment (69).

Herpes Zoster

Herpes zoster is a disease of the skin and nervous system caused by the recrudescence of varicella-zoster virus replication from a previously latent infection of dorsal sensory or cranial ganglia. Herpes zoster occurs almost exclusively in the elderly population and immunosuppressed persons. Although the prevalence or incidence of her-

pes zoster in nursing home residents is not known, it is known that the disease increases in frequency with age (71). Furthermore, the dreaded complication of postherpetic neuralgia also increases with age, affecting 50% and 75% of persons aged 60 to 69 years old and greater than 70 years old, respectively (72).

Acute herpes zoster begins as a prodrome of pain or paresthesia over a specific dermatome (3 to 5 days), followed by an erythematous maculopapular rash that is unilateral and dermatomal (1 to 2 days), and evolving into multiple vesicles that last for 7 to 10 days (71). The most common sites involved are the T-3 to L-3 dermatomes and the area of the face innervated by the ophthalmic division of the trigeminal nerve. Diagnosis is made clinically. Laboratory confirmation is best made by detection of varicella-zoster virus antigen in the vesicle by immunofluorescence method (71). Postherpetic neuralgia is characterized by pain at the site of the herpes zoster lesions that lasts for or recurs 1 month or more after the acute eruption (73). Allodynia (pain caused by a nonpainful stimulus—for example, rubbing of clothes against the skin) also occurs in over 90% of patients with postherpetic neuralgia (73).

Management of herpes zoster includes analgesics for pain, local wound care for vesicles, and antiviral drugs. Recent data indicate that elderly patients with herpes zoster who have significant pain can benefit from antiviral therapy if they receive treatment within 48 hours of rash onset. However, 72 hours or more after onset of rash, antiviral treatment offers no significant benefit. Clinical benefits from antiviral drugs include reducing acute pain and shortening the duration of postherpetic neuralgia (71,73,74). The antiviral agents recommended include oral acyclovir, 800 mg five times daily for 7 days; and famciclovir, 500 mg three times daily for 7 days (dose adjustment for renal dysfunction). Routine use of corticosteroids is not indicated in elderly herpes zoster patients, and there is no evidence that it reduces the frequency of postherpetic neuralgia (75).

Postherpetic neuralgia is difficult to treat, and no intervention has proved to be uniformly effective. Treatment should start with tricyclic antidepressants (nortriptyline and desipramine are preferred in elderly persons because they have fewer side effects). Topical agents such as lidocaine (5% or 10%) or capsaicin have mixed and limited results (73).

IMMUNIZATION

Influenza Vaccine

Nursing homes are common settings for outbreaks of influenza, with attack rates of up to 60% and case-to-fatality rates as high as 30%. All nursing home residents and employees, as well as health care providers who have contact with nursing home residents, should receive the trivalent influenza vaccine (76). The vaccine preparation for the 1995–1996 season, as established by the Centers for Disease Control and Prevention, included the following influenza antigens: A/Texas/36/91-like (H1/N1), A/Johannesburg/33/44-like (H3/N2), and B/Beijing/184/93-like (77). In the United States, the optimal time for influenza vaccine administration is between mid-October and mid-November. The vaccine should be administered annually. Amantadine or rimantadine, antiviral agents that are effective in preventing and treating (if given within 24 hours of symptom onset) type A influenza (but not type B influenza), should be administered to all unvaccinated nursing home residents who are exposed to other residents with influenza. Recently vaccinated residents should also receive chemoprophylaxis for at least 2 weeks after vaccination during the exposure. However, to control an *outbreak* of influenza A in an institution such as a nursing home, *all* residents, regardless of their vaccination status, should receive chemoprophylaxis. Chemoprophylaxis should also be offered to all unvaccinated staff who provide care to nursing home residents. During conditions in which no outbreak of influenza A occurs, chemoprophylaxis is continued until the influenza vaccination becomes effective—that is, for at least 2 weeks. During an outbreak in the nursing home, chemoprophylaxis is continued until the outbreak is controlled. The dose of amantadine or rimantadine for elderly persons is generally 100 mg/d, but if significant renal dysfunction is present, dose reduction may be necessary. The major side effects seizures and confusion should be carefully monitored.

Pneumococcal Vaccine

Although several important organizations such as the Immunization Practice Advisory Committee of the U.S. Public Health Service and the World Health Organization have recommended immunization of elderly persons with the pneumococcal vaccine (78, 79), controversy exists regarding the protective efficacy of the vaccine (80). Only three prospective, randomized, placebo-controlled trials of pneumococcal vaccine have been conducted in the United States during the past 50 years; all three studies, which consisted of elderly persons, did not show any significant benefit from the vaccine (80). Two of the studies, which were sponsored by the National Institutes of Health, were done in the Dorothea Dix Hospital for the mentally ill, Raleigh, North Carolina, and in the San Francisco Kaiser Permanante Health Plan; neither study was published (80). The third study was conducted in the Department of Veterans Affairs and consisted of veterans ≥55 years of age, many of whom had diabetes mellitus; cardiac, renal or hepatic diseases; or alcoholism (81).

In contrast, several studies using a case-control method and matching vaccinated and unvaccinated persons showed high rates of vaccine efficacy or clinical effectiveness, ranging from 60% to 70% in their study-participants, who included a large number of elderly persons (82–84). What explains the differences in the outcomes of all these studies? It appears that the pneumococcal vaccine is most effective in the healthy and immunocompetent elderly population (85). Thus, it would appear that among the geriatric age group, nursing home residents would experience a lesser benefit from the vaccine than healthy older adults.

Nevertheless, like the influenza vaccine, the pneumococcal vaccine is recommended for all persons who are ≥65 years of age (78), which would include practically all nursing home residents. The 23-serotype purified capsular polysaccharide antigen from *S. pneumoniae* is the recommended vaccine. It is administered on a one-time basis for most persons; however, persons with splenectomy or those who have been shown to have a rapid decline in pneumococcal antibody levels (for example, patients with nephrotic syndrome or renal failure, or recipients of transplants) should be revaccinated in 6 years (78). The pneumococcal vaccine may be administered at the same time that the influenza vaccine is given, but should be given at a different site.

Tetanus Toxoid Vaccine

Although tetanus cases in the United States are few in number (approximately 50 per year), most patients with tetanus are ≥60 years of age and 60% of all deaths due to tetanus occur in this age group

(86). The lack of adequate vaccination in the older adults explains this high incidence and mortality. It has been recommended that all persons, including elderly persons, who have not been previously immunized or inadequately immunized receive the primary series of three doses of tetanus toxoid and a booster every 10 years (86). However, it is unclear if routine tetanus immunization of nursing home residents is necessary or cost effective (87). Virtually no data are available on the incidence of tetanus or the cost effectiveness of tetanus immunization in nursing home residents, despite the fact that routine administration of tetanus toxoid to this population has been advocated (88). It would appear that nursing home residents with cutaneous ulcers associated with gangrene or pressure ulcers should be considered for tetanus immunization.

REFERENCES

1. Alvarez S. Incidence and prevalence of nosocomial infections in nursing homes. In: Verghese A, Berk SL, eds. Infections in Nursing Homes and Long-Term Care Facilities. Basel, Switzerland: Karger; 1990:41-54.

2. Smith PW, Daly PB, Roccaforte JS. Current status of nosocomial infection control in extended care facilities. Am J Med. 1991;91(Suppl 3B):281S-5S.

3. Norman DC, Castle SC, Cantrell M. Infections in the nursing home. J Am Geriatr Soc. 1987;35:796-805.

4. McGeer A, Campbell B, Emori TG, Hierholzer WJ, Jackson MM, Nicolle LE, et al. Definitions of infection for surveillance in long-term care facilities. Am J Infect Control. 1991;19:1-7.

5. Tresch DD, Simpson WM Jr, Burton JR. Relationship of long-term and acute-care facilities. The problem of patient transfer and continuity of care. J Am Geriatr Soc. 1985;33:819-26.

6. Gordon WZ, Kane RL, Rothenberg R. Acute hospitalization in a home for the aged. J Am Geriatr Soc. 1985;33:519-23.

7. Setia U, Serventi I, Lorenz P. Bacteremia in a long-term care facility. Spectrum and mortality. Arch Intern Med. 1984;144:1633-5.

8. Rudman D, Hontanasas A, Cohen Z, Mattson DE. Clinical correlates of bacteremia in a Veteran Administration extended care facility. J Am Geriatr Soc. 1988;36:726-32.

9. Muder RR, Brennen C, Wagener MM, Goetz AM. Bacteremia in a long-term care facility: a five-year prospective study of 163 consecutive episodes. Clin Infect Dis. 1992;14:647-54.

10. Marrie TA. Bacteremia in the nursing-home patient. In: Verghese A, Berk SL, eds. Infections in Nursing Homes and Long-Term Care Facilities. Basel, Switzerland:Karger;1990:77-94.

11. Yoshikawa TT. Pneumonia, UTI, and decubiti in the nursing home: optimal management. Geriatrics. 1989;44:32-43.

12. Nicolle LE, McIntyre M, Zacharias H, MacDonnell JA. Twelve-month surveillance of infections in institutionalized elderly men. J Am Geriatr Soc. 1984;32:513-9.

13. Farber BF, Brennen C, Puntereri AJ, Brody JP. A prospective study of nosocomial infections in a chronic care facility. J Am Geriatr Soc. 1984;32:499-502.

14. Finnegan TP, Austin TW, Cape RT. A 12-month fever surveillance study in a veterans' long-stay institution. J Am Geriatr Soc. 1985;33:590-4.

15. Alvarez S, Shell CG, Woolley TW, Berk SL, Smith JK. Nosocomial infections in long-term facilities. J Gerontol. 1988;43:M9-17.

16. Jackson MM, Fierer J, Barrett-Connor E, Fraser D, Klauber MR, Hatch R, et al. Intensive surveillance for infections in a three-year study of nursing home infections. Am J Epidemiol. 1992; 135:685-96.

17. Norman DC, Toledo SD. Infections in elderly persons. An altered clinical presentation. Clin Geriatr Med. 1992;8:713-9.

18. Norman DC, Yoshikawa TT. Clinical features of infection and the significance of fever in the elderly nursing-home patient. In: Verghese A, Berk SL, eds. Infections in Nursing Homes and Long-Term Care Facilities. Basel, Switzerland: Karger; 1990:32-40.

19. Keating HJ III, Klimek JJ, Levine DS, Kiernan FJ. Effect of aging on the clinical significance of fever in ambulatory adult patients. J Am Geriatr Soc. 1984;32:282-7.

20. Marrie TJ, Haldane EV,Faulkner RS, Durant H, Kwan C. Community-acquired pneumonia requiring hospitalization. Is it different in the elderly? J Am Geriatr Soc. 1985;33:671-80.

21. Alvarez S, Shell C, Berk SL. Pulmonary tuberculosis in elderly men. Am J Med. 1987; 82:602-6.

22. Terpenning MS, Buggy BP, Kauffman CA. Infective endocarditis: clinical features in young and elderly patients. Am J Med. 1987;83:626-34.

23. Gleckman R, Hibert D. Afebrile bacteremia. A phenomenon in geriatric patients. JAMA. 1982;248:1478-81.

24. Castle SC, Norman DC, Miller D, Yeh M, Yoshikawa TT. Fever response in elderly nursing home residents. Are the older truly colder? J Am Geriatr Soc. 1991;39:853-7.

25. Kluger MJ. The adaptive value of fever. In: Mackowiak P, ed. Fever: Basic Mechanisms and Management. New York:Raven Press; 1991:105-24.

26. Rockwood K. Acute confusion in elderly medical patients. J Am Geriatr Soc. 1989;37:150-4.

27. Wasserman M, Levinstein M, Keller E, Lee S, Yoshikawa TT. Utility of fever, white blood cells, and differential count in predicting bacterial infections in the elderly. J Am Geriatr Soc. 1989;37:537-43.

28. Marrie TJ, Durant H, Kwan C. Nursing home-acquired pneumonia. J Am Geriatr Soc. 1986;34:697-702.

29. Verghese A, Berk SL. Bacterial pneumonia in the elderly. Medicine (Baltimore). 1983;62:271-85.

30. Valenti WM, Trudell RG, Bentley DW. Factors predisposing to oropharyngeal colonization with gram-negative bacilli in the aged. N Engl J Med. 1978;298:1108-11.

31. Yoshikawa TT. Treatment of nursing home–acquired pneumonia. J Am Geriatr Soc. 1991;39:1040-1.

32. Bentley DW. Bacterial pneumonia in the elderly: clinical features, diagnosis, etiology, and treatment. Gerontology. 1984;30:297-307.

33. Garb JL, Brown RB, Garb JR, Tuthill RW. Differences in etiology of pneumonias in nursing home and community patients. JAMA. 1978;240:2169-72.

34. Peterson PK, Stein D, Guay DR, Logan G, Obaid S, Gruninger R, et al. Prospective study of lower respiratory tract infections in an extended-care nursing home program: potential role of oral ciprofloxacin. Am J Med. 1988;85:164-71.

35. Alvarez S, Shell CG, Woolley TW, Berk SL, Smith JK. Nosocomial infections in long-term facilities. J Gerontol. 1988;43:M9-17.

36. Marrie TJ. Community-acquired pneumonia. Clin Infect Dis. 1994;18:501-15.

37. Phillips SL, Phillips J. The use of intramuscular cefoperazone versus intramuscular ceftriaxone in patients with nursing-home acquired pneumonia. J Am Geriatr Soc. 1993;41:1071-4.

38. Dontas AS. Urinary tract infection in nursing home residents. In: Verghese A, Berk SL, eds. Infections in Nursing Homes and Long-Term Care Facilities. Basel, Switzerland: Karger; 1990:126-42.

39. Nicolle LE. Urinary tract infection in the institutionalized elderly. Infect Dis Clin Pract. 1992;1:68-71.

40. Boscia JA, Kobasa WD, Abrutyn E, Levinson ME, Kaplan AM, Kaye D. Lack of association between bacteriuria and symptoms in the elderly. Am J Med. 1986;81:979-82.

41. Nicolle LE, Muir P, Harding GK, Norris M. Localization of urinary tract infection in elderly institutionalized women with asymptomatic bacteriuria. J Infect Dis. 1988;157:65-70.

42. Warren JW, Muncie HL Jr, Hall-Craggs M. Acute pyelonephritis associated with bacteriuria during long-term catheterization: a prospective clinicopathological study. J Infect Dis. 1988;158:1341-6.

43. Warren JW, Muncie HL Jr, Hebel Jr, Hall-Craggs M. Long-term urethral catheterization increases risk of chronic pyelonephritis and renal inflammation. J Am Geriatr Soc. 1994;42:1286-90.

44. Nicolle LE, Bjornson J, Harding GK, MacDonnell JA. Bacteriuria in elderly institutionalized men. N Engl J Med. 1983;309:1420-5.

45. Warren JW. Catheter-associated bacteriuria. Clin Geriatr Med. 1992;8:805-19.

46. Breitenbucher RB. Bacterial changes in the urine samples of patients with long-term indwelling catheters. Arch Intern Med. 1984;144:1585-8.

47. Boscia JA, Abrutyn E, Kaye D. Asymptomatic bacteriuria in elderly persons: treat or do not treat? Ann Intern Med. 1987;106:764-6.

48. Nicolle LE, Mayhew JW, Bryan L. Prospective randomized comparison of therapy and no therapy for asymptomatic bacteriuria in institutionalized elderly women. Am J Med. 1987;83:27-33.

49. Grahn D, Norman DC, White ML, Cantrell M, Yoshikawa TT. Validity of urinary catheter specimen for diagnosis of urinary tract infection in the elderly. Arch Intern Med. 1985;145:1858-60.

50. Yoshikawa TT. Chronic urinary tract infections in elderly patients. Hosp Pract. 1993;28:103-18.

51. Yoshikawa TT, Norman DC. Aging and Clinical Practice: Infectious Diseases. Diagnosis and Treatment. New York: Igaku-Shoin; 1987:185-92.

52. Ginsberg MB. Cellulitis: analysis of 101 cases and review of the literature. South Med J. 1981;74:530-34.

53. Brandeis GH, Morris JN, Nash DJ, Lipsitz LA. History of pressure ulcers in elderly nursing home residents. JAMA 1990;264:2905-9.

54. Deloach ED, DiBenedetto RJ, Womble L, Gilley JD. The treatment of osteomyelitis underlying pressure ulcers. Decubitus 1993;5:32-41.

55. Bryan CS, Dew CE, Reynolds KL. Bacteremia associated with decubitus ulcers. Arch Intern Med. 1983;143:2093-5.

56. Kertesz D, Chow AW. Infected pressure and diabetic ulcers. Clin Geriatr Med. 1992;8:835-52.

57. Meyers LH. Clinical presentation of scabies in a nursing home population. J Am Acad Dermatol. 1988;18:396-7.

58. Yonkosky D, Ladia L, Gackenheimer L, Schultz MW. Scabies in nursing homes: an eradication program with permethrin 5% cream. J Am Acad Dermatol. 1990;23:1133-6.

59. Bradley SF: Methicillin-resistant *Staphylococcus aureus* infection. Clin Geriatr Med. 1992;8:853-68.

60. Bradley SF, Terpennning MS, Ramsey MA, Zarins LT, Jorgensen KA, Sottile WS, et al. Methicillin-resistant *Staphylococcus aureus* colonization and infection in a long-term care facility. Ann Intern Med. 1991;115:417-22.

61. Muder RR, Brennen C, Wagener MM, Vickers RM, Rihs JD, Jamcpcl GA, et al. Methicillin-resistant staphylococcal colonization and infection in a long-term care facility. Ann Intern Med. 1991;114:107-12.

62. Yoshikawa TT. Managing tuberculosis in today's nursing home. Nurs Home Practitioner. 1993;1:38-41.

63. Stead WW. Tuberculosis control in nursing homes. Resp Management. 1992;21:84-9.

64. Finucane TE. Clinical Practice Committee: The American Geriatrics Society statement on two-step PPD testing for nursing home patients on admission. J Am Geriatr Soc. 1988;36:77-8.

65. Bass JB Jr, Farer LS, Hopewell PC, O'Brien R, Jacobs RF, Ruben F, et al. Treatment of tuberculosis and tuberculosis infection in adults and children. American Thoracic Society and The Centers for Disease Control and Prevention. Am J Respir Crit Care Med. 1994;149:1359-74.

66. Centers for Disease Control. Prevention and control of tuberculosis in facilities providing long-term care of the elderly. Recommendations of the Advisory Committee for Elimination of Tuberculosis. MMWR Morb Mortal Wkly Rep. 1990;39:7-13.

67. Bentley DW. *Clostridium difficile*–associated disease in long-term care facilities. Infect Control Hosp Epidemiol. 1990;11:434-8.

68. Walker KJ, Gilliland SS, Vance-Bryan K, Moody JA, Larsson AJ, Rotschafer JC. Clostridium difficile colonization in residents of long-term care facilities: prevalence and risk factors. J Am Geriatr Soc. 1993;41:940-6.

69. Kelly CP, Pothoulakis C, LaMont JT. *Clostridium difficile* colitis. N Engl J Med. 1994; 330:257-62.

70. Bartlett JG. The 10 most common questions about *Clostridium difficile*–associated diarrhea/colitis. Infect Dis Clin Pract. 1992;1:254-9.

71. Schmader K. Herpes zoster management in elderly patients. Infect Dis Clin Pract. 1995;4:293-9.

72. deMoragas JM, Kierland RR. The outcome of patients with herpes zoster. Arch Dermatol. 1957; 75:193-6.

73. Bowsher D. Postherpetic neuralgia in older patients. Incidence and optimal treatment. Drugs Aging. 1994;5:411-8.

74. Bowsher D. The effects of acyclovir therapy for herpes zoster in treatment outcome in post-herpetic neuralgia: a randomized study. Eur J Pain. 1994; 15:9-12.

75. Wood MJ, Johnson RW, McKendrick MW, Taylor J, Mandal BK, Crooks J, et al. A randomized trial of acyclovir for 7 days or 21 days with and without prednisone for treatment of acute herpes zoster. N Engl J Med. 1994;330:896-900.

76. Centers for Disease Control and Prevention: Update: influenza activity—United States and Worldwide, and composition of the 1993–1994 influenza vaccine. MMWR Morb Mortal Wkly Rep. 1993; 42:177-80.

77. Centers for Disease Control and Prevention. Prevention and control of influenza. Recommendations of the Advisory Committee on Immunization Practice (ACIP). 1995;44:1-21.

78. Recommendations of the Immunization Practices Advisory Committee: Pneumococcal polysaccharide vaccine. MMWR Morb Mortal Wkly Rep. 1989; 33(No.5):64-76.

79. Fedson D, Henrichsen J, Makela, Austrian R. Immunization of elderly people with polyvalent pneumococcal vaccine. Infection. 1989;17:437-41.

80. Hirschmann JV. The pneumococcal vaccine after 15 years of use. Arch Intern Med. 1994;154:373-7.

81. Simberkoff MS, Cross AP, Al-Ibrahim M, Baltch AI, Geiseler PJ, Nadler J, et al. Efficacy of pneumococcal vaccine in high-risk patients: results of a Veterans Administration Cooperative Study. N Engl J Med. 1986;315:1318-27.

82. Bolan G, Broome CV, Facklam RR, Plikaytis BD, Fraser DW, Schlech WF III. Pneumococcal vaccine efficacy in selected populations in the United States. Ann Intern Med. 1986;104:1-6.

83. Sims RV, Steinmann WC, McConville JH, King LR, Zwick WC, et al. The clinical effectiveness of pneumococcal vaccine in the elderly. Ann Intern Med. 1988;108:653-7.

84. Shapiro E, Berg AT, Austrian R, Schroeder D, Parcells V, Margolis A, et al. The protective efficacy of polyvalent pneumococcal polysaccharide vaccine. N Engl J Med. 1991;325:1453-60.

85. LaForce FM, Eickoff TC. Pneumococcal vaccine: an emerging consensus. Ann Intern Med. 1988; 108:757-9.

86. Centers for Disease Control. Tetanus—United States, 1987 and 1988. MMWR Morb Mortal Wkly Rep. 1990;39:37-41.

87. Bentley DW. Vaccinations. Clin Geriatr Med. 1992;8(4):745-60.

88. Richardson JP, Knight AL, Stafford DT. Beliefs and policies of Maryland nursing home medical directors regarding tetanus immunization. J Am Geriatr Soc. 1990;38:1316-20.

5

Pressure Ulcers

David M. Smith, MD, FACP

**Now the bedsore on his buttock has come from
having been too long a time lying on it, without moving himself (1).**
Ambroise Paré, circa 1569

Although many advances have been made in the prevention and treatment of pressure ulcers, some principles implicit in the cure were recommended in 1569, including concern for the total welfare of the sickest and most dependent persons (1). For the physician caring for nursing home residents, this principle implies an understanding of the causes, epidemiology, effective methods for the prevention and treatment of pressure ulcers, and the role of the physician within a multidisciplinary team. This review focuses on these areas.

METHODS

The MEDLINE database was searched for English-language articles published between 1980 and October 1994 using the terms decubitus ulcer and elderly. Articles identified through this search were excluded if the title clearly indicated that the article pertained to one of the following:

1. Patients other than nursing home residents, except in articles for which data on nursing home residents were limited or unavailable

2. Patients younger than age 65 years

3. Ulcers related to peripheral vascular disease or neuropathy

4. Specific surgical interventions. Pertinent articles cited as references in the identified papers were also reviewed. Reviewed articles were excluded if they did not meet the above criteria, described

methods without patient data, or were reviews without meta-analyses.

Prevalence studies were required to have an identifiable denominator. Cohort (prospective and retrospective) studies of risk factors were selected in preference to cross-sectional studies. Incidence studies had to have an inception cohort and a specified follow-up period. If incidence figures were not provided, incidence was computed from the mean or median duration of follow-up. Preventive and therapeutic interventions were required to have an identifiable control group; preference was given to randomized controlled trials.

DEFINITIONS

A pressure ulcer is a localized area of soft-tissue injury resulting from compression between a bony prominence and an external surface. There is now consensus on the use of the term pressure ulcer rather than synonyms such as decubitus ulcer or bed sore (2). In the nursing home population, pressure ulcers are frequent, largely preventable, and, in the early stages, readily responsive to treatment. In the advanced stages, pressure ulcer treatment is problematic and associated with substantial morbidity and complications.

There is also consensus that four ulcer stages are useful for reporting prevalence and guiding therapy

(2). Stage 1 consists of nonblanchable erythema with intact skin. Erythema is redness of the skin produced by congestion of the capillaries. The difference between redness caused by capillary congestion and extravasation of blood with tissue damage is the blanching characteristic. Erythema is the initial reactive hyperemia caused by pressure, and nonblanchable erythema represents a stage 1 pressure ulcer. Reactive hyperemia completely disappears within 24 hours of relief of pressure; this characteristic helps to distinguish it from stage 1 pressure ulcers (3). However, many believe that reactive hyperemia can be distinguished from non-blanchable erythema within 2 hours of relief of pressure. The latter condition represents tissue injury and heralds skin ulceration.

Stage 2 is characterized by partial-thickness skin loss, that is, the epidermis is interrupted as an abrasion, blister, or shallow crater. Stage 3 features full-thickness skin loss involving damage or necrosis of subcutaneous tissue that may extend to, but not through, the underlying fascia. The ulcer appears as a crater, with or without undermining of adjacent tissue. In stage 4, there is full-thickness skin loss with extensive destruction; tissue necrosis; or damage to muscle, bone, or supporting structures (for example, a tendon or joint capsule).

These staging definitions have two limitations: 1) Assessment of stage 1 is difficult in patients with darkly pigmented skin; and 2) accurate staging of a pressure ulcer with an eschar is difficult until the eschar has sloughed or the wound is debrided (2).

CAUSES

The amount and duration of pressure are the primary contributing factors to the development of pressure ulcers. This time–pressure relation was shown in dogs, in which ischemic ulcers developed with 500 mm Hg of pressure applied for only 2 hours or 150 mm Hg applied for 10 hours. However, microscopic changes occurred in tissues when they were subjected to as little as 60 mm Hg of pressure for only 1 hour (4). These pressures are clinically relevant: Healthy persons seated on a flat board generate pressures of 300 to 500 mm Hg under their buttocks. A 2-inch deep foam pad reduced this pressure only to 160 mm Hg (5). Just lying in a hospital bed generates heel-to-bed pressures of 50 to 94 mm Hg when the patient lies supine (6–8) and femoral trochanter-to-bed pressures of 55 to 95 mm Hg when the patient lies on one side (6,7,9,10). These pressures exceed the normal intracapillary pressures of 12 to 32 mm Hg (11) and thus are sufficient to produce local occlusion, ischemia, and hypoxia. Lying on the sacrum or femoral trochanter can decrease the transcutaneous oxygen tension from 80 mm Hg to 13 mm Hg (12). Thus, the amount of pressure needed to produce tissue damage and pressure ulcers is readily present in all patients confined to a bed or chair.

Other factors proposed as etiologic agents include shearing force and friction. Friction is the rubbing of one body against another; it occurs when the patient is dragged across the bed and may result in an abrasion or skin tear. Shear is the stress from applied force that causes two parts of a body to slide on each other. This can be generated when the skin remains stationary and the underlying tissue moves. Shear occurs when the head of the bed is raised and the patient slips down and when the patient slides down in a chair. In elderly patients, the sitting mechanics result in shear that is on average three times that generated in healthy young adults (13). The force of stretching or bending blood vessels may produce ischemia. It has been shown that with shear, less pressure is needed to produce ischemic occlusion (14,15).

Recent reports suggest that acute illness and systemic and local circulatory conditions may also be etiologic factors in the development of pressure ulcers. For example, blood flow recovery time was delayed in elderly nursing home residents who developed pressure ulcers compared with residents without ulcers (16). In addition, ulcer development was associated with lower diastolic blood pressures and other risk factors in a cohort of nursing home residents (3). Finally, among a cohort of patients admitted to an intensive care unit, Acute Physiology and Chronic Health Evaluation II (APACHE II) scores were found to be markers of a high risk for developing pressure ulcers (17). In APACHE II, 12 routine physiologic measurements and previous health status are used to provide a general measure of disease severity (18). Thus, acute illness and associated hemodynamic factors may play a casual role in pressure ulcer development. The postulate, which deserves further study, is that decreased perfusion may cause ischemia and lead to ulcers.

EPIDEMIOLOGY

Data on the epidemiology of pressure ulcers in the nursing home (Table 5.1) show the magnitude of the problem and help guide prevention and therapy. Seventeen percent to 35% of patients have ulcers when admitted to the nursing home (3,19–22). Most of these patients are transferred from acute-care hospitals (19,21,22). Because of this high prevalence, a complete examination of each patient for ulcers at the time of admission to the nursing home is essential. The reported prevalence of pressure ulcers among residents in nursing homes ranges from 7% to 23% (19, 21,23–25). One study reported an average prevalence of 8.9% among 51 nursing homes in 11 states (19). Even at the lower range of prevalence, pressure ulcers are one of the more common problems facing physicians in nursing homes. Among patients with ulcers, the average prevalence of each stage (19) is shown in Table 5.1. The combined prevalence of stage 1 and stage 2 ulcers is 65%. When patients are followed very closely (such as in an incidence study [3]), as many as 98% of the developing ulcers are first detected at stages 1 and 2. With careful assessment, most ulcers can be identified in early stages, when they can be treated most easily.

Ulcers develop over the buttocks (ischial tuberosities) more frequently in patients who are chair-bound. The other sites of bony prominence are subjected to pressure when patients are lying supine or on their side (Figure 5.1). Pooled data reported from three nursing homes indicate that about 80% of ulcers develop over the sacrum or coccyx, hips (femoral trochanter), buttocks (ischium), and heels (25–27). Thus, for bed- and chair-bound patients, it is important to examine sites below the waist. The average number of ulcers reported per patient ranged from 1.6 to 2.5 (25–27).

Several reports on the incidence of pressure ulcers from nursing home databases are now available (19,28,29). These data were obtained by assessing all residents at 3- to 6-month intervals. The computed incidence from these studies of 0.20 to 0.56/1000 patient-days (Table 5.1) may be low because stage 1 ulcers were not included. Some investigators exclude stage 1 pressure ulcers from their studies because of the potential difficulty of reliable identification for research purposes (19,30–32). In a 2-week prospective cohort study of patients at risk (Braden Scale score <17), the incidence of pressure

TABLE 5.1. Epidemiologic data on pressure ulcers in the nursing home

Variable	Observation
Patients admitted with ulcers, %	17–35
Prevalence among residents, %	7–23
Of patients with ulcers, prevalence by ulcer stage, %	
Stage 1	24
Stage 2	41
Stage 3	22
Stage 4	13
Common ulcer sites, %	
Sacrum or coccyx	36
Hips (over trochanter)	17
Buttocks (over ischium)	15
Heels	12
Ankles (over malleolus)	7
Other	13
Range of ulcers per resident	1.6–2.5
Range of incidence computed from databases, *n/1000 patient-days*	0.20–0.56
Incidence in high-risk patients, *n/1000 patient-days*	14
Proportion of initial ulcers developing in high-risk patients, %	
By 7 days	53
By 14 days	82

ulcers (including stage 1) was 14/1000 patient-days (3). For comparison, the incidence among all admissions to an adult intensive care unit was 28/1000 patient-days (33); high-risk patients (APACHE II score >15) admitted to an intensive care unit had an incidence of 52/1000 patient-days (17). Among patients destined to develop ulcers after nursing home admission, most ulcers occur in the first 7 to 14 days (3), perhaps because the patients were still recovering from an acute event. Thus, it is imperative that patients at risk be recognized at admission to the nursing home and that preventive interventions be started as soon as is feasible.

PREVENTION

Good evidence suggests that many pressure ulcers are preventable. The following are three general guidelines for prevention:

1. Identify patients at higher risk for developing ulcers

2. Implement preventive measures appropriate for the level of risk

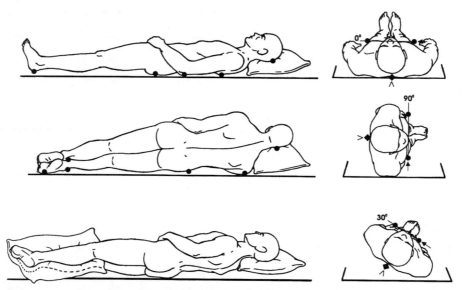

FIGURE 5.1. Positions of the bed-bound patient. In the supine position (*top*), the body weight is placed on the bony prominence of sacrum or coccyx and heels. In the lateral position (*middle*), the weight is placed on the prominence of the hips and malleoli of the ankles. These exposures can be avoided by propping the patient in the 30-degree lateral position (*bottom*) with pillows.

3. Follow high-risk patients closely and reassess patients when functional status decreases.

Identifying Patients at Risk

Because pressure ulcers rarely develop in ambulatory patients, those who are bed- or chair-bound are targeted for assessment of risk factors. Risk factors for developing ulcers, derived from cohort studies (3,28,34–37), are listed in Box 5.1. Each risk factor has varying levels of severity, and many patients will have more than one risk factor. Thus, both the severity of a risk factor and the number of risk factors characterize the level of risk.

Because the development of pressure ulcers depends on the length of time pressure is applied, immobility is the major risk factor. Although all patients who are bed- or chair-bound have some degree of mobility impairment, the severity ranges from complete immobility to the ability to reposition independently. Patients may not reposition themselves because they cannot move or cannot sense the discomfort associated with not moving. Patients who cannot move include those with spinal cord injury, fracture, Parkinson disease, stroke, and deconditioning from a severe illness. Physical restraints used in the bed or chair impair movement

and also may directly cause pressure (34). Examples of sensory loss that impair sensing the need to reposition include peripheral neuropathy, spinal cord injury, stroke, and coma from any cause. Sedated patients, such as those who are chemically restrained, also may not sense a need to reposition themselves. Although inability to move and inability to sense the need to move are separated in these examples, it is more common to find patients who have both immobility and sensory loss, such as a patient with hip fracture who is sedated to relieve pain.

Malnutrition has been linked to the development of pressure ulcers. In prospective cohorts with multivariate analyses, lower dietary protein intake (3) and inability to feed oneself (28) have been found to be independent predictors of ulcer development. Although these clinical findings of nutritional intake are clinically obvious, they are not only independent predictors but also the earliest signs of malnutrition. With continued poor intake, other markers of malnutrition, such as hypoalbuminemia or low vitamin C levels, may later occur. This observation is supported by the relation of hypoalbuminemia to the presence of pressure ulcers that has been seen in cross-sectional studies (37,38) but has not been an independent predictor in the longitudinal cohort

BOX 5.1. Risk factors for pressure ulcers among bed- or chair-bound elderly persons

Immobility
Limited ability to reposition because of the following:
Disease, such as paralysis, fracture, Parkinson disease
Physical restraints
Limited ability to sense need to reposition because of the following:
Disease, such as neuropathy, spinal cord lesions, stroke, or coma
Chemical restraints
Combinations of these losses
Malnutrition as manifested by poor dietary intake or inability to feed oneself

investigations (3,37). Thus, when identifying patients at risk for developing pressure ulcers, physicians should concentrate on assessing intake rather than other traditional markers, such as the serum albumin level.

Urinary and fecal incontinence have been considered to be predictive of pressure ulcers, at least since the development of the early predictive instruments (39). However, the independent contribution of incontinence in predicting pressure ulcers has not been consistently shown in three cohort studies (3,28,37). Urinary incontinence was not found to be a significant risk factor in these studies except as a component of skin moisture in the Braden Scale, which includes five other factors (3). Fecal incontinence was significant in one of the three studies (28), not independently observed in another (3), and not significant in the third (37). The lack of consistency may be related to the use of different measures of fecal incontinence (28,37) or confounding with mobility measures. Despite these findings, it would seem prudent to consider patients with mobility problems and fecal incontinence as being at higher risk for tissue damage than patients not exposed to moisture and bacterial contamination.

In most nursing homes, assessment of risk for pressure ulcer is a routine component of interdisciplinary patient care. In many nursing homes, part of the required admission protocol is the Minimum Data Set for Nursing Home Resident Assessment and Care Screening (40). The Minimum Data Set includes determination of the presence or absence of pressure ulcers and risk factors on admission, and it provides a mechanism for communicating risk assessment among members of the care team.

Some nursing homes prefer using standardized risk assessment instruments (39,41). The Braden Scale (41) has six items (sensory perception, activity, mobility, skin moisture, friction, and nutrition) that contain three to four grades each. Scores are continuous; those of 16 or 17 indicate mild risk, and those of 12 or below indicate high risk (3). The Braden Scale has been compared with the Norton Scale (39) in the same population, with a Cohen kappa statistic for agreement in classification of 0.73 (42). These scales provide a systematic method for quantitative risk assessment and a method for interdisciplinary team communication. When used in cohorts of high-risk patients in hospitals (in whom the incidence of developing ulcers is about 20% over 10 to 14 days or about 14/1000 patient-days), the sensitivity of both scales was 83%, the specificity was 63% and 64%, respectively, and the calculated positive predictive value was 36% and 37%, respectively (43). When used alone, these scales may not be helpful in populations at much lower risk. For example, among the nursing home population, the incidence of patients developing ulcers may average 0.5/1000 patient-days (Table 5.1), or about 1% over 14 days. If the same sensitivity and specificity are used, the positive predictive value would be 2%. Thus, the information gained from using these scales in low-risk populations (all residents) is limited. For this reason, many physicians choose to use these scales only for higher-risk populations, such as bed-bound patients.

Preventive Measures

Choosing the number and intensity of preventive measures appropriate for the level of risk requires clinical judgment. Preventive measures include reducing or eliminating factors contributing to the development of ulcers: prolonged pressure, amount of pressure, friction, shear forces, malnutrition, and fecal incontinence.

Physicians treating patients with mobility problems need to completely assess the medical conditions that limit the patients' ability to reposition or to sense the need for repositioning. This includes obtaining relevant history, physical examination, and laboratory data and then treating identified conditions or risks. Although the process of complete evaluation and management of medical conditions is important, any prolonged pressure must be relieved immediately. The choice of methods to relieve prolonged pressure depends on the extent of sensory loss and immobility. For patients with severe sensory losses, a standard method is turning the patient every 2 to 3 hours (39) so that the patient's weight does not rest on bony prominences (12). The objective is to prevent the patient from lying supine (a position in which the sacrum and heels bear weight) and on one side (a position in which the femoral trochanter bears weight) (Figure 5.1). Pillows are used to prop the patient at a 30-degree lateral position (Figure 5.1, *bottom*), and positions are rotated from side to side every 2 to 3 hours. Although protecting the sacrum and hips, 30-degree lateral turning places pressure on the knees and the medial and lateral malleoli. To protect these areas, pillows should be inserted between the ankles and knees.

The intervention prevents prolonged pressure and relieves the amount of pressure by using pillows. Pillows are one example of devices that relieve pressure over prominent bony surfaces by distributing the weight over a wider area using the principle of displacement. The wider the area of weight distribution, the less pressure will be exerted on one point. Thus, the best pressure-relieving device may be a water bed, but this is impractical in care settings.

Categories of pressure-relieving devices are listed in Box 5.2 (44,45). Static overlays and pressure-reducing mattresses are not attached to motors and do not contain moving parts. They are made of or contain gel, foam, water, or air. A 2-inch deep foam mattress does not significantly reduce pressure over the trochanter (6,10); however, a 4-inch deep foam mattress reduces pressure by 30% (10) compared with regular hospital beds. Among elderly patients in three different settings, a 4-inch deep solid foam mattress reduced the incidence of pressure ulcers compared with 3- or 4-inch deep convoluted foam mattresses (46). In addition, compared with a regular hospital bed, a 6.5-inch deep foam mattress reduced the incidence of pressure ulcers (68% and 24%, respectively) among elderly patients admitted to the hospital with femoral neck fractures (47). Other static mattresses reduce pressure by 40% to 70% (6,7,10) but are more expensive (48); in addition, little information on efficacy in actual prevention of ulcers is available.

Dynamic (alternating air) mattresses relieve pressure by the use of multiple air cushions with alter-

BOX 5.2. Devices and dressings available for preventing and treating pressure ulcers

Pressure-relieving devices
  Static mattresses or overlays made of or containing foam, gel, water, or air
  Static devices for special areas, such as heel protectors or chair or wheelchair cushions
  Dynamic mattresses or overlays, such as those with alternating air pressure
  Kinetic or oscillating beds
  Low-air-loss beds, with air cushions that allow some air to escape
  Air-fluidized or high-air-loss beds, with air blown through ceramic beads
Dressings
  Transparent membranes, such as polyurethane
  Hydrocolloid dressings
  Saline wet-to-dry dressings for debridement
  Minimally absorptive dressing, such as hydrogels and continuous saline-soaked gauze
  Absorptive dressings, such as calcium alginate, hydrophilic foam, and saline-impregnated gauze

nating air pressure controlled by a pump. These mattresses are more costly than static mattresses and are more complex to operate, but those with 6-inch diameter air tubes were effective in preventing pressure ulcers (43). Kinetic or oscillating beds can rotate the patient in a complete circle and are used for high-risk patients with spinal cord injury. Low-air-loss beds provide pressure relief using air cushions that allow air to escape through multiple pores. These beds reduced the incidence of pressure ulcers among patients admitted to an intensive care unit (17) but have not been compared with solid foam mattresses. Thus, for high-risk patients in the nursing home, the most inexpensive and effective pressure-relieving products for prevention are 4- to 6-inch deep solid foam mattresses.

The bony prominences of the heels are vulnerable, frequently neglected areas. When the patient is in the 30-degree lateral position (Figure 5.1, *bottom*), the heels can be protected with pillows. When the patient is lying supine, pillows can be placed under the legs to elevate the heels and relieve pressure. Special heel protectors and other pressure-relieving devices are appropriate for patients who cannot change the position of their lower extremities. Some of these heel protectors are constructed of foam and are inexpensive, but their effectiveness in prevention has not been shown. More expensive heel protectors (or boots) have posterior splints for the leg that lift the heel off of contact surfaces; these protectors are more appropriate for treatment or prevention in very-high-risk patients.

Chair-bound patients who cannot sense the need for repositioning require intensive efforts for relieving pressure. The pressures located over ischial prominences are larger, and the potential area for distributing weight is smaller. Measures of pressure reduction of cushions varied so widely among patients that specific recommendations could not be made (49,50). Thus, cushions need to be individually selected and prescribed for each patient (51). Many rehabilitation therapists and nurse specialists have been trained to evaluate patients and prescribe these devices. Doughnut-type devices or ring cushions are to be avoided because they compromise blood flow to areas of bony prominence. Seated patients should be repositioned frequently (that is, every hour) or, if feasible, trained to shift weight every 15 minutes.

Preventive measures for shear and friction include maintaining the head of the bed at the lowest elevation consistent with medical conditions, using a trapeze or bed linen (lift sheet) for moving the patient, and paying careful attention when the patient is being positioned. The use of skin moisturizers for dry skin may be considered. Advances have been made in ways to assess and manage fecal incontinence and malnutrition. Detailed discussion of these problems and interventions is beyond the scope of this review.

Follow-up and Reassessment

Patients should be followed up to determine whether the preventive interventions are working, that is, to observe whether pressure ulcers develop. In high-risk patients, pressure points should be monitored daily. If ulcers develop and are recognized early (for example, at stage 1), the number or intensity of preventive interventions can be increased and therapy can be begun immediately with expectations that the ulcers will resolve within days. The objective is to avoid advanced stages of ulcers associated with major morbidity.

Changes in patients' medical conditions may affect their level of risk for developing pressure ulcers. Thus, risk factors for pressure ulcers should be reassessed after any change in condition to decide whether the intensity of preventive measures must

be increased or decreased. Even patients not previously at risk should be periodically assessed (3 to 6 months) for the presence of risk factors for pressure ulcers. This is a routine staff procedure in most nursing homes.

TREATMENT

Therapeutic measures should be appropriate for each stage and should be consistent with the therapeutic goals for the patient. Many therapeutic interventions are the same as preventive interventions.

Stage 1: Nonblanchable Erythema

Perhaps the most important facet of therapy is shifting the attitudinal approach from "this is the minimal stage of disease" to "this is the warning that advanced stages will soon appear unless interventions are immediately implemented." Interventions initiated early may produce a cure within days, whereas delay may result in progression to advanced stages within the same period; cure may then take months. Thus, careful examination of patients to detect early stages of disease is imperative. On the basis of the epidemiology of pressure ulcers (Table 5.1), the careful examination process should start on the day of admission to the nursing home. The common sites below the waist deserve special attention.

To treat stage 1 ulcers, risk factors and current preventive measures should be reassessed. When preventive measures are in place, the intensity or number of measures discussed above for prevention should be increased (for example, increased frequency of turning, a more potent pressure-relieving device [Box 5.2], increased mobility through trapeze bars or physical therapy, or increased nutritional repletion). These measures alone may be sufficient for stage 1. As an alternative, polyurethane dressings applied every 1 to 10 days can protect the area from additional friction. The transparent polyurethane dressings are evenly coated on one side with a synthetic adhesive. These semipermeable films are permeable to water vapor, oxygen, and other gases and are impermeable to water and bacteria. They maintain a moist interface for healing but allow some exudate to be lost by transmission of water vapor. With appropriate treatment, most nonblanchable erythema lesions can be expected to heal by 2 weeks.

Stage 2: Partial-Thickness Skin Loss

All therapeutic interventions for nonblanchable erythema are also appropriate for stage 2 pressure ulcers. Because a defect is present in this stage, the wound should be inspected and monitored for signs of secondary infection (surrounding erythema, warmth). For stage 2 ulcers, polyurethane dressings are more effective and less costly than saline wet-to-dry dressing (52). Further, saline wet-to-dry dressings (a debridement dressing) are rarely indicated for this stage.

Stage 3: Full-Thickness Skin Loss

A difficulty with stage 3 (and stage 4) lesions is that the extent of disease may not be evident because of covering necrotic material or eschar. To establish the extent of disease and promote healing, the necrotic material must be removed. Debridement may be done by experienced primary care physicians when the eschar is small. When the eschar is large, surgical consultation should be considered. Because physical debridement can be associated with bacteremia (53), prophylactic antibiotic agents should be used for patients with implanted prosthetic devices. For smaller eschars, topical application of enzymatic debriding agents is effective (54). The eschar should be scored so that the penetration and effectiveness of topical debriding agents are increased. These enzymes must not touch the surrounding area because they irritate healthy skin. Applications should be stopped when the eschar sloughs.

Loose material can be effectively debrided by applying wet-to-dry saline dressings every 8 hours. Wet-to-dry dressings are primarily used for debridement. Although ulcers may heal with these dressings, the dry dressing may remove or disrupt the granulation tissue and delay healing when the lesion is clean with a granulating base. Polyurethane and hydrocolloid dressings are more effective for healing stage 3 pressure ulcers (52,55–58). Hydrocolloid dressings are impermeable to gas and moisture. In contrast to polyurethane, hydrocolloid dressings absorb exudate and are changed more frequently, that is, every 1 to 4 days. Hydrocolloid dressings are less costly (57,58) and more effective (55,56,58) than the wet-to-dry dressings, which are changed three times a day.

In the deeper stage 3 and stage 4 wounds, hydrocolloid dressings alone are not appropriate. These deeper wounds need to be packed with materials according to the amount of exudate. For dry wounds with minimal exudate, the less absorptive hydrogels are recommended. Continuous moist soaks with normal saline may be used, with care taken to ensure that the dressing does not become dry; healthy tissue is removed when dried dressing is changed. For wounds with significant exudate, the more absorptive dressings, hydrophilic foam, alginates, or saline-impregnated gauze are indicated for packing. Packings are changed daily.

Among patients with several or large ulcers, there is no consensus on the use of costly but effective specialized beds, that is, low-air-loss or air-fluidized beds (Box 5.2), for treatment in the nursing home. In hospitalized patients, the relative odds for showing improvement were 5.6-fold greater with air-fluidized beds compared with air mattresses covered with a 1.9-cm deep foam pad after a follow-up of 13 days (59). In nursing home residents, low-air-loss beds compared with 10-cm deep corrugated foam pads resulted in a threefold reduction in the ulcer area during a follow-up of 37.5 days (60). Among patients receiving home care, air-fluidized beds did not improve healing compared with usual care (that is, various pressure-reducing mattresses), but the costs of the beds were offset by reduced hospital days (61).

However, in nursing homes not using low-air-loss beds, 20% to 30% of stage 3 and stage 4 ulcers completely heal (19). Bennett and colleagues (62) advocated not prescribing specialized beds for most patients within the first 30 days of admission to a nursing home. This review showed that many patients, who are prescribed special beds shortly after admission, were extremely ill at that time, died of unrelated conditions during the first 30 days, and received no discernible benefit. A trial of intensive total-patient therapy with close monitoring (weekly linear measurements of size and depth) would provide objective evidence of healing, nonhealing, or worsening and the need or absence of need for special beds. Further, if specialized beds are prescribed, they should be used for at least 60 days before their use is discontinued because of a lack of therapeutic response (62).

If aggressive therapy is consistent with the overall goals for the patient, and if the severe ulcers do not heal or worsen with intensive but conservative therapy, specialized beds should be seriously considered. The constraint for not prescribing specialized beds earlier is the expense ($50 to $100 per day) (62). The degree to which these costs can be offset by potential benefits of avoiding surgery, reducing nursing home stay, or avoiding hospital readmission requires further clinical trials with long follow-up periods.

If patients with large defects are candidates for surgery, consultation with plastic surgeons for consideration of skin grafting is appropriate, depending on the goals for the patient and response to conservative therapy. Patients with large defects in the sacral area and urinary incontinence may require catheterization. Both venous and arterial insufficiency need to be assessed for pressure ulcers on the lower extremity.

Stage 4: Full-Thickness Skin Loss with Extensive Destruction

Stage 4 ulcers usually require surgical consultation for initial physical debridement. Completion of debridement can be done with wet-to-dry dressings or repeated debridement. For some patients, whirlpool baths facilitate debridement. Clean, deep ulcers require packing, as discussed for stage 3 ulcers.

When the wound is clean and granulation tissue evident, grafting procedures may be considered. The selection of patients for surgical procedures to close pressure ulcers is difficult. In elderly patients with severe cognitive dysfunction and other chronic disabilities, the rates of surgical complications, recurrences, and new ulcer formation can outweigh any benefit of surgery (63). Moss and La Puma (64) reported that aggressive treatment of advanced pressure ulcers is often inconsistent with the overall goals for the patient. Because elderly patients with advanced pressure ulcers are often terminally ill, Moss and La Puma emphasized the importance of defining the overall goals of therapy for the patient: Is the goal to prolong life, restore normal function, avoid burdensome therapies, or relieve pain and suffering? Alternatively, in patients with moderate dysfunction and comorbid conditions, surgical treatment may be preferred (65) if it is compatible with treatment goals and the patient's ability to tolerate surgery.

Careful attention to serious wounds should not detract from the continued assessment and management of the other factors, including general medical conditions, immobility, fecal incontinence, and malnutrition. Too frequently, aggressive care interventions are used without attention to basic care, such as nutritional assessment (66). This latter aspect of care is important, and recent good clinical trials have shown the effect of specific nutrients. For example, at least two studies have shown that a higher protein intake is related to faster healing of pressure ulcers (59,67). In addition, ascorbic acid supplements have been shown in a randomized, double-blind clinical trial to significantly improve healing (68).

Newer Forms of Therapy

Recent clinical trials of low-intensity direct current (69) for treating pressure ulcer in stages 2 and 3 and of topical growth factor (70,71) for treating ulcers in stages 3 and 4 have shown increased healing rates. These studies suggest promising new areas for clinical investigation.

OUTCOMES

Local Infection

Pressure ulcers are chronically contaminated wounds. Local infection is usually well controlled by relief of pressure, debridement, dressings, and other general measures of care. Although higher bacterial counts per gram of tissue are associated with delayed healing, unproven antiseptic or antibiotic topical applications should be avoided because they may be toxic to fibroblasts and impair formation of granulation tissue (72). Few studies have shown efficacy of topical antibiotic agents. One study reported that gentamicin cream applied to ulcers reduced bacterial counts and improved healing (73). Ulcers with a foul odor are probably infected with anaerobic organisms. Some reports suggest that topical metronidazole may be effective in reducing the foul odor and bacterial counts of these ulcers (74,75). However, until efficacy is better shown, topical antibiotic agents should have no role (72).

Sepsis

Among hospitalized patients, the combination of bacteremia and pressure ulcers has been associated with a mortality rate of 50% (76). Thus, if sepsis is suspected in nursing home residents, the patient should be transferred to the hospital when this move is consistent with the patient's treatment goals. In patients with stage 3 and 4 pressure ulcers and clinical manifestations of sepsis (fever, chills, confusion, and hypotension) without a definable cause, it must be assumed that the primary source of infection is from the wound. Because swab specimens frequently reflect surface colonization, a deep-tissue biopsy specimen for culture should be obtained when feasible (77), in addition to blood cultures.

Blood cultures frequently grow multiple microbial organisms (72) and have included *Pseudomonas aeruginosa, Bacteroides fragilis, and Staphylococcus aureus*. Thus, when sepsis is thought to be related to the pressure ulcer before culture results are obtained, antibiotic therapy should cover anaerobic organisms, gram-negative bacilli, and gram-positive cocci.

Osteomyelitis

Because ulcers develop over bony prominences, osteomyelitis is a potential complication (78). The diagnosis is more likely when the ulcer involves bone surface or when healing is delayed. However, clinical evaluation for osteomyelitis is often inaccurate. Appropriate diagnostic procedures, which may include pathologic examination of bone tissue (79), should be pursued to justify a prolonged course of antibiotic therapy. Ulcers located over joints also merit close attention for potential development of septic arthritis.

Mortality

Patients admitted to nursing homes with pressure ulcers have a mortality rate of 50% at 1 year compared with a 27% mortality rate in those without ulcers. Thirty-five percent of patients developing an ulcer within 3 months of admission die within 1 year compared with 25% who do not develop ulcers (19). In patients with pressure ulcers, death is more likely to be related to cardiovascular disease, respiratory disease, or cancer than a complication of the pressure ulcer (26). These data show the frailty of patients with or developing ulcers and the need for total patient care.

Costs

In an acute-care facility, the average variable costs (additional costs incurred to treat pressure ulcers) have been estimated to be $1 300 per patient or $80 per day (80). If the patient was admitted specifically for treatment of pressure ulcers, room costs were included; the average variable costs then increased to $3 746 per patient. In the nursing home, the average variable costs were estimated to be $751 per patient and $5.35 per day (range, $0 to $128 per day) (81). For some individual nursing home residents, costs may range from $4 255 to $23,300 per patient (82). These costs were estimated from the institutional perspective and are conservative from the patient perspective. For example, costs of the primary physician are not included, nor are the costs before or after institutionalization at that facility or the costs of the stay being prolonged because of the ulcer. Also, the costs not directly related to pressure ulcer treatment, such as costs of physical therapy to improve mobility, were not included. Further, the estimates from the nursing home did not include pressure-relieving devices nor hospitalizations for pressure ulcers (81). Thus, from the patient perspective, treatment costs can be significantly higher, thus providing incentive for early prevention and treatment.

MULTIDISCIPLINARY CARE AND OTHER RESOURCES

Pressure ulcers are a multidisciplinary care problem. Before-and-after studies have shown effective prevention with multidisciplinary teams for systematic risk assessment, implementation of preventive and therapeutic measures, education of patients and staff, and monitoring of incidence (24, 83). The teams include medicine, surgery, nursing, rehabilitative therapy, dietetics, and surgical subspecialties. Nursing staff play a major role in coordinating systematic preventive interventions. Nursing homes have established protocols for these interventions using the steps outlined above. Some interventions require physician orders, whereas others are automatically implemented. Dietitians are valuable resources for nutritional assessments and recommendations for supplements and methods for providing nutrition. Rehabilitation therapists are resources for improving mobility and devising or recommending protective and pressure-relieving devices. Physicians should be familiar with team function and organization and with established protocols. This will facilitate their roles as team participants, as more effective communicators, and as leaders in therapeutic interventions.

Recent and excellent resources for risk assessment, prevention, and treatment are the clinical practice guidelines Pressure Ulcers in Adults: Prediction and Prevention and Treatment of Pressure Ulcers. These booklets contain descriptions of risk assessment tools, further details on skin care, an algorithm for prevention, details of treatment, and an extensive list of references. Both of these booklets have illustrated companion pamphlets for patient education that explain pressure ulcers, their prevention, and treatment in lay language. These resources were developed by the Agency for Health Care Policy and Research (AHCPR) and the National Pressure Ulcer Advisory Panel. They can be obtained by calling the AHCPR Clearinghouse at (800)-358-9295.

TRENDS OVER TIME

As shown in this review, considerable information is now available on effective preventive and therapeutic interventions for pressure ulcers. It could be postulated that application of current knowledge and skills to practice sites would eventually reduce the prevalence and incidence of pressure ulcers. However, data from the National Hospital Discharge Survey (43,84–87) show that among persons 65 years of age and older, the prevalence of pressure ulcers (ICD-9-CM code 707.0), as any of all listed diagnoses, has more than doubled over the past 10 years (Figure 5.2), whereas the total number of discharges for older persons is constant or decreasing. The increasing prevalence of pressure ulcer diagnoses among discharged patients may be due to the following:

1. Coding changes when the prospective payment system was implemented in 1983

2. An increased proportion of very old persons (those aged 85 years)

3. More invasive procedures being done in older persons at risk for complications

4. The ineffectiveness of preventive and therapeutic interventions for pressure ulcers

5. The lack of implementation of effective interventions. Whatever the reason, these data do not

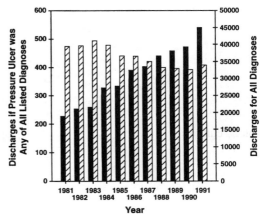

FIGURE 5.2. Pressure ulcer prevalence at hospital discharge over time. The bar graph shows the trend over time for discharges from short-stay hospitals in the United States for persons age 65 years and older per 100,000 persons. The total discharges for all diagnoses are indicated by the hatched bars wiith reference to the right vertical axis. The discharges for which a pressure ulcer (ICD-9-CM code 707.0) was any of all listed diagnoses are indicated by the solid black bars with reference to the left vertical axis.

provide evidence for a reduction in the prevalence in hospitals.

Whether the prevalence of pressure ulcers on admission to nursing homes or the prevalence among nursing home residents nationally is increasing or decreasing over time is unknown. A brief report from a multifacility group involving as many as 68 nursing homes suggests that the prevalence of pressure ulcers has remained stable over 10 years despite the increasing acuity of admissions (88). Thus, application of current knowledge and skills may be having an effect. With the development of large databases for nursing homes (19,29), more data on the prevalence for nursing home residents will become available. Such data will allow further judgments on the effectiveness of current practices in reducing the prevalence of pressure ulcers throughout the nation.

Acknowledgments. The author thanks Drs. Christopher Callahan, Jeffrey Darnell, Terrance Drake, and David Wilcox for review of drafts; David Gregory for the illustrations; and Jane Egan, RN, Terryl Adams, RN, Gayle Redmon, the Skin Care Resource Team of Wishard Memorial Hospital, and Rebecca York for technical assistance.

REFERENCES

1. Levine JM. Historical notes on pressure ulcers: the cure of Ambroise Paré. Decubitus. 1992;5:23-6.
2. Pressure ulcer prevalence, cost and risk assessment: consensus statement The National Pressure Ulcer Advisory Panel. Decubitus. 1989;2:24-8.
3. Bergstrom N, Braden B. A prospective study of pressure sore risk among institutionalized elderly. J Am Geriatr Soc. 1992;40:747-58.
4. Kosiak M. Etiology and pathology of ischemic ulcers. Arch Phys Med Rehab. 1959;40:62-71.
5. Kosiak M, Kubicek WG, Olson M, Danz JN, Kottke FJ. Evaluation of pressure as a factor in the production of ischial ulcers. Arch Phys Med Rehab. 1958;39:623-9.
6. Maklebust J, Mondoux L, Sieggreen M. Pressure relief characteristics of various support surfaces used in prevention and treatment of pressure ulcers. J Enterostomal Ther. 1986;13:85-9.
7. Thompson-Bishop JY, Mottola CM. Tissue interface pressure and estimated subcutaneous pressures of 11 different pressure reducing support surfaces. Decubitus. 1992;5:42-8.
8. Guin P, Hudson A, Gallo J. The efficacy of six heel pressure reducing devices. Decubitus. 1991;4:15-23.
9. Stewart TP, McKay MG, Magnano S. Pressure relief characteristics of an alternating pressure system. Decubitus. 1990;3:26-9.
10. Krouskop TA, Williams R, Krebs M, Herszkowicz I, Garber S. Effectiveness of mattress overlays in reducing interface pressures during recumbency. J Rehabil Res Dev. 1985;22:7-10.
11. Landis EM. Micro-injection studies of capillary blood pressure in human skin. Heart. 1930;15:209-28.
12. Seiler WO, Allen S, Stahelin HB. Influence of the 30 degree laterally inclined position and the 'super-soft' 3-piece mattress on skin oxygen tension on areas of maximum pressure implications for pressure sore prevention. Gerontology. 1986;32:158-66.
13. Bennett L, Kavner D, Lee BY, Trainor FS, Lewis JM. Skin blood flow in seated geriatric patients. Arch Phys Med Rehabil. 1981;62:392-8.
14. Bennett L, Kavner D, Lee BK, Trainor FA. Shear vs pressure as causative factors in skin blood flow occlusion. Arch Phys Med Rehabil. 1979;60:309-14.
15. Goossens RH, Zegers R, Hoek van Dijke GA, Snijders CJ. Influence of shear on oxygen tension. Clin Physiol. 1994;14:111-8.
16. Meijer JH, Germs PH, Schneider H, Ribbe MW. Susceptibility to decubitus ulcer formation. Arch Phys Med Rehabil. 1994;75:318-23.
17. Inman KJ, Sibbald WJ, Rutledge FS, Clark BJ. Clinical utility and cost-effectiveness of an air suspension bed in the prevention of pressure ulcers. JAMA. 1993;269:1139-43.
18. Knaus WA, Draper EA, Wagner DP, Zimmerman JE. APACHE II: a severity of disease classification. Crit Care Med. 1985;13:818-29.
19. Brandeis GH, Morris JN, Nash DJ, Lipsitz LA. The epidemiology and natural history of pressure ulcers in elderly nursing home residents. JAMA. 1990;264:2905-9.
20. Spector WD, Kapp MC, Tucker RJ, Sternberg J. Factors associated with presence of decubitus ulcers at admission to nursing homes. Gerontologist. 1988;28:830-4.
21. Reed JW. Pressure ulcers in the elderly: prevention and treatment utilizing the team approach. Md State Med J. 1981;30:45-50.
22. Shepard MA, Parker D, DeClercque N. The underreporting of pressure sores in patients transferred between hospital and nursing home. J Am Geriatr Soc. 1987;35:159-60.
23. Pinchcofsky-Devin GD, Kaminski MV Jr. Correlation of pressure sores and nutritional status. J Am Geriatr Soc. 1986;34:435-40.
24. Dimant J, Francis ME. Pressure sore prevention and management. J Gerontol Nurs. 1988;14:18-25.
25. Young L. Pressure ulcer prevalence and associated patient characteristics in one long-term care facility. Decubitus. 1989;2:52.
26. Michocki RJ, Lamy PP. The problem of pressure sores in a nursing home population: statistical data. J Am Geriatr Soc. 1976;24:323-8.
27. Frantz RA, Gardner S, Harvey P, Specht J. Adoption of research-based practice for treatment of pressure ulcers in long-term care. Decubitus. 1992; 5:44-54.
28. Brandeis GH, Ooi WL, Hossain M, Morris JN, Lipsitz LA. A longitudinal study of risk factors associated with the formation of pressure ulcers in nursing homes. J Am Geriatr Soc. 1994;42:388-93.
29. Rudman D, Mattson DE, Alverno L, Richardson TJ, Rudman IW. Comparison of clinical indicators in two nursing homes. J Am Geriatr Soc. 1993;41:1317-25.
30. Lyder CH. Conceptualization of the stage 1 pressure ulcer. J ET Nurs. 1991;18:162-5.
31. Abruzzese R. Quality care and staging of ulcers [Editorial]. Decubitus. 1991;4:6-7.
32. Salvadalena GD, Snyder ML, Brogdon KE. Clinical trial of the Braden Scale on an acute care medical unit. J ET Nurs. 1992;19:160-5.
33. Bergstrom N, Demuth PJ, Braden BJ. A clinical trial of the Braden Scale for Predicting Pressure Sore Risk. Nurs Clin North Am. 1987;22:417-26.
34. Lofgren RP, MacPherson DS, Granieri R, Myllenbeck S, Sprafka JM. Mechanical restraints on the medical wards: are protective devices safe? Am J Public Health. 1989;79:735-8.
35. Kemp MG, Keithley JK, Smith DW, Morreale B. Factors that contribute to pressure sores in surgical patients. Res Nurs Health. 1990;13:293-301.
36. Marchette L, Arnell I, Redick E. Skin ulcers of elderly surgical patients in critical care units. Dimensions Crit Care Nurs. 1991;10:321-9.
37. Berlowitz DR, Wilking SV. Risk factors for pressure sores. A comparison of cross-sectional and cohort-derived data. J Am Geriatr Soc. 1989;37:1043-50.
38. Allman RM, Laprade CA, Noel LB, Walker JM, Moorer CA, Dear MR, et al. Pressure sores among

hospitalized patients. Ann Intern Med. 1986;105: 337-42.

39. Norton D, McLaren R, Exton-Smith AN. An Investigation of Geriatric Nursing Problems in Hospital. London: Churchill Livingstone; 1962:193-224.

40. Morris JN, Hawes C, Fries BE, Phillips CD, Mor V, Katz S, et al. Designing the national resident assessment instrument for nursing homes. Gerontologist. 1990;30:293-307.

41. Bergstrom N, Braden BJ, Laguzza A, Holman V. The Braden Scale for Predicting Pressure Sore Risk. Nurs Res. 1987;36:205-10.

42. Xakellis GC, Frantz RA, Arteaga M, Nguyen M, Lewis A. A comparison of patient risk for pressure ulcer development with nursing use of preventive interventions. J Am Geriatr Soc. 1992;40:1250-4.

43. Smith DM, Winsemius DK, Besdine RW. Pressure sores in the elderly: can this outcome be improved? J Gen Intern Med. 1991;6:81-93.

44. Specialized Beds Technical Advisory Group. National Specialized Beds Study and Other Support Surface Guidelines. Washington, DC: National Center for Cost Containment, Department of Veterans Affairs; 1992.

45. Holzapfel SK. Support surfaces and their use in the prevention and treatment of pressure ulcers. J ET Nurs. 1993;20:251-60.

46. Kemp MG, Kopanke D, Tordecilla L, Fogg L, Shoot S, Matthieson V, et al. The role of suppport surfaces and patient attributes in preventing pressure ulcers in elderly patients. Res Nurs Health. 1993;16:89-96.

47. Hofman A, Geelkerken RH, Wille J, Hamming JJ, Hermans J, Breslau PJ, et al. Pressure sores and pressure-decreasing mattresses: controlled clinical trial. Lancet. 1994;343:568-71.

48. Hedrick-Thompson J, Halloran T, Strader MK, McSweeney M. Pressure-reduction products: making appropriate choices. J ET Nurs. 1993;20:239-44.

49. DeLateur BJ, Berni R, Hongladarom T, Giaconi R. Wheelchair cushions designed to prevent pressure sores: an evaluation. Arch Phys Med Rehabil. 1976;57:129-35.

50. Garber SL, Krouskop TA, Carter RE. A system for clinically evaluating wheelchair pressure-relief cushions. Am J Occup Ther. 1978;32:565-70.

51. Ferguson-Pell MW. Seat cushion selection. J Rehab Res Dev Clin Suppl. 1990; 2:49-73.

52. Kraft MR, Lawson L, Pohlmann B, Reid-Lokos C, Barder L. A comparison of Epi-Lock and saline dressings in the treatment of pressure ulcers. Decubitus. 1993;6:42-8.

53. Glenchur H, Patel BS, Pathmarajah C. Transient bacteremia associated with debridement of decubitus ulcers. Mil Med. 1981;146:432-3.

54. Varma AO, Bugatch E, German FM. Debridement of dermal ulcers with collagenase. Surg Gynecol Obstet. 1973;136:281-2.

55. Oleske DM, Smith XP, White P, Pottage J, Donovan MI. A randomized clinical trial of two dressing methods for the treatment of low-grade pressure ulcers. J Enterostomal Ther. 1986;13:90-8.

56. Gorse GJ, Messner RL. Improved pressure sore healing with hydrocolloid dressings. Arch Dermatol. 1987;123:766-71.

57. Xakellis GC, Chrischilles EA. Hydrocolloid versus saline-gauze dressings in treating pressure ulcers: a cost-effective analysis. Arch Phys Med Rehabil. 1992;73:463-9.

58. Colwell JC, Foreman MD, Trotter JP. A comparison of the efficacy and cost-effectiveness of two methods of managing pressure ulcers. Decubitus. 1993; 6:28-36.

59. Allman RM, Walker JM, Hart MK, Laprade CA, Noel LB, Smith CR. Air-fluidized beds or conventional therapy for pressure sores. A randomized trial. Ann Intern Med. 1987;107:641-8.

60. Ferrell BA, Osterweil D, Christenson P. A randomized trial of low-air-loss beds for treatment of pressure ulcers. JAMA. 1993;269:494-7.

61. Strauss MJ, Gong J, Gary BD, Kalsbeek WD, Spear S. The cost of home air-fluidized therapy for pressure sores. A randomized controlled trial. J Fam Pract. 1991;33:52-9.

62. Bennett RG, Bellantoni MF, Ouslander JG. Air-fluidized bed treatment of nursing home patients with pressure sores. J Am Geriatr Soc. 1989;37:235-42.

63. Disa JJ, Carlton JM, Goldberg NH. Efficacy of operative cure in pressure sore patients. Plast Reconstr Surg. 1992;89:272-8.

64. Moss RJ, La Puma J. The ethics of pressure sore prevention and treatment in the elderly: a practical approach. J Am Geriatr Soc. 1991;39:905-8.

65. Siegler EL, Lavizzo-Mourey R. Management of stage III pressure ulcers in moderately demented nursing home residents. J Gen Intern Med. 1991; 6:507-13.

66. Pieper B, Adams W, Mikols C, Mance B. Visceral protein nutritional assessment of patients placed on a high or low air-loss bed. J Enterostomal Ther. 1990;17:145-9.

67. Breslow RA, Hallfrisch J, Guy DG, Crawley B, Goldberg AP. The importance of dietary protein in healing pressure ulcers. J Am Geriatr Soc. 1993;41:357-62.

68. Taylor TV, Rimmer S, Day B, Butcher J, Dymock IW. Ascorbic acid supplementation in the treatment of pressure-sores. Lancet. 1974;2:544-6.

69. Wood JM, Evans PE 3d, Schallreuter KU, Jacobson WE, Sufit R, Newman J, et al. A multicenter study on the use of pulsed low-intensity direct current for healing chronic stage II and stage III decubitus ulcers. Arch Dermatol. 1993;129:999-1009.

70. Robson MC, Phillips LG, Lawrence WT, Bishop JB, Youngerman JS, Hayward PG, et al. The safety and effect of topically applied recombinant basic fibroblast growth factor on the healing of chronic pressure sores. Ann Surg. 1992;216:401-8.

71. Mustoe TA, Cutler NR, Allman RM, Goode PS, Deuel TF, Prause JA, et al. A phase II study to evaluate recombinant platelet-derived growth factor-BB in the treatment of stage 3 and 4 pressure ulcers. Arch Surg. 1994;129:213-9.

72. Kertesz D, Chow AW. Infected pressure and diabetic ulcers. Clin Geriatr Med. 1992;8:835-52.

73. Bendy RH, Nuccio PA, Wolfe E, Collins B, Tamburro C, Glass W, et al. Relationship of quantitative wound bacterial counts to healing of decubiti: effect of topical gentamicin. Antimicrob Agents Chemother. 1964;1:147-55.

74. Gomolin IH, Brandt JL. Topical metronidazole therapy for pressure sores of geriatric patients. J Am Geriatr Soc. 1983;31:710-2.

75. Witkowski JA, Parish LC. Topical metronidazole gel. The bacteriology of decubitus ulcers. Int J Dermatol. 1991;30:660-1.

76. Bryan CS, Dew CE, Reynolds KL. Bacteremia associated with decubitus ulcers. Arch Intern Med. 1983;143:2093-5.

77. Rudensky B, Lipschits M, Isaacsohn M, Sonnenblick M. Infected pressure sores: comparison of methods for bacterial identification. South Med J. 1992;85:901-3.

78. Sugarman B, Hawes S, Musher DM, Klima M, Young EJ, Pircher F. Osteomyelitis beneath pressure sores. Arch Intern Med. 1983;143:683-8.

79. Darouiche RO, Landon GC, Klima M, Musher DM, Markowski J. Osteomyelitis associated with pressure sores. Arch Intern Med. 1994;154:753-8.

80. Alterescu V. The financial costs of inpatient pressure ulcers to an acute care facility. Decubitus. 1989;2:14-23.

81. Frantz RA, Gardner S, Harvey P, Specht J. The cost of treating pressure ulcers in a long-term care facility. Decubitus. 1991;4:37-45.

82. Frantz RA. Pressure ulcer costs in long term care. Decubitus. 1989;2:56-7.

83. Ameis A, Chiarcossi A, Jimenez J. Management of pressure sores. Comparative study in medical and surgical patients. Postgrad Med. 1980;67:177-84.

84. Graves EJ. Detailed diagnoses and procedures, National Hospital Discharge Survey, 1988. Vital Health Stat [13]. 1991;107:1-239.

85. Graves EJ. Detailed diagnoses and procedures, National Hospital Discharge Survey, 1989. Vital Health Stat [13]. 1991;108:1-236.

86. Graves EJ. Detailed diagnoses and procedures, National Hospital Discharge Survey, 1990. Vital Health Stat [13]. 1992;113:1-225.

87. Graves EJ. Detailed diagnoses and procedures. National Hospital Discharge Survey, 1991. Vital Health Stat [13] 1994;115:1-290.

88. Powell JW. Increasing acuity of nursing home patients and the prevalence of pressure ulcers: a ten year comparison. Decubitus. 1989;2:56-8.

PART III

Drugs in the Nursing Home

6

Drug Use

Jerry Avorn, MD, and Jerry H. Gurwitz, MD, FACP

With increasing pressure on hospitals to shorten acute-care stays, and the unprecedented aging of the population in industrialized societies, pharmacotherapy for the nursing home patient has become an area of increasing importance. The demographic changes are most pronounced in the age group older than 85 years, which is the fastest-growing segment of the U.S. population; this is also the group with the greatest likelihood of requiring institutional care.

MEDICATION USE IN LONG-TERM CARE

Not surprisingly, nursing home residents receive more medication than noninstitutionalized older persons (1,2). One study of 12 nursing homes in a large U.S. city reported that the 1106 residents studied were prescribed an average of 7.2 medications (3). Another study of more than 800 residents in 12 representative intermediate care facilities in another state indicated that residents were prescribed an average of 8.1 medications (4). The most commonly prescribed medications found in our study are listed in Table 6.1.

Although it has been cause for some concern, this frequent prescribing of medication does not necessarily indicate poor quality of care. The use of numerous medications in the care of a complex, elderly nursing home resident can be appropriate and may be necessary to optimize medical and functional status. Further, determining the magnitude of inappropriate drug use in the nursing home is not a straightforward process. Defining ideal or even acceptable prescribing is limited by controversy and by the absence of adequate data. Therapy that is proper for a middle-aged patient may have greater risks and lower benefits for an institutionalized patient with several impairments.

The challenges of defining criteria for inappropriate medication use in nursing home residents have been underscored in a study that used a national panel of experts in an attempt to reach a consensus on guidelines for medication use in the elderly population (5–7). The panelists agreed about many aspects of medication use, but they could not agree on issues such as the use of antipsychotic medications in nonpsychotic patients, the use of diphenhydramine as a hypnotic agent, and the safety of cimetidine relative to other histamine-2 (H_2)–receptor antagonists. The criteria developed through this consensus were applied to actual patterns of drug use in the nursing home setting. More than 40% of 1106 nursing home residents studied were reported to have at least one "inappropriate" prescription (3) using these conservative criteria. Box 6.1 summarizes the most common types of "problematic" prescribing according to the criteria.

DRUG REGIMEN ACCRETIONS AND DRUG HOLIDAYS

Although it is often an occasion of turmoil and perceived loss for residents and families, admission to

TABLE 6.1. Most commonly prescribed medications for 823 residents of 12 intermediate care facilities in Massachusetts

Medication	Orders per 100 Residents
Gastrointestinal medication	
Laxatives and enemas	179
Acid peptic medication*	36
Other†	41
Analgesic agents	
Acetaminophen	96
Aspirin	26
Opioids	15
Nonsteroidal anti-inflammatory drugs	12
Cardiovascular medication	
Digoxin	27
Loop diuretics	26
Nitrates	23
Thiazide diuretics	15
β-blockers	10
Calcium channel blockers	5
Antiarrhythmic agents	3
Other‡	9
Vitamins and supplements	
Multivitamins	45
Potassium	19
Iron	15
Calcium	4
Psychoactive medication	
Sedatives and hypnotics§	29
Antipsychotics	28
Antidepressants	16
Diphenhydramine	9
Antibiotic and antifungal agents	20
Endocrine and metabolic medication	
Hypoglycemic agents	12
Thyroid replacement drugs	8
Respiratory medication	
Theophylline	7
β-sympathomimetics	6
Neurologic medication	
Antiseizure drugs	8
Antiparkinsonian drugs	5
Anticoagulant and antiplatelet medication	
Dipyridamole	6
Warfarin	4
Ophthalmic medication	
Artificial tears	6
Glaucoma	4
Steroids	4
Urinary medication	1

* Includes antacids, histamine-2 blockers, and sucralfate.
† Includes attapulgite, simethicone, and metoclopramide.
‡ Includes angiotensin-converting enzyme inhibitors and potassium-sparing diuretics.
§ Excluding diphenhydramine.

a nursing home presents an ideal opportunity for comprehensive drug regimen review, an exercise too often neglected in the care of elderly patients in all clinical settings. Over many years and through many care providers, the elderly patient can accumulate a regimen of many drugs; admission to a nursing home provides an opportunity for a fresh look at each one. The need for this review is heightened for residents who enter the nursing home from the hospital, where additional medications may have been added to treat acute problems that may not persist beyond the hospital stay (8). In some patients, routine administration of many medications is continued, even though the indication that initially prompted the use of these drugs is no longer present (or never was). For example, digoxin is one of the drugs most commonly prescribed to nursing home patients (Table 6.1), but considerable controversy surrounds its role in elderly patients with diagnoses of compensated congestive heart failure (9), especially in the setting of preserved systolic ventricular function. Forman and coworkers (10) studied 47 nursing home residents (mean age, 87 years) receiving long-term digoxin therapy. Thirty-five had normal ejection fractions (50% or greater), and 23 of these had normal sinus rhythm. The physicians of 14 of these 23 patients were willing to discontinue digoxin therapy. None of the patients in whom therapy was discontinued had ejection fractions decrease to less than 50%, and none showed signs of clinical deterioration during 2 months of follow-up. Although these were the first such data to come from a long-term-care setting, they replicated findings from studies done in community settings. In contrast, more recent findings suggest that withdrawal of digoxin in patients with impaired systolic function can be detrimental (11).

The stable, supervised environment of the nursing home allows for the slow, cautious withdrawal of medications of uncertain benefit in a given patient. It is possible to watch closely for clinical signs that the drug may indeed be necessary (for example, a slow increase in blood pressure may indicate the need to restore an antihypertensive drug). Although some practitioners advocate keeping a "time-tested" regimen intact even if the validity of its original indications is obscure, we take a different view of the risks and benefits involved. A patient taking a medication without a clear ongoing indication for its use remains at risk for all potential toxicities (particularly at a time of intercurrent

BOX 6.1. Most common types of inappropriate prescribing in 12 nursing homes in California*

Drugs to be avoided
  Long-acting benzodiazepines
  Dipyridamole
  Propoxyphene
  Amitriptyline
  Methyldopa
  Propranolol
  Trimethobenzamide
  Pentazocine
  Chlorpropamide
  Muscle relaxants
  Indomethacin
  Cerebral vasodilators
  Gastrointestinal antispasmodic agents
  Meprobamate
  Reserpine
Excessive duration of treatment
  Histamine-2–receptor antagonists
  Short-acting benzodiazepines
  Oral antibiotics
Excessive drug dosage
  Iron supplements
  Histamine-2–receptor antagonists
  Antipsychotic agents

* Adapted from Beers and colleagues (3).

illness or other metabolic insult) without deriving any benefit.

Aside from a comprehensive annual examination or visit to a geriatric assessment unit, few elderly patients have the opportunity for a thorough reassessment of every medication in their regimen; this reassessment can be done soon after admission to a nursing home. Such assessment must be done more gradually if the patient is still recovering from an acute illness. As many as 50% of residents entering from the community who have been prescribed long-term medications have not been taking them as prescribed (12). Thus, it is all the more important to thoroughly review the drug regimen early in the nursing home stay: Diligent dispensing of every medication the resident is thought to have been taking before admission could result in toxicity in those who had been substantially nonadherent.

In response to concerns about the overuse of medications in long-term-care facilities, some nursing homes have instituted policies of complete cessation of most or all medications on admission, or they implement regularly scheduled "drug holidays," particular intervals in the week or month during which no medications are administered. Although

well intentioned, such simplistic solutions can be counterproductive. Drug regimen review and drug withdrawal should be done systematically and selectively, altering the use of one agent at a time; this will minimize the risk for hard-to-trace withdrawal symptoms or other deterioration. Excessively rapid cessation of some drugs can precipitate withdrawal symptoms ranging from extreme discomfort in the case of benzodiazepines (13,14) to severe cardiovascular compromise and even death in the case of β-blockers (15).

UNIQUE ASPECTS OF THE NURSING HOME AS A SETTING FOR DRUG USE

The use of medication in the nursing home represents a complex blending of issues from several diverse realms of medical practice. At its foundation lie basic concepts from the practice of clinical geriatrics, such as the atypical presentation of disease in the elderly; the propensity of elderly persons to manifest central nervous system dysfunction as a "final common pathway" for various metabolic insults; and the reduced physiologic reserve, or "homeostenosis," that marks the response of the aging organism to stressors of various kinds. Built on this are the pharmacokinetic and pharmacodynamic differences seen with senescence: the reduced renal and hepatic function that occur even in healthy aging persons; the increased proportion of body fat at the expense of skeletal muscle, which together with reduced drug clearance can result in the marked elevation of drug half-lives and serum concentrations; and age-related increases in intrinsic sensitivity to medications such as benzodiazepines and opioids and reduced sensitivity to others, such as ß-adrenergic agonists and antagonists (16).

Layered on top of these general aspects of geriatric pathophysiology and pharmacology are the special circumstances of the long-term-care facility. Drug use in the nursing home occurs in some of the frailest patients in the elderly population in institutions with the potential for 24-hour clinical observation in a supervised setting. Paradoxically, however, the nursing home environment may also include little physician input, particularly in relation to the severity and complexity of the patients cared for in these facilities. Nursing homes are what sociologists refer to as "total institutions," places in which residents live, eat, socialize, and spend their leisure time; they often do not leave its walls. They are complex social institutions in which physicians, nurses, consultant pharmacists, other health professionals, aides, and administrators interact to make decisions about drug prescribing and drug administration.

These interactions often play themselves out in unconventional ways in relation to medication use. The physician writes a prescription, but a nurse (or an aide) in much closer contact with the nursing home resident often spurs the decision to prescribe and guides the physician's prescribing decisions by telephone or in brief visits. Furthermore, although the physician authorizes the prescription of a drug for pro re nata use (such as psychoactive medications, analgesics, and laxatives), it is the nursing staff or their assistants who frequently make the crucial decision about whether the drug will actually be administered and how often, and even in what dose and by what route (17).

This decision-making process is further complicated by the unique role of the pharmacist in nursing homes. Since 1974, the Health Care Financing Administration (18) has required that a consultant pharmacist periodically review the drug regimens of all residents of skilled nursing facilities. Thus, the nursing home is the only component of the health care system in which regular pharmacist involvement in monitoring drug use is required. Although often dramatically beneficial in specific clinical instances, the overall effect of this mandated review has been more modest than originally anticipated (17).

Recently, medication regulation has been extended to apply to prescribing decisions made for individual patients in nursing homes. Federal legislation requiring the regulation of the use of antipsychotic medication in Medicare- and Medicaid-certified nursing homes became law in 1987 as the Nursing Home Reform Amendments of the Omnibus Budget Reconciliation Act (OBRA '87) (19,20). Guidelines to assist regulators in evaluating nursing homes were developed by the Health Care Financing Administration. Intended to limit psychoactive drug use to specific indications, they require explicit documentation in the medical record to justify psychoactive therapy. After public review and comment, guidelines for antipsychotic drug use were implemented in October 1990, and guidelines for anxiolytics and sedatives were implemented in April 1992. For the first time, the federal government issued explicit medical practice criteria defin-

ing the proper use of particular medications in individual clinical situations. This occurred in part because of the widespread perception that only a powerful regulatory approach could control what was seen as the excessive use of psychoactive medications in long-term care facilities. Unfortunately, the implementation of these regulations on a national scale was done without concurrent provision for the evaluation of their effect on patient outcomes; thus, this is one of the largest uncontrolled health care experiments of modern times. Nonetheless, some post hoc evaluations of drug use patterns have been done since implementation, albeit without benefit of before and after comparisons of residents' actual clinical status. The use of antipsychotics in nursing homes was substantially reduced after implementation of the guidelines for use of this class of drugs (21). The effect of the guidelines for anxiolytic and sedative drug use remains to be determined.

Adding still another dimension to drug use in the nursing home is the fiscal situation of the nursing home. Most hospitals in the United States are nonprofit institutions, but most long-term care facilities in the United States are for-profit entities. Both nonprofit and for-profit institutions face reimbursement constraints that influence many aspects of care: Because Medicaid programs are the main payers for about half of the nation's nursing home residents, even nonprofit facilities must confront the limited per diem reimbursement rate provided by these state programs. Although drugs are generally covered separately and in full, limited reimbursement to the institution can constrain the level of staffing in both nonprofit and for-profit homes. Insufficient staffing, in turn, can influence the incentive for the use of psychoactive medications, as well as the capacity for monitoring both the therapeutic and the adverse consequences of drug use.

Thus, as a setting for care, the nursing home lies in a vortex of forces and relations that heavily influence the ways in which medications are used. In addition, nursing home residents are far more likely than noninstitutionalized elderly persons to be chronically ill, to have more than one functional impairment, to lack economic resources and family caregivers, to be older than 85 years of age, and to be burdened by cognitive deficits (22). Taken together, all of these factors make the nursing home one of the most complex and challenging pharmacotherapeutic settings in all of medicine.

THE SPECIAL CASE OF PSYCHOACTIVE DRUGS

Sedation of Residents with Dementia

For decades, the use of psychotropic drugs has remained extensive in nursing homes. Although recent regulatory changes have had a marked effect, numerous studies done through the early 1990s indicated that about half of all nursing home residents were regularly being given one or more psychoactive drugs. Antipsychotic drugs were, until recently, given to about one fourth of all nursing home residents (4). A few studies suggest that antipsychotic drugs may be effective in the treatment of agitation in geriatric patients with dementia (23), but the literature on this topic is both limited and ambiguous. Clear evidence, however, links the use of these drugs with extrapyramidal symptoms, gait instability, falls, and hip fractures (24–26). Benzodiazepines, frequently used for agitation associated with dementia, can also be troublesome; benzodiazepines with long elimination half-lives pose their own risks for falls, fractures (27,28), and other side effects, including daytime somnolence, confusion, and ataxia (29), although not for parkinsonian symptoms.

Cross-national studies indicate that patients with dementia are managed in long-term care facilities in Western Europe and Japan with much less reliance on sedating medications than in the United States; these facilities apparently maintain good control of agitated behavior. A retrospective review of the medical records of 1996 residents of 60 nursing homes in the United States from 1976 through 1985 suggested that half of the recorded uses of neuroleptic therapy would be considered improper under regulations mandated by OBRA '87 (30). Concern has been raised over whether these regulations might result in increases in behavioral problems or agitation in residents and over whether a shift would occur from antipsychotic drugs to potentially hazardous sedating agents that are not regulated. Initial reports indicate that the prescribing of antipsychotic drugs in nursing homes has been substantially reduced coincident with the implementation of the regulations and that the use of other psychotropic drugs (cyclic antidepressants, benzodiazepines, and nonbenzodiazepine sedatives) has not concomitantly increased (21,31).

In a randomized trial, a comprehensive educational outreach program ("academic detailing") was directed at physicians, nurses, and aides to reduce the use of psychoactive drugs in nursing homes. The use of antipsychotic drugs was subsequently discontinued in more residents in nursing homes receiving the intervention (32%) than in those in control homes (14%); these reductions did not adversely affect the overall behavior and level of functioning of the residents (32) or the level of distress among staff (33). In a similar study, designed to train nursing home caregivers in the proper use of psychoactive drugs, Ray and colleagues (34) reported somewhat larger reductions, although their sample of homes was smaller.

Considerably more needs to be learned about the relative clinical efficacy of interpersonal interventions, benzodiazepine therapy, and antipsychotic agents in calming agitated, demented nursing home residents. Some studies have found that reliance on sedative drugs is more common in larger nursing homes, in facilities with lower staff-to-patient ratios, and among physicians with larger nursing home practices (35,36), but these findings have not been consistently replicated. The interplay among economic constraints, staffing patterns, and sedative use is a crucial topic for further investigation.

In deciding whether pharmacologic intervention is required to manage agitated behavior in an elderly nursing home resident, two basic facts should be considered. Unusual behavior in the elderly is not necessarily an indication for drug intervention. Incoherent babbling or constant repetition of inappropriate requests may require increased tolerance from staff members rather than sedation. Other problems, such as wandering, might have environmental solutions—for example, a facility design that enables disoriented patients to move about freely while remaining under staff supervision. If intervention is warranted, the safest therapeutic approach is personal attention and support, which can be highly effective and is often preferable to sedation.

Among antipsychotic drugs used in the nursing home setting (Table 6.2), high-potency drugs such as haloperidol have side-effect profiles that differ from those of agents with lower potency, such as thioridazine. Low-potency antipsychotic medications tend to be strongly sedating, hypotensive, and anticholinergic, but they produce less marked extrapyramidal symptoms. Commonly used doses of high-potency agents produce more prominent extrapyramidal symptoms but are less anticholiner-

TABLE 6.2. Side effects of antipsychotic drugs*

Agent	Potency	Sedation	Hypotension	Extrapyramidal Symptoms	Anticholinergic Symptoms
Chlorpromazine	Low	Marked	Marked	Moderate	Marked
Chlorprothixene	Low	Marked	Marked	Moderate	Marked
Thioridazine	Low	Marked	Marked	Mild/moderate	Moderate
Acetophenazine	Moderate	Moderate	Moderate	Moderate	Moderate
Perphenazine	Moderate	Moderate	Moderate	Moderate	Moderate
Loxapine	Moderate	Moderate	Moderate	Moderate	Moderate
Molindone	Moderate	Moderate	Moderate	Moderate	Moderate
Trifluoperazine	Moderate	Moderate	Moderate	Moderate/marked	Moderate/mild
Thiothixene	Moderate	Moderate	Moderate	Moderate/marked	Moderate/mild
Fluphenazine	High	Mild	Mild	Marked	Mild
Haloperidol	High	Mild	Mild	Marked	Mild

* Reprinted with permission from Lohr and colleagues. Treatment of disordered behavior. In: Salzman C, ed. Clinical Geriatric Psychopharmacology. Second edition. Baltimore: Williams & Wilkins; 1992:79-113.

gic, sedating, and hypotensive. However, two recent studies document that, in moderate to high doses, the "low-potency" antipsychotics are still important causes of extrapyramidal side effects (25,26). New data suggest that at least some of the frequently observed propensity for extrapyramidal side effects associated with haloperidol may be attributable to its use in relatively higher doses compared with other antipsychotic drugs, after correction for potency differences (26).

One particularly important extrapyramidal symptom is akathisia, in which the patient develops an irresistible urge to move about. Patients may repeatedly cross and uncross their legs, stamp their feet, change posture, rock, sway, or pace. These actions may be misinterpreted as signaling a need for a higher, rather than a lower, dose of the offending antipsychotic drug. Tardive dyskinesia is another important consequence of antipsychotic drug use; its frequency is more common in elderly persons, particularly institutionalized elderly persons. It may be irreversible even after cessation of the offending agent (37).

A new antipsychotic agent, respiridone, is gaining increasing popularity for use in elderly persons. Extrapyramidal symptoms may be less common with this agent, but they do occur: Sedation, orthostatic hypotension, and reflex tachycardia are among the reported side effects of this drug.

Use of Hypnotics

Hypnotics are among the drugs most frequently prescribed in long-term-care settings. However, the long-term daily use of any hypnotic agent is associated with tachyphylaxis in most patients after several weeks to months. After this time, the drug primarily prevents withdrawal symptoms if the patient has become habituated to the long-term use of benzodiazepines. Such withdrawal is often misinterpreted as evidence for the ongoing need for hypnotic drugs, when in fact it is continuing evidence of the hazards of the routine use of these drugs. It is preferable to institute a more biologically appropriate approach to sleep hygiene that would include the following elements.

ALLOW APPROPRIATE SLEEP HOURS

The organizational constraints of nursing home life may require that patients be put to bed in the evening to reduce the need for care by the night staff. As a result, a patient may be put to bed at 9:00 p.m. and may need only 6 hours of sleep. If this is the case, the resident will awaken at 3:00 a.m., may be diagnosed as "having insomnia," and may be prescribed a hypnotic drug. It is far more reasonable to allow the patient to remain awake later, as many community-dwelling elderly persons do, and thus to remain asleep until later in the morning.

OMIT COFFEE AFTER 1:00 PM

Caffeine is a stimulant and can have as disproportionally strong an effect on elderly persons as other psychoactive drugs. It makes little sense to offer a resident a stimulant at one point in the evening and a depressant an hour or two later.

PROMOTE EXERCISE AND DISCOURAGE
DAYTIME NAPPING

Normal sleep is unlikely in a resident who remains immobile all day, particularly if daytime sleep comes to replace nighttime sleep. Although plasma benzodiazepine concentration and clinical effect are not always clearly related (38), the problem of daytime somnolence can be exacerbated if a hypnotic with a long elimination half-life is routinely administered (Box 6.2). This drug may remain at therapeutic levels well into the following afternoon, potentially reducing activity, causing lethargy, and inducing daytime somnolence. Unfortunately, the further deterioration of sleep that results may, in turn, provoke additional use of the offending hypnotic at night, creating a vicious cycle.

When pharmacologic intervention is required, the altered pharmacokinetics and pharmacodynamics of the elderly patient suggest that low doses of short-acting agents should be used initially whenever possible. Oxazepam is a benzodiazepine with a satisfactorily short half-life. Triazolam has been advocated as ideal for the elderly because of its ultra-short half-life, but it may cause more cognitive impairment and anterograde amnesia in the elderly than similar doses of other drugs (39). The hypnotic drug flurazepam, like its anxiolytic cousins chlordiazepoxide and diazepam, has a long half-life and should rarely be used in the care of institutionalized elderly persons. No compelling evidence indicates that the clinical outcomes of the newer nonbenzodiazepine hypnotic zolpidem differ from those of older, less costly benzodiazepines. Although diphenhydramine is commonly used as a hypnotic, its strong anticholinergic side effects make it undesirable for use in nursing home residents (40).

Antidepressants

Despite questions about the excessive use of antipsychotic drugs and hypnotic agents in the nursing home setting, concern exists over the possible underuse of another class of medications, antidepressants. Clinical depression is common among nursing home residents, and, in many cases, it goes undiagnosed and untreated (41–43). In a study based on data collected between 1976 and 1983, Heston and colleagues (44) reported that only 10% of 868 nursing home residents with a diagnosis of

BOX 6.2. Elimination half-lives of benzodiazepines

Long elimination half-life
Chlorazepate
Chlordiazepoxide
Clonazepam
Diazepam
Flurazepam
Halazepam
Prazepam
Medium to short elimination half-life
Alprazolam
Lorazepam
Oxazepam
Temazepam
Very short elimination half-life
Triazolam

depression equivalent to DSM-III-R major depression were being treated with antidepressant drugs. Residents more often received antipsychotics or benzodiazepines than antidepressants, but most (52%) were receiving no psychoactive drug therapy. Although awareness of depression in the elderly has increased somewhat, continued vigilance is still needed. Symptoms of depression can be inappropriately dismissed as reasonable reactions to chronic illness or as an understandable response to institutionalization (45,46). This is particularly unfortunate because depression in the elderly often responds well to therapy. In contrast, untreated depression is associated with increased mortality and causes an obvious decrement in quality of life.

Older tertiary amine antidepressants, such as amitriptyline, are generally not recommended for most depressed nursing home residents because of their sedative and highly anticholinergic properties. Secondary amines, such as desipramine or nortriptyline, are preferable because of their lower rate of side effects. Remarkably little evidence exists to guide the use of any of these agents in very elderly patients, and the characteristics of geriatric patients who participate in and complete studies of these agents often cast doubt on the generalizability of research findings (47–49). Few studies have been attempted in institutional settings. Recently, concern has been raised about the possible arrhythmogenic role of tricyclic antidepressants in elderly patients with cardiac ischemia, but little information exists from clinical or epidemiologic studies to guide the clinician in this difficult area (50). The absence of relevant data on efficacy is particularly acute for newer agents, such as fluoxetine and other selective serotonin re-uptake inhibitors; they are often promoted as much better tolerated than tricyclic antidepressants in older patients, despite some reports to the contrary (51,52). Data on their efficacy or side effects in frail, institutionalized, elderly persons are inadequate.

MILD TO MODERATE PAIN

Apart from insomnia and constipation *(see* below), the treatment of mild to moderate pain is one of the most common issues in pharmacotherapy in the long-term care setting. Nonsteroidal anti-inflammatory drugs (NSAIDs) are among the most popular agents for this ubiquitous problem; however, two important lines of research have begun to emerge, suggesting an alternative approach. The first is the increasing body of data documenting the hazards of NSAID therapy in very old persons; these hazards include renal insufficiency, gastrointestinal hemorrhage, and blood pressure elevations. The second is the demonstration that in many residents with degenerative joint disease (probably the most common indication for analgesics in the nursing home), acetaminophen often provides satisfactory pain relief with a much lower risk for side effects than is produced by NSAID therapy (53).

The NSAIDs all inhibit the biosynthesis of prostaglandins, some of which mediate various important protective physiologic effects. Prostaglandins maintain renal blood flow and glomerular filtration in the face of reduced effective or actual circulatory volume (such as that caused by congestive heart failure or volume depletion due to diuretic therapy). Under such conditions, the vasoconstrictive effects on renal blood flow are mitigated by the effects of vasodilatory renal prostaglandins, preserving renal perfusion. When this prostaglandin-mediated compensatory mechanism is suppressed by NSAID therapy, impairment in renal function can result. A prospective study of 114 elderly residents of a large long-term care facility who were newly treated with NSAIDs showed that 13% developed azotemia over a short course of therapy (Figure 6.1) (54). It is of clinical relevance that the factors associated with this adverse effect included higher NSAID doses and concomitant loop diuretic therapy.

Prostaglandins also mediate several effects that protect the gastric and duodenal mucosa. Reduction

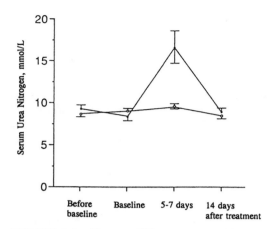

FIGURE 6.1. Mean ± SE serum urea nitrogen levels for patients receiving nonsteroidal anti-inflammatory drugs (NSAIDs) before baseline, at baseline, after 5 to 7 days of therapy, and 14 days after discontinuation of therapy. Of 114 patients studied, 15 (13%) had an increase in serum urea nitrogen levels of more than 50% during NSAID therapy *(closed circles)* (42).

of the biosynthesis of prostaglandins induced by NSAIDs can lead to impaired mucosal defense, and acid and peptic activity can then overpower mucosal protective mechanisms to produce ulcers. Epidemiologic studies investigating the association between NSAIDs and severe upper gastrointestinal bleeding have suggested that older patient age may be associated with a higher risk for gastrointestinal toxicity (55). In addition, prostaglandins play a role in modulating two major determinants of blood pressure vasoconstriction of arteriolar smooth muscle and control of extracellular fluid volume, thus raising concerns about the effect of NSAIDs on blood pressure control (56). A recently published study of drug use in a very large population of Medicaid enrollees indicated that NSAIDs increased the risk for the initiation of antihypertensive therapy in this population (57). To limit the occurrence of side effects, NSAID therapy should be limited to those clinical situations in which it is absolutely required. Inflammation is a rare cause of pain in chronic osteoarthritis, and thus an analgesic with limited or no anti-inflammatory properties (such as acetaminophen or nonacetylated salicylates) may be appropriate to manage this condition in many older patients. A study comparing the analgesic effects of acetaminophen (4 g/d) with those of ibuprofen (1.2 g/d and 2.4 g/d) in patients with osteoarthritis of the knee found no difference in pain relief (53). Although acetaminophen is free of NSAID-related side effects, its dose should not exceed 4 g/d and its toxicity is increased in the presence of hepatic insufficiency, heavy alcohol intake, or fasting (58). When NSAID therapy is required, the lowest feasible dose should be prescribed for the shortest time necessary to achieve the desired therapeutic effect. The best treatment of NSAID-associated nephrotoxicity, gastropathy, or hypertension is discontinuation of NSAID therapy.

BOWEL FUNCTION

Laxatives and stool softeners are among the drugs most commonly prescribed in long-term care facilities (Table 6.1). Yet, despite their widespread use and the firm belief many residents have in their benefits, it is often difficult to assess the efficacy of such therapy in institutional geriatric practice. In long-term care, the evaluation of constipation is often inadequate (59); it is frequently considered the domain of the nursing staff rather than of the physician. As with psychoactive drugs, excessive reliance on pharmacologic solutions sometimes occurs even when these solutions are not necessary and may be counterproductive. For example, the long-term use of stimulant laxatives has been reported to damage the myenteric plexus, leading to the "cathartic syndrome," which is characterized by impairment of motility, dilatation of the colon, worsening constipation, and the diminished effectiveness of laxatives (60).

Although good progress has been made in many institutions, some nursing home diets tend to be low in fiber, adding to the risk for constipation already generated by reduced exercise, modest dehydration, changes in gut motility, and the effects of constipating medications. Although the importance of medications as a cause of constipation is frequently emphasized, few studies have evaluated such associations. Medications with strong anticholinergic properties (such as some antipsychotics and tricyclic antidepressants), narcotics, diuretics, calcium channel blockers, iron supplements, antacids containing aluminum, and calcium supplements require careful evaluation.

In contrast to almost every other area of pharmacotherapy, laxative treatment has had few advances during the past 50 years. Further, few well-controlled, comparative trials of laxatives have been done in the elderly (61); management strategies are necessarily empiric. One randomized, double-blind, crossover trial comparing sorbitol with lactulose in the treatment of elderly men (65 to 86 years of age) with chronic constipation found no clinically significant differences in laxative effect between the two osmotic agents (62). Sorbitol is an effective and much less costly alternative to lactulose for the treatment of constipation in the elderly. Although stool softeners are popular treatments for constipation in some nursing homes, evidence suggests that they often work poorly in this clinical setting (61,63). As with insomnia, the most rational mainstays of therapy are behavioral rather than pharmacologic: a high-fiber diet, adequate hydration, and as much physical activity as possible.

OPPORTUNITIES FOR PREVENTION

Although the treatment of acute problems or the management of chronic disease often absorbs most of the staff's attention, the nursing home can be an ideal setting in which to practice preventive care. Protection against infectious disease is one example. The objectives of the Department of Health and Human Services, as summarized in *Healthy People 2000* (64), include having at least 80% of nursing home residents immunized for pneumococcal pneumonia and influenza. Data on pneumococcal vaccine coverage are not available, although a study describing vaccination levels among elderly Medicare beneficiaries (institutionalized and noninstitutionalized) suggests that the current proportion of nursing home residents immunized for pneumococcal pneumonia is low and is far lower than the proportion immunized for influenza (65).

Along with homeless persons and patients with the acquired immunodeficiency syndrome, nursing home residents have become an important population at risk for the resurgence of tuberculosis (66). Immunosenescence, frailty, and close contact between institutionalized elderly patients can enhance contagion, and the clinical manifestations of tuberculosis in the elderly may be missed by the unwary physician. It has been recommended that new tuberculin converters in the nursing home be treated, because 10% to 20% of them will develop clinical tuberculosis if left untreated, resulting in additional cases and spread of infection (67). Although the risk for isoniazid-induced hepatic toxicity does increase with advancing age, most elderly patients can tolerate isoniazid therapy without difficulty (68).

Hip fractures are a major problem in the nursing home population and are associated with high long-term morbidity and mortality. Until recently, approaches to prevention in the nursing home focused primarily on reducing the risk for falls. Chapuy and colleagues (69) recently published the results of a randomized clinical trial in 3270 ambulatory elderly women living in nursing homes; they compared a regimen of 1.2 g/d elemental calcium and 20 µg (800 U) of vitamin D_3 with placebo. After 18 months, the women receiving treatment had 43% fewer hip fractures and 32% fewer vertebral fractures. As summarized by Heaney (70), persuasive evidence now indicates that some age-related bone loss in elderly women is due to insufficient intake of calcium and vitamin D and that some osteoporotic fractures can be prevented by ensuring higher intake of both nutrients. It is never too late to consider such treatment. The effectiveness of other pharmacologic measures (such as estrogens and thiazide diuretics) in preventing risk for fracture in elderly nursing home residents requires further study (71–76).

Cardiovascular disease presents two contrasting opportunities for the preventive use of drugs in the nursing home. On the positive side, the ubiquity of nursing personnel means that detection of hypertension (including isolated systolic hypertension) should be universal. The nursing home provides an ideal opportunity for the identification, treatment, and surveillance of this important cause of preventable morbidity in the elderly (77). On the negative side, the ready availability of blood chemistry analysis makes it possible to identify hundreds of thousands of cases of mild hypercholesterolemia and to initiate treatment with lipid-lowering drugs. Before seizing this apparent opportunity to practice preventive care, it should be recognized that almost all data on the efficacy of lipid-lowering medications are derived from interventions in middle-aged men. No compelling data exist to justify the widespread treatment of mild to moderate hyperlipidemia in very old persons, particularly for primary prevention (78,79).

REDUCING MEDICATION USE TO CONTAIN COSTS: HISTAMINE-2 BLOCKERS

As pressures mount in all sectors of health care to control expenditures, the cost of drugs used in long-term care has come under increasing scrutiny. This is particularly true of expensive drugs that are often used for extended periods without evidence of clinical benefit; H_2-receptor antagonists are one example.

Since cimetidine was introduced in the 1970s as a breakthrough drug, H_2-receptor antagonists have become the primary mode of treatment of many acid peptic disorders, including peptic ulcer disease and gastroesophageal reflux. However, as with many other categories of medication, overuse of these agents has become apparent in all settings of care (80). A survey of H_2-receptor antagonist use in one large long-term care facility indicated that more than 40% of patients receiving these agents were receiving them for reasons unsubstantiated by the medical literature (81). These reasons included treatment of nonulcer dyspepsia; treatment of and prophylaxis for gastropathy associated with NSAID therapy; gastrointestinal prophylaxis in the setting of steroid therapy; and the ongoing empiric treatment of occult gastrointestinal bleeding of undetermined cause. In an intervention trial done in that facility, educational interventions involving group discussions with the medical staff, printed educational materials, and physician-specific listings of patients receiving H_2-blockers did result in substantial and therapeutically appropriate reductions in the use of these agents. However, inappropriate discontinuation of H_2-blocker therapy was also seen in some patients for whom such therapy was indicated and necessary. Unintended consequences of well-intentioned interventions to improve prescribing always need to be considered when the effects of such interventions are evaluated (82).

When prescribed in proper doses, H_2-blockers have relatively few side effects (83); drug interaction problems can generally be addressed through product selection and adequate monitoring (84). Therefore, the continued use of these agents despite the lack of a substantiated clinical indication or obvious therapeutic benefit is primarily an issue of economics rather than of quality of care. However, no drug is risk-free, and an adverse reaction in a frail elderly patient is particularly unfortunate if no therapeutic benefit was derived from the offending drug in the first place. Additionally, bad therapy can drive out good therapy if reflexive use of an H_2-blocker displaces an adequate work-up of abdominal pain or the finding of fecal occult blood that prompted its use. At a time when such drugs may consume as much as 10% of a state's Medicaid drug expenditure, it is reasonable to ask whether the resources thus used could not be deployed more effectively elsewhere in nursing homes.

MAKING PHARMACOTHERAPEUTIC DECISIONS IN THE NURSING HOME

The following questions should be asked in evaluating any medication use in a nursing home resident:

1. What is the target problem being treated?
2. Is the drug necessary?
3. Are nonpharmacologic therapies available?
4. Is this the lowest practical dose?
5. Could discontinuing therapy with a medicine help reduce symptoms?
6. Does this drug have adverse effects that are more likely to occur in an older patient?
7. Is this the most cost-effective choice?
8. By what criteria, and at what time, will the effects of therapy be assessed?

CONCLUSIONS AND RECOMMENDATIONS FOR RESEARCH

Pharmacotherapy in the nursing home represents a particular challenge for the physician and for all who care for the institutionalized patient, combining as it does all of the complexities of geriatric pharmacology with the unique features of the institutional setting. Although improvements in quality of care could be achieved by the application of currently established principles of geriatric pharmacology, enormous gaps still exist in the knowledge base necessary to guide this aspect of geriatric practice. Prerelease clinical trials of many agents underrepresent the elderly populations who eventually receive them; this problem is even more intense in the assessment of the risks and benefits of drugs in complex, frail, older patients typical of the nursing home population (85). The problem is pervasive in geriatric pharmacology, but some aspects of it are particularly urgent in relation to nursing home care.

First, despite the large volume of drugs dispensed for managing agitated behavior in nursing home patients with dementing illness, surprisingly little is known about the relative efficacy and risks of alternative approaches to this problem. Researchers in this area should emphasize nonpharmacologic interventions as well as the examination of newer pharmacologic therapies.

Second, little is known about the best ways to treat depression in very old persons; this is a problem of particular importance in long-term care. Parallel comparisons of several kinds of therapeutic approaches, including interpersonal approaches, pharmacologic approaches, or a combination of these, need to be made in depressed, elderly nursing home residents. Within pharmacology, more needs to be learned about the relative benefits and risks of tricyclic agents, monoamine oxidase inhibitors, and selective serotonin re-uptake inhibitor drugs in elderly depressed nursing home residents.

Third, given the proliferation of federal regulations governing drug use in the long-term setting, research on the optimal mix of regulation, credentialing, and education is needed to improve the outcomes of drug therapy in nursing home residents. It is particularly important to document the clinical consequences of changes in prescribing rather than simply considering the end point of an intervention to be the changes themselves.

Fourth, further attention should be directed to the potential underuse of beneficial drug therapies, including antidepressant, antihypertensive, and antithrombotic agents, vaccines, and opioid analgesics in patients with metastatic cancer.

Fifth, practical guidelines for the safe discontinuation of unneeded chronic therapy in the nursing home setting, including therapy with antihypertensives, digoxin, psychoactive drugs, and laxatives, should be developed, tested, and disseminated.

Sixth, more institutionalized elderly persons need to be enrolled in clinical trials of new drug therapies that will be widely used in this population.

Seventh, systematic postmarketing surveillance studies should be done for currently used drugs to better define their risks and benefits in this unique population. Despite important methodologic hurdles, Medicaid claims data are well suited for such pharmacoepidemiologic research because of their detailed depiction of drug use in nursing home care.

Eighth, cost-effective drug choices should be defined for the nursing home setting to specifically address the special patterns of illnesses found there, the unique nature of reimbursement (usually capitated), and the mix of health care professionals available.

Ninth, as prescribing authority is given to nurse practitioners and physicians' assistants caring for institutionalized elderly persons in several states, it is crucial to monitor the effect of such policy changes in prescribing practices and to evaluate the best means of improving decisions about drug use in this setting by both traditional and new prescribers.

In the past, being admitted to a nursing home was often referred to pejoratively as "being put in an institution." Today, a greater understanding of geriatric pharmacology and a move to acknowledge long-term care as a vital and increasingly important component of the health care system make it possible to take advantage of the institutional setting to enhance the way medications are used within it.

Acknowledgments: The authors thank Mark Monane, MD, MS, for providing data used in Table 6.1 and Ms. Rita Bloom for assistance in the manuscript preparation.

Grant Support: In part by a grant from the Medications and Aging Program of the John A. Hartford Foundation of New York. Dr. Gurwitz is the recipient of a Clinical Investigator Award (K08 AG00510) from the National Institute on Aging, Bethesda, Maryland.

REFERENCES

1. Ostrom JR, Hammarlund ER, Christensen DB, Plein JB, Kethley AJ. Medication usage in an elderly population. Med Care. 1985;23:157-64.
2. Chrischilles EA, Foley DJ, Wallace RB, Lemke JH, Semla TP, Hanlon JT, et al. Use of medications by persons 65 and over: data from the established populations for epidemiologic studies of the elderly. J Gerontol. 1992;47:M137-44.
3. Beers MH, Ouslander JG, Fingold SF, Morgenstern H, Reuben DB, Rogers W, et al. Inappropriate medication prescribing in skilled-nursing facilities. Ann Intern Med. 1992;117:684-9.
4. Beers M, Avorn J, Soumerai SB, Everitt DE, Sherman DS, Salem S. Psychoactive medication use in intermediate-care facility residents. JAMA. 1988; 260:3016-20.
5. Beers MH, Ouslander JG, Rollingher I, Reuben DB, Brooks J, Beck JC. Explicit criteria for determining inappropriate medication use in nursing home residents. Arch Intern Med. 1991;151:1825-32.
6. Willcox SM, Himmelstein DU, Woolhandler S. Inappropriate drug prescribing for the community-dwelling elderly. JAMA. 1994;272:292-6.
7. Gurwitz JH. Suboptimal medication use in the elderly. The tip of the iceberg [Editorial]. JAMA. 1994; 272:316-7.
8. Beers MH, Dang J, Hasegawa J, Tamai IY. Influence of hospitalization on drug therapy in the elderly. J Am Geriatr Soc. 1989;37:679-83.
9. Yusuf S, Garg R, Held P, Gorlin R. Need for a large randomized trial to evaluate the effects of digitalis on morbidity and mortality in congestive heart failure. Am J Cardiol. 1992;69:64G-70G.
10. Forman DE, Coletta D, Kenny D, Kosowsky BD, Stoukides J, Rohrer M, et al. Clinical issues related to discontinuing digoxin therapy in elderly nursing home patients. Arch Intern Med. 1991;151:2194-8.
11. Packer M, Gheorghiade M, Young JB, Costantini PJ, Adams KF, Cody RJ, et al. Withdrawal of digoxin from patients with chronic heart failure treated with angiotensin-converting-enzyme inhibitors. RADIANCE Study. N Engl J Med. 1993;329:1-7.
12. Sackett DL, Snow JC. The magnitude of compliance and noncompliance. In: Haynes RB, Taylor DW, Sackett DL, eds. Compliance in Health Care. Baltimore: Johns Hopkins Univ Pr; 1979.
13. Greenblatt DJ, Harmatz JS, Zinny MA, Shader RI. Effect of gradual withdrawal on the rebound sleep disorder after discontinuation of triazolam. N Engl J Med. 1987;317:722-8.
14. Busto U, Sellers EM, Naranjo CA, Cappell H, Sanchez-Craig M, Sykora K, et al. Withdrawal reaction after long-term therapeutic use of benzodiazepines. N Engl J Med. 1986;315:854-9.
15. Psaty BM, Koepsell TD, Wagner EH, LoGerfo JP, Inui TS. The relative risk of incident coronary heart disease associated with recently stopping the use of beta-blockers. JAMA. 1990;263:1653-7.
16. Gurwitz JH, Avorn J. The ambiguous relation between aging and adverse drug reactions. Ann Intern Med. 1991;114:956-66.
17. Gurwitz JH, Soumerai SB, Avorn J. Improving medication prescribing and utilization in the nursing home. J Am Geriatr Soc. 1990;38:542-52.
18. Conditions of participation pharmaceutical services. Federal Register. 1974;39:12-7.
19. Winograd CH, Pawlson LG. OBRA 87 a commentary. J Am Geriatr Soc. 1991;39:724-6.
20. Elon R, Pawlson LG. The impact of OBRA on medical practice within nursing facilities. J Am Geriatr Soc. 1992;40:958-63.
21. Shorr RI, Fought RL, Ray WA. Changes in antipsychotic drug use in nursing homes during implementation of OBRA-87 regulations. JAMA. 1994;271: 358-62.
22. Hing E, Bloom B. Long-term care for the functionally dependent elderly. Vital Health Stat. 1990;13:1-50.
23. Schneider LS, Pollock VE, Lyness SA. A meta-analysis of controlled trials of neuroleptic treatment in dementia. J Am Geriatr Soc. 1990;38:553-63.
24. Ray WA, Griffin MR, Schaffner W, Baugh DK, Melton LJ 3d. Psychotropic drug use and the risk of hip fracture. N Engl J Med. 1987;316:363-9.
25. Avorn J, Monane M, Everitt DE, Beers MH, Fields D. Clinical assessment of extrapyramidal signs in nursing home patients given antipsychotic medication. Arch Intern Med. 1994;154:1113-7.
26. Avorn J, Bohn RL, Mogun H, Gurwitz JH, Monane M, Everitt DE, et al. Neuroleptic drug exposure and treatment of parkinsonism in the elderly: a case-

control study. Am J Med. 1995;99:48-54.

27. Ray WA, Griffin MR, Downey W. Benzodiazepines of long and short elimination half-life and the risk of hip fracture. JAMA. 1989;262:3303-7.

28. Cummings SR, Nevitt MC, Browner WS, Stone K, Fox KM, Ensrud KE, et al. Risk factors for hip fracture in white women. Study of Osteoporotic Fractures Research Group. N Engl J Med. 1995;332: 767-73.

29. Greenblatt DJ, Allen MD, Shader RI. Toxicity of high-dose flurazepam in the elderly. Clin Pharmacol Ther. 1977;21:355-61.

30. Garrard J, Makris L, Dunham T, Heston LL, Cooper S, Ratner ER, et al. Evaluation of neuroleptic drug use by nursing home elderly under proposed Medicare and Medicaid regulations. JAMA. 1991; 265:463-7.

31. Rovner BW, Edelman BA, Cox MP, Shmuely Y. The impact of antipsychotic drug regulations on psychotropic prescribing practices in nursing homes. Am J Psychiatry. 1992;149:1390-2.

32. Avorn J, Soumerai SB, Everitt DE, Ross-Degnan D, Beers MH, Sherman D, et al. A randomized trial of a program to reduce the use of psychoactive drugs in nursing homes. N Engl J Med. 1992;327:168-73.

33. Everitt DE, Fields DR, Soumerai SS, Avorn J. Resident behavior and staff distress in the nursing home. J Am Geriatr Soc. 1991;39:792-8.

34. Ray WA, Taylor JA, Meador KG, Lichtenstein MJ, Griffin MR, Fought R, et al. Reducing antipsychotic drug use in nursing homes. A controlled trial of provider education. Arch Intern Med. 1993;153: 713-21.

35. Ray WA, Federspiel CF, Schaffner W. A study of antipsychotic drug use in nursing homes: epidemiologic evidence suggesting misuse. Am J Public Health. 1980;70:485-91.

36. Svarstad BL, Mount JK. Nursing home resources and tranquilizer use among the institutionalized elderly. J Am Geriatr Soc. 1991;39:869-75.

37. Lohr JB, Jeste DV, Harris MJ, Salzman C. Treatment of disordered behavior. In: Salzman C, ed. Clinical Geriatric Psychopharmacology. Second edition. Baltimore: Williams & Wilkins; 1992:79-113.

38. Greenblatt DJ. Benzodiazepine hypnotics: sorting the pharmacokinetic facts. J Clin Psychiatry. 1991; 52(Suppl):4-10.

39. Greenblatt DJ, Harmatz JS, Shapiro L, Engelhardt N, Gouthro TA, Shader RI. Sensitivity to triazolam in the elderly. N Engl J Med. 1991;324:1691-8.

40. Monane M, Avorn J, Beers MH, Everitt DE. Anticholinergic drug use and bowel function in nursing home patients. Arch Intern Med. 1993;153:633-8.

41. Parmelee PA, Katz IR, Lawton MP. Depression among institutionalized aged: assessment and prevalence estimation. J Gerontol. 1989;44:M22-9.

42. Parmelee PA, Katz IR, Lawton MP. Incidence of depression in long-term care settings. J Gerontol. 1992;47:M189-96.

43. Rovner BW, German PS, Brant LJ, Clark R, Burton L, Folstein MF. Depression and mortality in nursing homes. JAMA. 1991;265:993-6.

44. Heston LL, Garrard J, Makris L, Kane RL, Cooper S, Dunham T, et al. Inadequate treatment of depressed nursing home elderly. J Am Geriatr Soc. 1992;40:1117-22.

45. Psychotherapeutic medications in the nursing home. Board of Directors of the American Association for Geriatric Psychiatry, Clinical Practice Committee of the American Geriatrics Society, and Committee on Long-Term Care and Treatment for the Elderly, American Psychiatric Association. J Am Geriatr Soc. 1992;40:946-9.

46. Tallis R. How long should elderly patients take antidepressants? Lancet. 1993;341:1444-5.

47. Koenig HG, Goli V, Shelp F, Kudler HS, Cohen HJ, Meador KG, et al. Antidepressant use in elderly medical inpatients: lessons from an attempted clinical trial. J Gen Intern Med. 1989;4:498-505.

48. Gerson SC, Plotkin DA, Jarvik LF. Antidepressant drug studies, 1964 to 1986: empirical evidence for aging patients. J Clin Psychopharmacol. 1988;8:311-22.

49. How long should elderly take antidepressants? A double-blind placebo-controlled study of continuation/prophylaxis therapy with dothiepin. Old Age Depression Interest Group. Br J Psychiatry. 1993;162:175-82.

50. Glassman AH, Roose SP, Bigger JT Jr. The safety of tricyclic antidepressants in cardiac patients. Risk-benefit reconsidered. JAMA. 1993;269:2673-5.

51. Brymer C, Winograd CH. Fluoxetine in elderly patients: is there cause for concern? J Am Geriatr Soc. 1992;40:902-5.

52. Song F, Freemantle N, Sheldon TA, House A, Watson P, Long A, et al. Selective serotonin reuptake inhibitors: meta-analysis of efficacy and acceptability. BMJ. 1993;306:683-7.

53. Bradley JD, Brandt KD, Katz BP, Kalasinski LA, Ryan SI. Comparison of an antiinflammatory dose of ibuprofen, an analgesic dose of ibuprofen, and acetaminophen in the treatment of patients with osteoarthritis of the knee. N Engl J Med. 1991; 325:87-91.

54. Gurwitz JH, Avorn J, Ross-Degnan D, Lipsitz LA. Nonsteroidal anti-inflammatory drug-associated azotemia in the very old. JAMA. 1990;264:471-5.

55. Bollini P, Rodriguez LA, Perez Gutthann SP, Walker AM. The impact of research quality and study design on epidemiologic estimates of the effect of nonsteroidal anti-inflammatory drugs on upper gastrointestinal tract disease. Arch Intern Med. 1992;152:1289-95.

56. Pope JE, Anderson JJ, Felson DT. A meta-analysis of the effects of nonsteroidal anti-inflammatory drugs on blood pressure. Arch Intern Med. 1993;153:477-84.

57. Gurwitz JH, Avorn J, Bohn RL, Glynn RJ, Monane M, Mogun H. Initiation of antihypertensive treatment during nonsteroidal anti-inflammatory drug therapy. JAMA. 1994;272:781-6.

58. Whitcomb DC, Block GD. Association of acetaminophen hepatotoxicity with fasting and ethanol

use. JAMA. 1994;272:1845-50.

59. Harari D, Gurwitz JH, Avorn J, Choodnovskiy I, Minaker KL. Constipation: assessment and management in an institutionalized elderly population. J Am Geriatr Soc. 1994;42:947-52.

60. Smith B. Effect of irritant purgatives on myenteric plexus in man and the mouse. Gut. 1968;9:139-43.

61. Harari D, Gurwitz JH, Minaker KL. Constipation in the elderly. J Am Geriatr Soc. 1993;41:1130-40.

62. Lederle FA, Busch DL, Mattox KM, West MJ, Aske DM. Cost-effective treatment of constipation in the elderly: a randomized double-blind comparison of sorbitol and lactulose. Am J Med. 1990;89:597-601.

63. Castle SC, Cantrell M, Israel DS, Samuelson MJ. Constipation prevention: empiric use of stool softeners questioned. Geriatrics. 1991;46:84-6.

64. United States Public Health Service. Healthy People 2000: National Health Promotion and Disease Prevention Objectives. Washington, DC: U.S. Department of Health and Human Services, Public Health Service; 1991: DHHS Publication (PHS) 91-50212.

65. McBean AM, Babish JD, Prihoda R. The utilization of pneumococcal vaccine among elderly Medicare beneficiaries, 1985 through 1988. Arch Intern Med. 1991;151:2009-16.

66. Stead WW, Lofgren JP, Warren E, Thomas C. Tuberculosis as an endemic and nosocomial infection among the elderly in nursing homes. N Engl J Med. 1985;312:1483-7.

67. Stead WW, Dutt AK. Tuberculosis: a special problem in the elderly. In: Hazzard WR, Andres R, Bierman EL, Blass JP, Ettinger WH, Halter JB, eds. Principles of Geriatric Medicine and Gerontology. Third edition. New York: McGraw-Hill; 1994:575-82.

68. Stead WW, To T, Harrison RW, Abraham JH 3d. Benefit-risk considerations in preventive treatment for tuberculosis in elderly persons. Ann Intern Med. 1987;107:843-5.

69. Chapuy MC, Arlot ME, Duboeuf F, Brun J, Crouzet B, Arnaud S, et al. Vitamin D_3 and calcium to prevent hip fractures in the elderly women. N Engl J Med. 1992;327:1637-42.

70. Heaney RP. Thinking straight about calcium [Editorial]. N Engl J Med. 1993;328:503-5.

71. Ray WA, Griffin MR, Downey W, Melton LG 3d. Long-term use of thiazide diuretics and risk of hip fracture. Lancet. 1989;1:687-90.

72. LaCroix AZ, Wienpahl J, White LR, Wallace RB, Scherr PA, George LK, et al. Thiazide diuretic agents and the incidence of hip fracture. N Engl J Med. 1990;322:286-90.

73. Heidrich FE, Stergachis A, Gross KM. Diuretic drug use and the risk for hip fracture. Ann Intern Med. 1991;115:1-6.

74. Ray WA. Thiazide diuretics and osteoporosis: time for a clinical trial? [Editorial] Ann Intern Med. 1991;115:64-5.

75. Felson DT, Zhang Y, Hannan MT, Kiel DP, Wilson PW, Anderson JJ. The effect of postmenopausal estrogen therapy on bone density in elderly women. N Engl J Med. 1993;329:1141-6.

76. Ettinger B, Grady D. The waning effect of postmenopausal estrogen therapy on osteoporosis [Editorial]. N Engl J Med. 1993:329:1192-3.

77. Prevention of stroke by antihypertensive drug treatment in older persons with isolated systolic hypertension. Final results of the Systolic Hypertension in the Elderly Program (SHEP). SHEP Cooperative Research Group. JAMA. 1991;265:3255-69.

78. Krumholz HM, Seeman TE, Merrill SS, Mendes de Leon CF, Vaccarino V, Silverman DI, et al. Lack of association between cholesterol and coronary heart disease mortality and morbidity and all-cause mortality in persons older than 70 years. JAMA. 1994; 272:1335-40.

79. Hulley SB, Newman TB. Cholesterol in the elderly. Is it important? [Editorial]. JAMA. 1994;272:1372-4.

80. Sherman DS, Avorn J, Campion EW. Cimetidine use in nursing homes: prolonged therapy and excessive doses. J Am Geriatr Soc. 1987;35:1023-7.

81. Gurwitz JH, Noonan JP, Soumerai SB. Reducing the use of H_2-receptor antagonists in the long-term-care setting. J Am Geriatr Soc. 1992;40:359-64.

82. Katz J. The use of H_2-receptor antagonists in the nursing home [Editorial]. J Am Geriatr Soc. 1992;40:425-6.

83. Richter JM, Colditz GA, Huse DM, Delea TE, Oster G. Cimetidine and adverse reactions: a meta-analysis of randomized clinical trials of short-term therapy. Am J Med. 1989;87:278-84.

84. Feldman M, Burton ME. Histamine$_2$-receptor-antagonists. Standard therapy for acid-peptic diseases. 1. N Engl J Med. 1990;323:1672-80.

85. Avorn J. Reporting drug side effects: signals and noise [Editorial]. JAMA. 1990;263:1823.

7

Pain Evaluation and Management

Bruce A. Ferrell, MD, FACP

In November 1990, a trial was held in North Carolina. After 3.5 days of testimony, a jury took less than an hour to find the owner and operator of a nursing home negligent in failing to give a patient adequate pain medication (1). The patient had been admitted to the nursing home with cancer of the prostate metastatic to the femur and spine and with a prognosis of less than 6 months to live. Although the attending physician had ordered morphine elixir to be given every 3 hours as needed, a nurse had assessed the patient as "addicted to morphine." On this basis, and without advice or orders from the physician, the administration of morphine was reduced, delayed, and withheld altogether; a minor tranquilizer was occasionally substituted. The lawsuit focused on the responsibilities of health care providers to ensure the proper administration of appropriate doses of pain medications. The patient's family was able to prove that the failure of health care providers to meet this responsibility had caused the patient physical pain and suffering as well as mental anguish. The jury awarded the estate $15 million ($7.5 million in compensatory and $7.5 million in punitive damages [2]). Later, the jury verdict was resolved by settlement for an undisclosed amount. In the summary statement approving the settlement, the judge emphasized the serious legal consequences health care providers face if they overlook or negligently underuse appropriate pain medication. This event suggests that a standard of practice is emerging that requires

more diligent attention to pain management in the nursing home setting.

Many nursing home residents endure prolonged efforts at disease modification, but supportive, symptomatic care is not approached aggressively enough. Residents of nursing homes often believe that pain is to be expected with aging and that complaining may negatively affect their care (3). Even when pain is identified, it is often not optimally managed (3,4).

Effective pain management has important implications for improving functional status, quality of life, and quality of care in nursing homes. Comfort and maximum independence are the most important goals for most nursing home residents (5). Pain management has become more successful in younger patients (6) and in patients with cancer (7), and it can also be improved in nursing home residents (8).

It has been suggested that age-related changes in pain sensation occur within the complex processing of nociperception by the central nervous system and in psychological responses to painful stimuli (9–12). Elderly persons are known to present with painless myocardial infarctions (13,14) and intra-abdominal catastrophes (15,16). Whether these clinical events result from altered pain reporting or from age-related changes in pain receptors, nerve transmission, or central nervous system processing remains to be seen. Studies using various methods to experimentally induce pain in volunteers have shown mixed results (8,11,17). More-over, the clinical relevance of these studies is questionable because experimentally induced pain may not be analogous to pain associated with disease. In the final analysis, the widespread belief of many clinicians that aging itself decreases pain sensitivity or increases pain tolerance lacks scientific support (6).

Finally, the Agency for Health Care Policy and Research (6,18) has stated that frail elderly persons, especially those in nursing homes, have special needs for acute and postoperative pain management as well as for pain management in chronic cancer. The Agency's guidelines have highlighted the fact that most pain research has systematically excluded elderly persons and that relatively little attention has been paid to pain management in geriatric medical and nursing textbooks and medical and nursing school curricula. Given the growing number of elderly persons requiring nursing home care, more research is clearly needed (6–18).

EPIDEMIOLOGY

In several selected nursing home populations, the overall prevalence of pain has been reported to be as high as 45% to 80% (2–4,19,20). Most pain in nursing home residents is related to arthritis and musculoskeletal problems, including degenerative arthritis, lower-back disorders, and crystal-induced arthropathies (3,19–21). The neuropathic pain syndromes, including diabetic neuropathy and herpes zoster, are also common (3). Cancer may be less common, but it is a source of severe pain in this setting (3,19). Other common pain problems include leg cramps, headaches, and claudication (3).

Complications of unrelieved pain are also widespread in the nursing home resident. Depression, decreased socialization, sleep disturbance, impaired ambulation, and increased health care use and costs have all been associated with the presence of pain in elderly patients and patients in nursing homes (3,22,23). Deconditioning, gait disturbances, falls, slow rehabilitation, polypharmacy, cognitive dysfunction, and malnutrition are among the many geriatric conditions potentially worsened by the presence of pain (8). These facts highlight the need to recognize pain as a complication with substantial potential to disrupt treatment goals and overall quality of life for nursing home residents.

ASSESSMENT OF PAIN

Typical nursing home residents present many challenges to an adequate assessment of pain. Multiple concurrent illnesses, under-reporting of symptoms, and a high prevalence of cognitive impairment make pain evaluation much more difficult in this compared with other adult populations (24). With no objective biological markers for pain, physicians must rely on patients' self-reports. Accurate pain assessment begins when the physician believes patients and takes their complaints of pain seriously.

Some elderly patients do not complain, despite severe pain that affects their mood and functional status. They see others around them that are worse off than themselves, and they expect pain to be associated with aging (3). They may fear the meaning of pain. For example, among patients with cancer, pain is a metaphor for advancing disease and approaching death (25). Elderly patients may also think that pain cannot be relieved. Nursing home residents often try to avoid being labeled a "complainer" because of the negative effects that this might have on their overall care (3). In this setting, functional decline, mood disturbances, and changes in behavior may be important in the evaluation of pain. The importance of nursing staff and family caregivers as sources of information about elderly patients cannot be overemphasized.

It has been estimated that more than 50% of nursing home residents have substantial cognitive impairment or dementia (19,26). Pain-assessment instruments such as visual-analog, word-descriptor, and numerical scales have been only partially validated in elderly populations (19,27). A high prevalence of visual, hearing, motor, and cognitive impairments may impede the direct adaptation of many of these instruments in nursing home populations. Behavioral scales based on facial grimace and posturing have been investigated in infants in postoperative recovery rooms (28), but they have not been well established for clinical use in patients with Alzheimer disease or other dementias common in the nursing home. Recently, Hurley and colleagues (29) presented a new multidimensional discomfort scale for use in noncommunicative patients with Alzheimer disease. Although this scale may eventually prove to be useful, it requires substantial training to administer.

Despite the difficulties involved in quantifying pain in patients with delirium or dementia, Parmelee and coworkers (30), in a study of more than 750 nursing home residents, found no evidence that cognitive impairment "masked" pain complaints. Data indicated that although cognitively impaired patients tended to under-report pain, the self-reports of such patients were no less valid than those of cognitively intact patients (30). We recently reported our experience with five unidimensional pain-intensity scales that had previously been established for younger patients (19). These included a visual-analog scale, three word-descriptor scales, and a graphic pictorial scale. Our results suggested that only one third of the patients who had pain could complete all of the scales but that 83% could complete at least one scale. These observations indicate that pain reports, even those of persons with moderate to severe cognitive impairment, are usually valid and reliable. Patients can report pain using existing scales that are tailored to individual patients' disabilities and preferences when questions are framed at the moment (for example, How much pain are you having right now?). On the other hand, whether these patients can accurately recall, integrate, and report pain over time (for example, in answers to questions such as, How much pain have you had over the last week?) has not been fully evaluated and needs further study.

Many nursing home residents with chronic pain will have substantial anxiety or depressive symptoms at some time and may benefit from psychological or psychiatric intervention (22). However, care must be taken to avoid attributing pain entirely to depression or psychogenic causes. Psychogenic pain (pain for which no cause other than a psychological origin can be identified) is unusual in this setting (3,19,22).

Nursing home residents often have multiple potential sources of pain (3,19,22), and care must be taken to avoid attributing acute pain to preexisting illness. Exacerbating this problem is the fact that chronic pain is usually not constant; both the character and the intensity of chronic pain fluctuate with time. Frail nursing home patients are particularly prone to falls and occult traumas that can be easily overlooked. Acute gout and calcium pyrophosphate can be mistaken for osteoarthritis (21). Therefore, new pain complaints or changes in the character of old pain complaints require careful evaluation in this population.

Physical examination in the evaluation of nursing home residents with pain should concentrate on the musculoskeletal and nervous systems because diagnoses in these systems are so common. It is important to palpate for trigger points and inflammation. Trigger points resulting from tendonitis, muscle strain, or nerve irritation may benefit from local injections or specific physical therapy. Maneuvers that reproduce the pain, such as straight-leg raising and joint motion, are often useful in both diagnosis and functional assessment. Neurologic examination should include attention to signs of autonomic, sensory, and motor deficits suggestive of neuropathic conditions and nerve injuries that may require specific treatments (24).

The evaluation of functional status is important as an outcome measure for pain management so that mobility and independence are maximized. Functional assessment may include information from the history and physical examination as well as the use of several available functional-assessment scales. Assessment of activities of daily living used in routine geriatric evaluation may be useful (31). For ambulatory patients, advanced activities of daily living and "elective" activities, such as ambulation, psychosocial function, and quality of life, may correlate clinically with the presence and severity of pain (8).

When risky or highly technical procedures are required to evaluate and treat severe pain problems, brief hospitalizations may be appropriate, because some nursing homes are not equipped to manage technical procedures or their acute complications (32). Most nursing homes do not have on-site laboratories, diagnostic facilities, or pharmacies; this frequently tempts physicians to send patients with acute distress to emergency rooms or distant facilities. It should be remembered that transportation to other facilities often results in missed meals and medications, making the trips physically exhausting, emotionally disruptive, and fraught with the potential for iatrogenic illness for most nursing home residents.

PAIN MANAGEMENT

Physicians have paid little attention to pain management in the nursing home; this is exemplified by the dearth of data-based information on this topic in medical textbooks (8). Fewer than 1% of the more than 4000 papers published on pain each year focus on pain in elderly persons (12), and almost no English-language studies describe the effectiveness of available pain-management strategies in the nursing home population. Pharmacologic pain research has largely been limited to single-dose studies or trials in young or middle-aged adults. Most reports from rehabilitation programs or specialized pain centers are flawed by biased referral sources for elderly patients that include only patients with easy access to transportation and other support (6,33,34).

Most pain problems encountered in the nursing home can be managed with the careful use of medications and effective nonpharmacologic pain-management strategies. A combination of pharmacologic and nonpharmacologic techniques results in more effective pain control and less reliance on medications that have major side effects in elderly persons (35). Nursing home residents may benefit most from physicians, nurses, and restorative care personnel who use an interdisciplinary approach to these complex problems.

Prescribing Analgesic Drugs

The analgesic drugs of choice for nursing home residents are those with the lowest side-effect profiles. Adverse effects of drugs are more common in elderly persons and nursing home residents, probably because these patients often have multiple medical problems and require multiple medications (36). Therefore, several things should be considered when prescribing analgesic drugs for nursing home residents.

Acetaminophen is the analgesic most often prescribed for elderly nursing home patients (3). Although it is safe in most cases, a recent case control report suggested that this drug causes a cumulative dose-dependent increase in the risk for end-stage renal disease (37). The investigators reported that, when persons who received less than 1000 acetaminophen pills in a lifetime were used as a reference, the odds ratio for developing end-stage renal disease was 2.0 for those who received 1000 to 4999 pills in a lifetime and 2.4 for those who received 5000 or more pills in a lifetime. Although this study can be criticized for its case-control design and for the investigators' reliance on self-reported past medication use, the risk for end-stage renal disease among long-term users of acetaminophen deserves consideration. Alternatives to acetaminophen (such as salicylates and pyrazolones) may induce less end-stage renal disease, but their own side-effect profiles for gastrointestinal

bleeding, platelet dysfunction, and other abnormalities must be considered.

Nonsteroidal anti-inflammatory drugs often work well for nursing home residents, whether given alone or in combination with opioid analgesics for metastatic bone pain and inflammatory conditions. However, these drugs have been associated with various adverse effects, including peptic ulcer disease, renal insufficiency, and bleeding diathesis (37–39), that may be more common in typical nursing home patients. Among frail elderly persons, these drugs have occasionally been reported to cause constipation, cognitive impairment, and headaches (38).

A recent review (40) has pointed out that older persons have generally been omitted from clinical trials of nonsteroidal anti-inflammatory drugs. Between 1987 and 1990, 83 randomized controlled trials including more than 9600 participants were found to have no patients more than 85 years of age. Only 2.3% of participants were more than 65 years of age (39). This is disturbing in light of the particularly high incidence of peptic ulcer disease and upper gastrointestinal bleeding in older persons. Griffin and colleagues (41) estimated that the relative risk for peptic ulcer disease among elderly persons who used nonsteroidal anti-inflammatory drugs other than aspirin was 4.1 (95% CI, 3.5 to 4.7) compared with persons who did not use them. These investigators showed that the relative risk increased with dose from 2.8 for the lowest dose to 8.0 for the highest dose.

Finally, the analgesic activity of nonsteroidal anti-inflammatory drugs is limited by a low ceiling effect. An agent that has a ceiling effect has a level beyond which increasing the dose of the agent does not further increase analgesia. Bradley and colleagues (42) showed that acetaminophen (4000 mg/d) resulted in analgesia similar to that of ibuprofen, whether administered as an analgesic dose (1200 mg/d) or as an anti-inflammatory dose (2400 mg/d) to patients with chronic osteoarthritis of the knee. Thus, acetaminophen may be the preferred choice for patients without substantial inflammation because of its lower side-effect profile.

Opiate drugs, such as morphine, have no ceiling and have been shown to relieve all types of pain (43). Short-term studies (44,45) have shown that elderly patients are more sensitive than younger patients to the pain-relieving properties of these drugs. Advanced age is associated with a prolonged serum half-life for most opiate drugs (46). Thus, elderly patients may achieve pain relief from doses of opiate drugs that are smaller than those required by younger patients.

The potential of opiate drugs to cause cognitive disturbances, respiratory depression, and constipation is increased in typical nursing home residents. These drugs may also produce paradoxical excitement and agitation. Morphine remains the standard with which other opiate drugs should be compared in elderly persons because its effects are the best understood and the most predictable. Thus, morphine is the opiate of choice for severe pain in most nursing home residents (6,18). In the nursing home setting, issues of drug dependency and drug tolerance are usually irrelevant (47). This is not to suggest that morphine and other opiates can be used indiscriminately; it means only that dependency and other side effects do not justify withholding effective pain relief.

Tolerance to some side effects of opiates has the beneficial effect of reducing the risk for respiratory depression and drowsiness. For this reason, these drugs should be administered on a continuous basis (as opposed to pro re nata or "as needed") whenever possible. Regular dosing results in reduced overall drug consumption, continuous analgesia, and tolerance to drowsiness and respiratory depression (35). On the other hand, some side effects of opiates, such as constipation and possibly nausea, do not diminish with time and make overall pain management more difficult. In nursing home patients, it is important to begin bowel regimens early, when opiate therapy is first started. Increased fluids, bulk agents, lubricating agents, and bowel stimulants may be required (8). Although antiemetic drugs such as antihistamines and phenothiazines have been mainstays in the prevention of opiate-induced nausea, no clinical trials on this point have been done in elderly or nursing home populations. It is important to remember that patients in these populations are especially sensitive to the anticholinergic side effects of many antiemetic drugs, including bowel or bladder dysfunction, delirium, and movement disorders. Thus, antiemetic drugs should be chosen with an eye to which ones have the lowest side-effect profiles.

Some opiates require special attention when used in the nursing home setting. Propoxyphene is a controversial drug that is probably overprescribed in elderly persons. Reports suggest that its efficacy is no better than that of aspirin or acetaminophen, and it has substantial potential for dependency and renal injury (48). Pentazocine is an opiate that should be avoided because it frequently causes delirium and agitation in elderly persons. This effect seems to be related to the drug's mixture of agonist and antagonist opiate-receptor activity (49). Meperidine is also particularly hazardous in the elderly; its unique toxicity has been seen in patients with renal impairment and in those receiving antidepressants of the monoamine oxidase-inhibitor class. The active metabolite normeperidine is particularly prone to accumulation and is often associated with delirium and seizure activity (50). Methadone should be used with caution because of its propensity to accumulate. More importantly, it may be a poor choice because its analgesic effect may be short in comparison with its serum half-life (51); this increases the potential for accumulation or overdosage in elderly persons. Finally, transdermal fentanyl citrate is an extremely potent drug (perhaps 50 times as potent as morphine) with a potential for complications (52). The transdermal delivery system for this drug forms a tissue reservoir that results in a serum half-life of 36 hours (53). Because of the drug's extreme potency and the potential for overdosage, transdermal fentanyl citrate should not be used in "opiate-naive" elderly patients or in those unaccustomed to the respiratory depression caused by opiates.

Some adjuvant drugs may be helpful in recalcitrant pain problems. It is important to remember that these drugs are usually only partially successful and that they work best when used with other analgesic drug and nondrug pain strategies (54). Various antidepressant drugs have been shown to alleviate the pain of diabetic and other neuropathies; it has been suggested that this occurs because pain relief is mediated by the prolonged synaptic activity of norepinephrine and serotonin, which inhibits neurons in pain transmission. Recent reports (55,56) have suggested that drugs with more selective norepinephrine inhibition (such as amitriptyline and imipramine) may be more effective than drugs that have mixed serotonergic inhibition (such as desipramine) or those that have more selective serotonergic inhibition (such as paroxetine and fluoxetine) (55,56). One recent study (56) found desipramine to be as effective as amitriptyline in the management of diabetic neuralgia; thus, desipramine is an alternative for patients unable to tolerate the high side-effect profile of amitriptyline. The same study found fluoxetine to be no better than placebo.

Some neuropathic pain syndromes, such as trigeminal neuralgia, have been found to respond to antiepileptic drugs, including carbamazepine, valproate, and clonazepam (54,57). Intravenously administered local anesthetics, such as lidocaine and procaine, may also ameliorate the neuropathic pain syndromes independently of conduction blockade (57–59). Randomized trials have found oral tocainide to be effective in trigeminal neuralgia (58) and mexiletine to be effective in diabetic neuralgia (59). Each of these drugs has a substantial risk for toxicity in nursing home residents and should be reserved for patients with severe pain in whom other treatments have failed.

Capsaicin is applied topically and has been shown to deplete free nerve endings of substance P by blocking its re-uptake. It may be useful as an anesthetic for herpes zoster (60), diabetic neuropathy (61), and postoperative neuropathies (62). Although now available without a prescription, its overall efficacy for arthritis and other painful syndromes remains controversial. It normally causes a burning sensation that may be intolerable to some patients and that has led to speculation that a gate-control mechanism may contribute to its action.

Finally, tramadol, a new analgesic recently released in the United States (Ultram, McNeil Consumer Products Company, Fort Washington, Pennsylvania) may be helpful to some nursing home residents. This non-narcotic analgesic may have a potency similar to that of codeine or oxycodone. It has some opiate-receptor activity and has been reported to cause drowsiness, nausea, and—rarely—respiratory depression. Tramadol has been available for some time in Europe, but long-term studies and experience in older populations have been only partially explored (63,64).

Physicians who care for nursing home residents must help to establish a plan of care that is reasonable given the resources and skills available in the nursing home setting. Medication regimens can often be simplified. Long-acting analgesics should be used to provide a longer duration of comfort for patients and fewer doses for nurses to administer. Pain should be prevented by routine analgesia, and pro re nata medications should be avoided if possible. Short-acting analgesics should be prescribed for breakthrough pain or for pain associated with phys-

ical therapy, bathing, or other potentially painful activities. Treatments should be simplified so that night-time monitoring requirements are minimized. It is important to remember that nursing homes usually have limited pharmacy resources that are not available on a 24-hour basis. Contingency plans for pain management must be anticipated so that delays do not occur during medication changes or dosage adjustments. Finally, state regulatory requirements for multiple-copy prescriptions may be a substantial barrier to effective pain management in this setting; careful planning is the only solution (65).

Nonpharmacologic Pain-Management Strategies

Many nonpharmacologic pain-management strategies are effective, especially when used in combination with drug strategies. Education programs for patients have been shown to significantly improve pain management and quality of life (66,67). The benefits of physical methods, including heat, cold, and massage, should not be underestimated. These methods are effective for many patients (67); they relax tense muscles and soothe many problems. Some of these techniques can be applied by the patient, providing a sense of control over symptoms and treatment, although precautions should be taken to avoid injury from the use of heat or ice by patients with cognitive impairment. Physical therapy directed at stretching and strengthening specific muscles and joints and maintenance exercise programs are available in most nursing homes; these are useful in improving muscle strength, reducing muscle spasm, and enhancing functional activity. Consultation and treatment by skilled therapists (available in many nursing homes) are appropriate for safe and effective rehabilitation from many painful conditions.

Transcutaneous nerve stimulation has been used successfully in various chronic pain conditions in older patients (68). Painful diabetic neuropathies, shoulder pain or bursitis, and fractured ribs have been shown to respond to transcutaneous nerve stimulation therapy. Although this therapy has relieved some patients for years, its effectiveness usually diminishes with time, and strong placebo effects have been associated with its use (69). The appropriate placement of electrodes and current adjustment are important to the success of this therapy. This involves meticulous searching, with the help of a trained physical therapist, for the best settings for an individual patient's optimum comfort. Care must also be taken to avoid skin irritation from the electrodes.

Some psychological maneuvers may be effective in controlling pain. Biofeedback, relaxation, and hypnosis may help some patients. These methods usually require high levels of cognitive function and may not be suitable for patients with substantial cognitive impairment. A trained psychologist or therapist should be consulted about these techniques.

Finally, various activities provided in the nursing home may be effective in decreasing the perception of pain. Many patients find comfort in prayer, meditation, or music. Activities, exercise, and recreation should be encouraged insofar as they can be tolerated. Inactivity and immobility may contribute extensively to depression and worsening of pain.

"High-Tech" Pain-Management Strategies

Recent developments in pain management have focused on various "high-tech" drug-delivery systems for the management of pain; these systems are being used in some nursing homes. With appropriate supervision and patient education, many techniques have become feasible for selected nursing home patients (70,71). A randomized trial (72) found that patient-controlled analgesia using morphine infusions is safe and effective for postoperative pain management among nondemented, frail elderly men. However, parenteral morphine infusions for chronic cancer pain are expensive and may cost several thousands of dollars a month to maintain (73).

These procedures have been effective in selected cases, but more work needs to be done to define expanded roles for these technologies in nursing home residents with pain. Because of cost and potential side effects, it is usual to consider "high-tech" strategies only after oral medications have failed or after all other treatments have been tried. Further study is needed to determine whether these technologies have risk-to-benefit ratios sufficient to justify their routine use for nonmalignant pain or the less intense pain syndromes. Although most of these techniques are expensive, they are often partially reimbursable by Medicare and other insurers. These issues have raised ethical questions about the application of "high-tech" pain-management technologies in patients who might be equally well managed with oral medications that, unfortunately, are not reimbursable (74,75).

SUMMARY AND FUTURE DIRECTIONS

Pain is a common problem that has tremendous potential to influence the physical function and quality of life of nursing home residents. It is unfortunate that so little geriatric research and education has focused on this important topic. Pain management in nursing homes can be improved, particularly through the careful use of appropriate pharmacologic and nonpharmacologic pain-management strategies. The incorporation of pain management into geriatric nursing and medical education at all levels will produce long-term-care professionals who are skilled in pain management and in comforting persons with chronic pain.

Substantial research is still needed to further our understanding of pain and its management among elderly persons. Valid and reliable pain measures, such as pain-intensity scales, functional scales, and behavioral observations need to be established for cognitively impaired persons. New drugs with milder side-effect profiles are urgently needed. Non-drug pain-management strategies, such as exercise and other physical methods, should be investigated. Indications for "high-tech" pain-management strategies, such as morphine pumps and chronic spinal infusions, need to be clarified in this population. And, finally, comparative studies of the long-term outcomes of pain-management strategies need to be done.

As the need for nursing home care continues, many residents will require effective pain management to maintain their dignity and quality of life. It is our obligation to do everything possible to provide comfort and effective pain management for these persons during their remaining years.

REFERENCES

1. Roark AC. How much painkiller is enough? (the quiet epidemic). Los Angeles Times. 10 Dec 1991: A1 (column 1).
2. Shapiro RS. Liability issues in the management of pain. Journal of Pain and Symptom Management. 1994;9:1-7.
3. Ferrell BA, Ferrell BR, Osterweil D. Pain in the nursing home. J Am Geriatr Soc. 1990;38:409-14.
4. Roy R, Michael T. A survey of chronic pain in an elderly population. Can Fam Physician Med Fam Can. 1986;32:513-16.
5. Ouslander JG, Osterweil D, Morley JE. Medical Care in the Nursing Home. New York: McGraw-Hill; 1991.

6. Acute Pain Management: Operative or Medical Procedures and Trauma. Rockville, MD: U.S. Department of Health and Human Services, Public Health Service, Agency for Health Care Policy and Research: 1992.

7. Foley KM. The treatment of cancer pain. N Engl J Med. 1985;113:84-95.

8. Ferrell BA. Pain management in elderly people. J Am Geriatr Soc. 1991;39:64-73.0

9. Wall PD, Melzack R, eds. Textbook of Pain. 2nd ed. New York: Churchill Livingstone; 1990.

10. Wall RT 3d. Use of analgesics in the elderly. Clin Geriatr Med. 1990;6:345-64.

11. Harkins SW, Price DD. Assessment of pain in the elderly. In: Turk DC, Melzack R, eds. Handbook of Pain Assessment. New York: Guilford Pr; 1992.

12. Melding PS. Is there such a thing as geriatric pain? [Editorial] Pain. 1991;46:119-21.

13. Bayer AJ, Chada JS, Farag RR, Pathy MS. Changing presentation of myocardial infarction with increasing old age. J Am Geriatr Soc. 1986;34:263-66.

14. Barsky AJ, Hochstrasser B, Coles NA, Zisfein J, O'Donnell C, Eagle KA. Silent myocardial ischemia. Is the person or the event silent? JAMA. 1990;264:1132-5.

15. Bender JS. Approach to the acute abdomen. Med Clin North Am. 1989;73:1413-22.

16. Norman DC, Yoshikawa TT. Intraabdominal infections in the elderly. J Am Geriatr Soc. 1983;31:677-84.

17. Harkins SW, Kwentus J, Price DD. Pain in the elderly. In: Benedetti C, Chapman CR, Moricca G, eds. Recent Advances in the Management of Pain. v. 7. New York: Raven; 1984.

18. Jacox A, Carr DB, Payne R, et al. Management of Cancer Pain. Rockville, MD: U.S. Department of Health and Human Services, Public Health Service, Agency for Health Care Policy and Research: 1994. Clinical Practice Guideline no. 9. AHCPR Publication no. 94-0592.

19. Ferrell BA, Ferrell BR, Rivera L. Pain in cognitively impaired nursing home patients. Journal of Pain and Symptom Management. 1995;10:591-8.

20. Lau-Ting C, Phoon WO. Aches and pains among Singapore elderly. Singapore Med J. 1988;29:164-7.

21. Davis MA. Epidemiology of osteoarthritis. Clin Geriatr Med. 1988;4:241-55.

22. Parmelee PA, Katz IR, Lawton MP. The relation of pain to depression among institutionalized aged. J Gerontol. 1991;46:P15-21.

23. Lavsky-Shulan M, Wallace RB, Kohout FJ, Lemke JH, Morris MC, Smith IM. Prevalence and functional correlates of low back pain in the elderly: the Iowa 65 + Rural Health Survey. J Am Geriatr Soc. 1985;33:23-8.

24. Nishikawa ST, Ferrell BA. Pain assessment in the elderly. Clinical Geriatrics and Issues in Long Term Care. 1993;1:15-28.

25. Ferrell BR, Rhiner M, Cohen MZ, Grant M. Pain as a metaphor for illness. Part I: Impact of cancer pain on family caregivers. Oncol Nurs Forum. 1991; 18:1303-9.

26. Kane RL, Ouslander JG, Abrass IB. Essentials of Clinical Geriatrics. 2nd ed. New York: McGraw Hill; 1989.

27. Herr KA, Mobily PR. Comparison of selected pain assessment tools for use with the elderly. Appl Nurs Res. 1993;6:39-46.

28. Barrier G, Attia J, Mayer MN, Amiel-Tison C, Shnider SM. Measurement of post-operative pain and narcotic administration in infants using a new clinical scoring system. Intensive Care Med. 1989;15(Suppl. 1):S37-9.

29. Hurley AC, Volicer BJ, Hanrahan PA, Houde S, Volicer L. Assessment of discomfort in advanced Alzheimer patients. Res Nurs Health. 1992;15: 369-77.

30. Parmelee PA, Smith B, Katz IR. Pain complaints and cognitive status among elderly institution residents. J Am Geriatr Soc. 1993;41:517-22.

31. Branch LG, Meyers AR. Assessing physical function in the elderly. Clin Geriatr Med. 1987;3:29-51.

32. Ouslander JG. Medical care in the nursing home. JAMA. 1989;262:2582-90.

33. Crook J, Tunks E, Rideout E, Browne G. Epidemiologic comparison of persistent pain sufferers in a specialty pain clinic and in the community. Arch Phys Med Rehabil. 1986;67:451-5.

34. Sorkin BA, Rudy TE, Hanlon RB, Turk DC, Stieg RL. Chronic pain in old and young patients: differences appear less important than similarities. J Gerontol. 1990;45:B64-8.

35. Melzack R. The tragedy of needless pain. Sci Am. 1990;262:27-33.

36. Gurwitz JH, Avorn J. The ambiguous relation between aging and adverse drug reactions. Ann Intern Med. 1991;114:956-66.

37. Perneger TV, Whelton PK, Klag MJ. Risk of kidney failure associated with the use of acetaminophen, aspirin, and nonsteroidal antiinflammatory drugs. N Engl J Med. 1994;331:1675-9.

38. Roth SH. Merits and liabilities of NSAID therapy. Rheum Dis Clin North Am. 1989;15:479-98.

39. Kantor TG. Peripherally-acting analgesics. In: Kuhar MJ, Pasternak GW, eds. Analgesics Neurochemical, Behavioral, and Clinical Perspectives. New York: Raven; 1984.

40. Rochon PA, Fortin PR, Dear KB, Minaker KL, Chalmers TC. Reporting of age data in clinical trials of arthritis. Arch Intern Med. 1993;153:243-8.

41. Griffin MR, Piper JM, Dougherty JR, Snowden M, Ray WA. Nonsteroidal anti-inflammatory drug use and increased risk for peptic ulcer disease in elderly persons. Ann Intern Med. 114;1991:257-63.

42. Bradley JD, Brandt KD, Katz BP, Kalasinski LA, Ryan SI. Comparison of an antiinflammatory dose of ibuprofen, an analgesic dose of ibuprofen, and acetaminophen in the treatment of patients with osteoarthritis of the knee. N Engl J Med. 1991; 325:87-91.

43. Portenoy RK. Opiate therapy for chronic noncancer pain: Can we get past the bias? American Pain Society Bulletin. 1991;1:4-7.

44. Kaiko RF. Age and morphine analgesia in cancer patients with postoperative pain. Clin Pharmacol Ther. 1980;28:823-6.

45. Bellville JW, Forrest WH Jr, Miller E, Brown BW Jr. Influence of age on pain relief from analgesics. A study of postoperative patients. JAMA. 1971;217:1835-41.

46. Kaiko RF, Wallenstein SL, Rogers AG, Grabinski PY, Houde RW. Narcotics in the elderly. Med Clin North Am. 1982;66:1079-89.

47. Wanzer SH, Federman DD, Adelstein SJ, Cassel CK, Cassem EH, Cranford RE, et al. The physician's responsibility toward hopelessly ill patients. A second look. N Engl J Med. 1989;320:844-9.

48. Beaver WT. Impact of non-narcotic oral analgesics on pain management. Am J Med. 1988;84:3-15.

49. Hanks GW. The clinical usefulness of agonist-antagonistic opioid analgesics in chronic pain. Drug Alcohol Depend. 1987;20:339-46.

50. Kaiko RF, Foley KM, Grabinski PY, Heidrich G, Rogers AG, Inturrisi CE, et al. Central nervous system excitatory effects of meperidine in cancer patients. Ann Neurol. 1983;13:180-5.

51. Foley KM, Inturrisi CE. Analgesic drug therapy in cancer pain: principles and practice. Med Clin North Am. 1987;71:207-32.

52. Steinberg RB, Gilman DE, Johnson F 3d. Acute toxic delirium in a patient using transdermal fentanyl. Anesth Analg. 1992;75:1014-6.

53. Payne R. Transdermal fentanyl: suggested recommendations for clinical use. J Pain Symptom Manage. 1992;7(3 Suppl):S40-4.

54. Portenoy RK. Drug treatment of pain syndromes. Semin Neurol. 1987;7:139-49.

55. Max MB. Antidepressants as analgesics. In: Fields HL, Liebeskind JC, eds. Progress in Pain Research and Management, v. 1. Seattle: International Society for the Study of Pain Pr; 1994: 229-46.

56. Max MB, Lynch SA, Muir J, Shoaf SE, Smoller B, Dubner R. Effects of desipramine, amitriptyline, and fluoxetine on pain in diabetic neuropathy. N Engl J Med. 1992;326:1250-6.

57. Swerdlow M. The use of local anaesthetics for relief of chronic pain. The Pain Clinic. 1988;2:3-6.

58. Lindstrom P, Lindstrom U. The analgesic effect of tocainide in trigeminal neuralgia. Pain. 1987;28:45-50.

59. Stracke H, Meyer UE, Schumacher HE, Federlin K. Mexiletine in the treatment of diabetic neuropathy. Diabetes Care. 1992;15:1550-5.

60. Watson CP, Evans RJ, Watt VR. Post-herpetic neuralgia and topical capsaicin. Pain. 1988;33:333-40.

61. Tandan R, Lewis GA, Badger GB, Fries TJ. Topical capsaicin in painful diabetic neuropathy. Effect on sensory function. Diabetes Care. 1992;15:15-8.

62. AMA Drug Evaluations Annual. Chicago: American Medical Association; 1992.

63. Lee CR, McTavish D, Sorkin EM. Tramadol. A preliminary review of its pharmacodynamic and pharmacokinetic properties, and therapeutic potential in acute and chronic pain states. Drugs. 1993;46:313-40.

64. Rauch RL, Ruoff GE, McMillen JI. Comparison of tramadol and acetaminophen with codeine for long-term pain management in elderly patients. Current Therapeutic Research. 1994;55:1417-31.

65. Zullich SG, Grasela TH Jr, Fiedler-Kelly JB, Gengo FM. Impact of triplicate prescription program on psychotropic prescribing patterns in long-term care facilities. Ann Pharmacother. 1992;26:539-46.

66. Ferrell BR, Rhiner M, Ferrell BA. Development and implementation of a pain education program. Cancer. 1993;72(11 Suppl):3426-32.

67. Rhiner M, Ferrell BR, Ferrell BA, Grant MM. A structured nondrug intervention program for cancer pain. Cancer Pract. 1993;1:137-43.

68. Thorsteinsson G. Chronic pain: use of TENS in the elderly. Geriatrics. 1987;42:75-7, 81-2.

69. Deyo RA, Walsh NE, Martin DC, Schoenfeld LS, Ramamurthy S. A controlled trial of transcutaneous electrical nerve stimulation (TENS) and exercise for chronic low back pain. N Engl J Med. 1990;322:1627-34.

70. Kerr IG, Sone M, Deangelis C, Iscoe N, MacKenzie R, Schueller T. Continuous narcotic infusion with patient-controlled analgesia for chronic cancer pain in outpatients. Ann Intern Med. 1988;108:554-7.

71. Sjogren P, Banning A. Pain, sedation and reaction time during long-term treatment of cancer patients with oral and epidural opioids. Pain. 1989;39:5-11.

72. Egbert AM, Parks LH, Short LM, Burnett ML. Randomized trial of postoperative patient-controlled analgesia vs intramuscular narcotics in frail elderly men. Arch Intern Med. 1990;150:1897-903.

73. Ferrell BR, Griffith H. Cost issues related to pain management: report from the Cancer Pain Panel of the Agency for Health Care Policy and Research. J Pain Symptom Manage. 1994;9:221-34.

74. Whedon M, Ferrell BR. Professional and ethical considerations in the use of high-tech pain management. Oncol Nurs Forum. 1991;18:1135-43.

75. Ferrell BR, Rhiner M. High-tech comfort: ethical issues in cancer pain management for the 1990s. J Clin Ethics. 1991;2:108-12.

PART IV

Special Considerations in the Nursing Home

—— 8 ——

Falls and Their Prevention

Laurence Z. Rubenstein, MD, MPH, FACP,
Karen R. Josephson, MPH, and Alan S. Robbins, MD

Falls are responsible for considerable morbidity, immobility, and mortality among older persons, especially those living in nursing homes. Falls have many different causes, and several risk factors that predispose patients to falls have been identified. To prevent falls, a systematic therapeutic approach to residents who have fallen is necessary, and close attention must be paid to identifying and reducing risk factors for falls among frail older persons who have not yet fallen. We review the problem of falls in the nursing home, focusing on identifiable causes, risk factors, and preventive approaches.

EPIDEMIOLOGY

Both the incidence of falls in older adults and the severity of complications increase steadily with age and increased physical disability. Accidents are the fifth leading cause of death in older adults, and falls constitute two thirds of these accidental deaths. About three fourths of deaths caused by falls in the United States occur in the 13% of the population aged 65 years and older (1,2). Approximately one third of older adults living at home will fall each year, and about 5% will sustain a fracture or require hospitalization. The incidence of falls and fall-related injuries among persons living in institutions has been reported in numerous epidemiologic studies (3–18). These data are presented in Table 8.1. The mean fall incidence calculated from these studies is about three times the rate for community-living

elderly persons (mean, 1.5 falls/bed per year), caused both by the more frail nature of persons living in institutions and by more accurate reporting of falls in institutions.

As shown in Table 8.1, only about 4% of falls (range, 1% to 10%) result in fractures, whereas other serious injuries such as head trauma, soft-tissue injuries, and severe lacerations occur in about 11% of falls (range, 1% to 36%). However, once injured, an elderly person who has fallen has a much higher case fatality rate than does a younger person who has fallen (1,2). Each year, about 1800 fatal falls occur in nursing homes. Among persons 85 years and older, 1 of 5 fatal falls occurs in a nursing home (19). Nursing home residents also have a disproportionately high incidence of hip fracture and have been shown to have higher mortality rates after hip fracture than community-living elderly persons (20). Furthermore, because of the high frequency of recurrent falls in nursing homes, the likelihood of sustaining an injurious fall is substantial.

In addition to injuries, falls can have serious consequences for physical functioning and quality of life. Loss of function can result from both fracture-related disability and self-imposed functional limitations caused by fear of falling and the "postfall anxiety syndrome." Decreased confidence in the ability to ambulate safely can lead to further functional decline, depression, feelings of helplessness, and social isolation. In addition, the use of physical or chemical restraints by institutional staff to pre-

TABLE 8.1. Incidence of falls and fall-related injuries in long-term-care facilities*

Study (Reference)	Site	Mean Age of Patients	Annual Incidence per 1000 Beds	Falls with Serious Injury	Falls with Fracture
		y		%	
Gryfe et al, 1977 (3)	BC	81% ≥ 75	650	17	6
Pablo, 1977 (4)	CC	72	730	17	0
Feist, 1978 (5)	NH	83	3300	4	3
Cacha, 1979 (6)	NH	82	2400	1	NA
Miller and Elliott, 1979 (7)	NH	82	1400	NA	1
Louis, 1983 (8)	NH	83	760	12	NA
Louis, 1983 (8)	NH	79	1100	14	NA
Colling and Park, 1983 (9)	NH	NA	2600	5	2
Blake and Morfitt, 1986 (10)	BC	≥ 60	3600	3	NA
Berry et al, 1981 (11)	CC	68% ≥ 70	1500	5	3
Berryman et al, 1989 (12)	NH	≥ 65	2000	NA	NA
Gross et al, 1990 (13)	NH and BC	82	220	15	10
Rubenstein et al, 1990 (14)	NH and BC	≥ 65	1200	NA	2
Gostynski, 1991 (15)	NH and BC	86	1300	6	2
Neufeld et al, 1991 (16)	NH and BC	84	630	NA	5
Svensson et al, 1991 (17)	NH	95% ≥ 65	350	35[†]	NA
Tinetti et al, 1992 (18)	NH	84	1530	3	3
Simple mean of all surveys			1450	11	4

* BC = board and care facility; CC = chronic care facility; NA = not available; NH = nursing home.
† Percentage of injurious falls in this study that were considered serious.

vent high-risk persons from falling also has negative effects on functioning.

CAUSES OF FALLS

The major reported immediate causes of falls and their relative frequencies as described in four detailed studies of nursing home populations (14,15,17,21) are presented in Table 8.2. The table also contains a comparison column of causes of falls among elderly persons not living in institutions as summarized from seven detailed studies (21–28). The distribution of causes clearly differs among the populations studied. Frail, high-risk persons living in institutions tend to have a higher incidence of falls caused by gait disorders, weakness, dizziness, and confusion, whereas the falls of community-living persons are more related to their environment.

In the nursing home, weakness and gait problems were the most common causes of falls, accounting for about a quarter of reported cases. Studies have reported that the prevalence of detectable lower-extremity weakness ranges from 48% among community-living older persons (29) to 57% among residents of an intermediate-care facility (30) to more than 80% of residents of a skilled nursing

facility (27). Gait disorders affect 20% to 50% of elderly persons (31), and nearly three quarters of nursing home residents require assistance with ambulation or cannot ambulate (32). Investigators of case-control studies in nursing homes have reported that more than two thirds of persons who have fallen have substantial gait disorders, a prevalence 2.4 to 4.8 times higher than the prevalence among persons who have not fallen (27,30).

The cause of muscle weakness and gait problems is multifactorial. Aging introduces physical changes that affect strength and gait. On average, healthy older persons score 20% to 40% lower on strength tests than young adults (33), and, among chronically ill nursing home residents, strength is considerably less than that. Much of the weakness seen in the nursing home stems from deconditioning due to prolonged bedrest or limited physical activity and chronic debilitating medical conditions such as heart failure, stroke, or pulmonary disease. Aging is also associated with other deteriorations that impair gait, including increased postural sway; decreased gait velocity, stride length, and step height; prolonged reaction time; and decreased visual acuity and depth perception. Gait problems can also stem from dysfunction of the nervous, musculoskeletal, circulato-

TABLE 8.2. Comparison of causes of falls in nursing home and community-living populations: summary of studies that carefully evaluated elderly persons after a fall and specified a "most likely cause."

Cause of Falls	Nursing Home (n = 4 studies* and 1076 falls)	Community-Living (n = 7 studies[†] and 2312 falls)
	% (range)	
Gait or balance disorder or weakness	26 (20–39)[‡]	13 (2–29)
Dizziness or vertigo	25 (0–30)	8 (0–19)
"Accident" or environment-related	16 (6–27)	41 (23–53)
Confusion	10 (0–14)	2 (0–7)
Visual disorder	4 (0–5)	0.8 (0–4)
Postural hypotension	2 (0–16)	1 (0–6)
Drop attack	0.3 (0–3)	13 (0–25)
Syncope	0.2 (0–3)	0.4 (0–3)
Other specified causes[§]	12 (10–34)	17 (2–39)
Unknown	4 (0–34)	6 (0–16)

* References 14, 15, 17, and 21.
† References 22 to 28.
‡ Mean percentage calculated from the total number of falls in the studies reviewed. Ranges indicate the percentage reported in each of the studies. Percentages do not total 100% because some studies reported more than one cause per fall.
§ This category includes arthritis, acute illness, drugs, alcohol, pain, epilepsy, and falling from bed.

ry, or respiratory systems, as well as from simple deconditioning after a period of inactivity.

Dizziness is commonly reported by elderly persons who have fallen and was the attributed cause in 25% of reported nursing home falls. This symptom is often difficult to evaluate because "dizziness" means different things to different people and has diverse causes. True vertigo, a sensation of rotational movement, may indicate a disorder of the vestibular apparatus such as benign positional vertigo, acute labyrinthitis, or Ménière disease. Symptoms described as "imbalance on walking" often reflect a gait disorder. Many residents describe a vague lightheadedness that may reflect cardiovascular problems, hyperventilation, orthostatic hypotension, drug side effect, anxiety, or depression.

Accidents, or falls stemming from environmental hazards, are a major cause of reported falls—16% of nursing home falls and 41% of community falls. However, the circumstances of accidents are difficult to verify, and many falls in this category may actually stem from interactions between environmental hazards or hazardous activities and increased individual susceptibility to hazards because of aging and disease. Among impaired residents, even normal activities of daily living might be considered hazardous if they are done without assistance or modification. Factors such as decreased lower-extremity strength, poor posture control, and decreased step height all interact to impair the abil-

ity to avoid a fall after an unexpected trip or while reaching or bending. Age-associated impairments of vision, hearing, and memory also tend to increase the number of trips. Studies have shown that most falls in nursing homes occurred during transferring from a bed, chair, or wheelchair (3,11). Attempting to move to or from the bathroom and nocturia (which necessitates frequent trips to the bathroom) have also been reported to be associated with falls (34,35) and fall-related fractures (9). Environmental hazards that frequently contribute to these falls include wet floors caused by episodes of incontinence, poor lighting, bedrails, and improper bed height. Falls have also been reported to increase when nurse staffing is low, such as during breaks and at shift changes (4,7,9,13), presumably because of lack of staff supervision.

Confusion and cognitive impairment are frequently cited causes of falls and may reflect an underlying systemic or metabolic process (for example, electrolyte imbalance or fever). Dementia can increase the number of falls by impairing judgment, visual-spatial perception, and ability to orient oneself geographically. Falls also occur when residents with dementia wander, attempt to get out of wheelchairs, or climb over bed siderails.

Orthostatic (postural) hypotension, usually defined as a decrease of 20 mm or more of systolic blood pressure after standing, has a 5% to 25% prevalence among "normal" elderly persons living at home (36). It is even more common among persons with certain predisposing risk factors, including autonomic dysfunction, hypovolemia, low cardiac output, parkinsonism, metabolic and endocrine disorders, and medications (particularly sedatives, antihypertensives, vasodilators, and antidepressants) (37). The orthostatic drop may be more pronounced on arising in the morning because the baroreflex response is diminished after prolonged recumbency, as it is after meals and after ingestion of nitroglycerin (38,39). Yet, despite its high prevalence, orthostatic hypotension infrequently causes falls, particularly outside of institutions. This is perhaps because of its transient nature, which makes it difficult to detect after the fall, or because most persons with orthostatic hypotension feel light-headed and will deliberately find a seat rather than fall.

Drop attacks are defined as sudden falls without loss of consciousness and without dizziness, often precipitated by a sudden change in head position. This syndrome has been attributed to transient vertebrobasilar insufficiency, although it is probably caused by more diverse pathophysiologic mechanisms. Although early descriptions of geriatric falls identified drop attacks as a substantial cause, more recent studies have reported a smaller proportion of persons who fall because of drop attacks. This probably reflects greater precision in diagnosis and a correction of an earlier tendency to attribute falls of unclear cause to drop attacks (40). Only one of the four nursing home studies we reviewed documented drop attack as a cause of falls.

Syncope, defined as a sudden loss of consciousness with spontaneous recovery, is a serious but relatively uncommon cause of falls that usually results from decreased cerebral blood flow or occasionally from metabolic disorders such as hypoglycemia or hypoxia. The most frequent causes in elderly persons are vasovagal reactions, cardiac arrhythmias, and orthostatic hypotension, although, in many cases, a clear cause is never determined (41). A history of syncope may be difficult to obtain because many residents do not remember exactly what occurred during the fall and because the resident may confuse drop attacks or dizziness with syncope. Many studies of falls do not identify syncope as causing a fall but rather as a separate syndrome. This perhaps explains the extremely low proportion of falls from syncope (*see* Table 8.2).

Other important causes of falls include visual problems, arthritis, acute illnesses, disorders of the central nervous system, drug side effects, and alcohol intake. Diseases of the central nervous system (for example, cerebrovascular disease, dementia, normal pressure hydrocephalus, and parkinsonism) often result in falls by causing dizziness, orthostatic hypotension, and gait disorders. Residents with cognitive deficits often cannot recognize and avoid hazards. Drugs frequently have side effects that result in impaired thinking, stability, and gait. Especially important are agents with sedative, antidepressant, and antihypertensive effects, particularly diuretics, vasodilators, and β-blockers (42,43). Alcohol may be an occult cause of instability, falls, and serious injury, although it is less likely to be a problem in the nursing home than in the community. Other less common causes of falls include seizures, anemia, hypothyroidism, unstable joints, foot problems, and severe osteoporosis with spontaneous fracture.

RISK FACTORS FOR FALLS

Studies have shown that among persons living in institutions, specific risk factors exist that significantly increase the likelihood of falling. Some of these risk factors are only temporary, whereas others may be related to a chronic condition. Risk factors that have been identified in case-control studies are presented in Table 8.3, along with an approximate mean relative risk of each factor. Of the 10 studies reviewed, 6 included physical examinations or tests for persons who have and have not fallen (21,27,30,39,44,45), and the other 4 studies relied on data abstracted from medical chart reviews (42,43,46,47).

Comparison of persons who have fallen with those who have not showed that lower-extremity weakness was a significant risk factor in all four of the studies that looked for it and increased the odds of falling about sixfold. Gait and balance impairments were found to be a significant risk factor associated with about a four- and fivefold increased risk for falling, respectively. Thus, gait and balance impairments are both the most important immediate causes and the most serious risk factors for falls in the nursing home.

Functional impairment has also been shown to be a significant risk factor for falls. Inability to do basic activities of daily living and the use of an assistive device were both associated with a threefold increased risk for falling. (Use of an assistive device

TABLE 8.3. Important individual risk factors for falls: summary of 10 controlled studies done in long-term care institutions*

Risk Factor	Significant/ Total[†], n	Mean Relative Risk and Odds Ratio (n)[‡]	Range
Physical Examination			
Weakness	4/4	6.2 (3)	4.9–8.4
Balance deficit	3/3	4.6 (2)	3.9–5.4
Gait deficit	4/4	3.6 (2)	2.4–4.8
Impaired mobility or use of walking aid	2/2	3.3 (2)	2.0–4.6
Functional impairment	2/2	3.1 (1)	NA
Visual deficit	3/4	2.7 (3)	1.1–4.5
Postural hypotension	2/3	2.1 (3)	1.0–3.4
Cognitive impairment	2/3	1.5 (2)	1.0–2.0
Drugs			
Number of drugs	4/4	NA	NA
Antidepressants	3/6	2.4 (6)	1.0–5.7
Sedative/hypnotic agents	4/7	2.0 (7)	1.0–3.2
Nonsteroidal anti-inflammatory drugs	2/6	1.6 (6)	1.0–2.4
Vasodilators	2/6	1.4 (6)	1.0–2.2
Diagnoses			
Arthritis	2/4	1.6 (4)	0.9–2.4
Depression	2/5	1.6 (5)	1.0–2.5

* References 21, 27, 30, 39, and 42 to 47.
† Number of studies with significant association/total number of studies looking at each factor.
‡ Relative risks of the prospective studies and odds ratios of the retrospective studies. The numbers in parentheses indicate the number of studies that reported relative risks or odds ratios.

is presumably a marker for impaired gait because when well-fitted, assistive devices should improve safety.) Visual impairment, postural hypotension, and cognitive impairment approximately doubled the risk for falls.

Several case-control studies have shown an association between falls and medication use, with reported odds ratios ranging from 1.0 to 5.7. In one study, residents taking four or more prescription medications had a significantly greater risk for falling (27). Specific classes of medications found to increase the risk for falling in nursing home residents include psychotropic drugs (42,43,48), sedatives (17,42,47), cardiac drugs (42,43,46,47), and nonsteroidal anti-inflammatory drugs (42,43).

A weak relation exists between medical diagnoses and falls. In two studies, persons who have

fallen had significantly more established medical diagnoses than persons who have not fallen (27,46). Specific medical diagnoses shown to be significant risk factors for falls include arthritis (42,43) and depression (42).

Appreciating the interaction and probable synergism among multiple risk factors is important in making a clinical assessment. Several studies have shown that the risk for falling increases dramatically as the number of risk factors increases (27,30,42). In one study, the predicted 1-year risk for falling ranged from 12% for persons with none of three risk factors (hip weakness assessed manually, unstable balance, and taking four or more prescribed medications) to 100% for persons with all three risk factors (27).

Most falls, even among frail elderly persons, do not result in serious injury. This observation has motivated several research groups to attempt to identify patients and specific risk factors associated with injurious falls. On the whole, the risk factors identified for injurious falls are the same as those for falls in general (that is, lower-extremity weakness, impaired balance, dizziness, poor vision and hearing, medications, and disorientation) (17,18,49,50). However, several additional risk factors among nursing home populations are particularly noteworthy. These include the female sex (probably largely related to osteoporosis), functional independence, the number of falls, and use of mechanical restraints. In one study (18), the risk for a fall-related injury was 10 times greater for residents who had been restrained at some time during a 1-year study period than that of those who had not been restrained. Both falls and serious injuries significantly increased as restraint use increased. This observation challenges the assumption that restraints protect patients from falls. The authors suggest that intermittent use of restraints in frail older persons may result in further deconditioning and actually increase the risk for falling.

In summary, it is possible to identify persons at substantially increased risk for sustaining a fall or fall-related injury by detecting the presence of selected risk factors.

DIAGNOSTIC APPROACH

The exact cause of a fall is frequently difficult to determine because most nursing home residents have more than one identifiable age-related change or medical condition that could constitute a risk factor for falling; frequently, the event is not witnessed or is poorly recalled. The diagnostic assessment of the resident who falls should focus on identifying risk factors that can be treated to reduce the likelihood of future falls. The basic components of this diagnostic approach are outlined in Box 8.1.

After any immediate injuries caused by the fall are treated, the diagnostic approach should begin with a well-directed history aimed at uncovering any specific cause and associated risk factors. Obtaining a full report of the circumstances and symptoms surrounding the fall is crucial; however, because the patient may poorly remember these events, reports from any witnesses are often important. Historical factors that can point to a specific cause or help to narrow the differential diagnosis include suddenly rising from a lying or sitting position (orthostatic hypotension), a trip or slip (gait, balance, or vision disturbance or an environmental hazard), antecedent cough or urination (reflex hypotension), a recent meal (postprandial hypotension), looking up or sideways (arterial or carotid sinus compression), and loss of consciousness (syncope or seizure).

Symptoms experienced near the time of falling may also indicate a potential cause—dizziness or giddiness (orthostatic hypotension, vestibular problem, hypoglycemia, arrhythmia, or a drug side effect), palpitations (arrhythmia), incontinence or tongue biting (seizure), asymmetric weakness (cerebrovascular disease), chest pain (myocardial infarction or coronary insufficiency), or loss of consciousness (any cause of syncope). Medications, especially those with hypotensive or psychoactive effects, and existence of concomitant medical problems may be important contributing factors (Box 8.1). Other points to elicit during the history that might be helpful in directing further work-up and care planning include the following: How long was the patient on the ground? What effect did the fall have on patient confidence, fear of further falls, and activity? Are there any effects on caregiver expectations, fears, and plans for future activities?

Pertinent items to be noted during the physical examination after the fall include orthostatic changes in pulse and blood pressure and presence of arrhythmias, carotid bruits, nystagmus, focal neurologic signs, confusion, musculoskeletal abnormalities, sensory impairments, and gait disturbances. It is often useful to attempt, under carefully monitored conditions, to reproduce the circum-

---

BOX 8.1. Key points of the clinical assessment of the patient who falls

History
  Ask the patient or witness about the following:
    Circumstances of the fall: trip or slip, environmental hazard, posture change, recent meal, urination or defecation, head turning, cough or sneeze, or other activity
    Associated symptoms: chest pain, palpitations, light-headedness, vertigo, fainting, weakness, confusion, incontinence, or dyspnea
    Relevant comorbid conditions: previous stroke, parkinsonism, osteoporosis, seizure disorder, cardiac disease, joint dysfunction, depression, or sensory deficit
    Medication review (note drugs that have hypotensive or psychoactive effects): antihypertensives, diuretics, autonomic blockers, antidepressants, hypnotics, auxiolytics, analgesics, or psychotropics
Physical examination
  Pay particular attention to the following:
    Vital signs: postural pulse and blood pressure changes, fever, or hypothermia
    Head and neck: visual impairment, hearing impairment, nystagmus, motion-induced imbalance, or bruit
    Heart: arrhythmia or valve dysfunction
    Neurologic signs: altered mental status, focal deficits, peripheral neuropathy, muscle weakness, instability, rigidity, or tremor
    Musculoskeletal signs: arthritic changes, motion limitations, podiatric problems, or deformities
Functional assessment
  Observe or inquire about the following:
    Functional gait or balance: Observe patient rising from chair, walking (note the stride length, velocity, and symmetry), turning, and sitting down
    Mobility: use of assistive device or personal assistance, extent of ambulation, or restraint use
    Activities of daily living: bathing, transferring, dressing, and continence

---

stances that might have precipitated the fall, such as changes in position, head turning, urination, or carotid pressure.

A careful assessment of gait and balance done as part of the assessment after the fall can provide meaningful information about impairments and functional abilities. Gait and balance should be assessed by close observation of how the patient rises from a chair, stands with eyes open and closed, walks, turns, and sits down. One should particularly note gait velocity and rhythm, stride length, symmetry, weakness, double-limb support time (the time spent with both feet on the floor), height of stepping, use of assistive devices, and degree of sway. Imbalance observed during head turning or flexion is an important finding associated with vestibular or vertebrobasilar pathologic conditions and an increased risk for falling. A useful clinical screening test for gait and balance described by Tinetti (51) provides a reproducible score helpful in detecting abnormalities, quantifying severity, localizing the type of problem, and serving as a baseline measure for assessing change over time.

The clinician should also assess the patient's mobility level and degree of independence in doing activities of daily living to realistically appraise the risk for falling. Patients with risk factors who engage in little independent physical activity may have a lower risk for falling than patients with risk factors who are ambulatory and try to do activities of daily living independently. If restraints are being used, the clinician should carefully review the rationale for their use and discuss alternative strategies with the resident and staff.

Laboratory evaluation should be considered on an individual patient basis and could include several key tests when the cause is not obvious: complete blood counts to search for anemia or infection; tests of serum sodium, potassium, glucose, and creatinine levels; electrocardiography to document arrhythmia; and thyroid function tests because occult thyroid disease may be difficult to diagnose clinically. Even then, the clinical evaluation and initial laboratory tests may not detect an intermittent problem that may have caused the fall (orthostatic changes, arrhythmias, and electrolyte disturbances, for example). More extensive testing may be indicated depending on the causes entertained after the initial history and physical examination.

An ambulatory cardiac (Holter) monitor is advisable when a transient arrhythmia is suspected by history, in cases of syncope, or when the patient with unexplained falls has a history of cardiac disease and receives cardiac medication; however, it should not be part of the routine evaluation after the fall. The likelihood of finding fall-relevant abnormalities on Holter monitoring in elderly residents, regardless of fall status, is particularly high. In one study done among nursing home residents, 82% of persons who had fallen and those who had not fallen had ventricular arrhythmias documented on Holter monitoring, and 100% had supraventricular

arrhythmias (52); none were symptomatic during the Holter monitoring. Because transient arrhythmias are so prevalent among the elderly, it is often unclear whether a monitored abnormality is related to the fall unless corresponding symptoms are noted during the monitoring process.

The value of assessing a patient after a fall has been reported by two study groups (14,53). In a descriptive study, an assessment done by a multidisciplinary falls consultation team in a nursing home uncovered new diagnoses and led to a reduction in the number of future falls (53). In a randomized trial of an intervention involving assessment after a fall (14), nursing home residents who received a comprehensive assessment after they fell by a nurse practitioner experienced significant reductions in the number of hospitalizations (26%) and days spent in the hospital (52%) over 2 years compared with controls. Although patients receiving intervention were found to have lower fall and mortality rates (9% fewer falls and 17% fewer deaths), these trends did not reach statistical significance. This study strongly suggests that falls are markers of underlying disorders easily identifiable by a careful assessment after the fall, which, in turn, can be treated with reduction in disability.

This type of assessment to detect risk factors for falls has also been frequently recommended for inclusion in the periodic physical examination of frail nursing home residents (27,30). Despite the logic and appeal of such an approach, the efficacy of screening residents for these risk factors on admission or periodically as a fall prevention strategy remains to be proven.

THERAPY AND PREVENTION

Once the clinician has uncovered the possible cause or causes of the fall and additional risk factors, the most challenging aspect of the fall evaluation process begins—prescribing effective treatments and interventions to prevent future falls. Because of the multifactorial nature of falls, it should be expected that there is no standard approach to treatment and prevention. The clinician must develop an individual plan for each patient, considering intrinsic risk factors, the patient's functional level, and how treatment will affect quality of life. When a fall is caused by an obvious acute problem, treatment may be relatively simple, direct, and effective (for example, discontinuing therapy with medication that causes postural hypotension). However, most patients fall because of chronic interacting conditions, and treatment will require a combination of medical, rehabilitative, environmental, and behavioral intervention strategies (for example, treating an underlying cause of syncope, lowering bed height, and advising a patient to wear safe footwear). In other cases, the intervention required to prevent falls (for example, limiting ambulation and using restraints) may be more detrimental to the patient than a possible fall.

The types of treatment interventions for major risk factors for falls that have been proposed or studied are discussed below. Although clinical and empirical evidence suggest that risk factors for falls can be treated, few data are available to confirm that such treatment interventions actually prevent falls. The ability to establish the efficacy of fall prevention interventions is undoubtedly limited by the fact that falls have multiple confounding causes that require many different interventions. Patient compliance with interventions, especially among frail and cognitively impaired patients, is also a potential problem. In addition, because many falls are probably not preventable, studies need a large sample size to show an effect. Another consideration complicating the formulation of fall prevention strategies is the two-edged effect of physical activity on falls. Activity is and should be encouraged as a positive goal that can lead to higher function and quality of life; however, activity also facilitates the opportunity for falling and injuries. Although not well studied, active persons may have more falls overall but may also have fewer falls per unit of activity. These interactions among falls, activity levels, frailty, and injury need to be studied much more carefully. Currently, many large randomized trials are being done to study fall prevention strategies for nursing home and community-dwelling older persons (54), and these should provide some additional results that can be translated into practice guidelines. Until that time, identification of risk factors, especially those associated with injurious falls, and focused treatment interventions appear to be the most sensible approach to fall prevention.

Weakness and Impaired Function

As noted previously, muscle weakness and functional impairments are important risk factors for

falls and are often interrelated. Treatment should focus on improving strength and endurance, which should improve functional ability. Unfortunately, rehabilitation efforts in the nursing home tend to focus on treating conditions after an acute event (for example, stroke and hip fracture) rather than on trying to maintain or improve strength and function. Several studies of exercise interventions to improve muscle strength have been done with mixed results in persons living in institutions. In one uncontrolled study of an 8-week exercise program among frail nursing home residents with a mean age of 90 years, remarkable increases in muscle strength, a 9% increase in the mid-thigh muscle area, and a 48% increase in mean tandem gait speed were seen (55). In addition, two patients no longer needed an assistive device for ambulation. In a randomized trial, frail nursing home residents received 4 months of physical therapy or friendly visits. Although the rates of falls did not decrease, the experimental group did show a 15% improvement in mobility and a reduced use of assistive devices and wheelchairs (56). Noteworthy in both studies is that mobility improved, which suggests that patients were more functionally independent.

In addition to physical therapy or exercise training programs, simple walking programs may also improve strength and function. Residents should be encouraged to be as physically active as possible, even if that only consists of walking with assistance a few minutes each day, as long as it can be done with reasonable safety.

Gait and Balance Impairments

Residents with gait and balance disturbances should be evaluated for the underlying process. This can usually be categorized after examination into problems with strength, sensation, pain, joint mobility, spasticity, or central processing or commonly a combination of these (57). Treatment approaches should be tailored accordingly but generally involve programs of gait training, specific exercises, and prescription of assistive devices. Gait training, usually under the supervision of a physical therapist, can be particularly helpful for persons with stroke, hip fracture, arthritis, or parkinsonism. Exercise interventions for weakness have been discussed above. Assistive devices include walkers, crutches, canes, orthotics, and shoe modification. Because the assistive device must be tailored individually, it should be prescribed in consultation with a physiatrist or physical therapist. Residents should be referred to a podiatrist for foot problems such as toe deformities and calluses.

Dizziness Syndromes

As with gait and balance problems, treatment approaches to dizziness depend on the underlying cause, whether it be hypofusion (from such things as hypotension, arrhythmias, or local ischemia), vestibular problems, drug effects, or other less common disorders. A thorough evaluation to determine the cause is thus imperative (58), and useful individualized treatments can usually be devised. For example, patients with benign positional vertigo may benefit from learning desensitization exercises (59). Antihistamines and antiemetic agents, which are often prescribed to treat vertigo, should be used with caution because of their tendency to sedate or cause confusion in older persons.

Postural Hypotension

As noted previously, postural hypotension can also stem from many causes. Hypotension caused by hypovolemia or drugs has obvious therapeutic approaches. More difficult is treating postural hypotension that is caused by autonomic dysfunction, which is particularly common among patients with diabetes and parkinsonism. Several techniques may help residents with persistent orthostatic hypotension caused by autonomic dysfunction: sleeping in a bed with the head raised to minimize a sudden decrease in blood pressure on rising; wearing elastic stockings to minimize venous pooling in the legs; rising slowly or sitting on the side of the bed for several minutes before standing up; and avoiding heavy meals and activity in hot weather. If such conservative measures are ineffective, the volume of circulating blood can be increased by liberalizing dietary salt, provided that associated medical conditions are not a contraindication. Rarely, if disabling postural hypotension persists, mineralocorticoid therapy can be initiated with low doses of fludrocortisone acetate (Florinef; Apothecon, Princeton, New Jersey); a dose of 0.1 to 0.2 mg/d will usually suffice in elderly patients. Extreme caution must be used to avoid precipitating congestive heart failure, fluid overload, hypokalemia, and hypertension.

Polypharmacy and Inappropriate Medications

The goal of the clinician should be to reduce the number of medications taken by the resident. When choosing medications, the clinician should consider drugs that are least associated with postural hypotension, are short-acting, and are less likely to have sedative effects. Numerous interventions to improve prescribing practices and reduce the incidence of polypharmacy in nursing homes have been studied (60). In most of these studies, the intervention has consisted of a consultant pharmacist reviewing medication orders and recommending treatment to physicians and nurses. Positive outcomes shown by these interventions include reductions in the number of drugs prescribed per patient and the number of doses taken per patient; however, a corresponding reduction in the number of falls has not been documented specifically.

Although we have focused on specific interventions for individual residents, fall prevention strategies have also been recommended and tested at the institutional level. These include environmental assessment, nursing interventions, and technological devices.

Environmental Assessment

The environmental assessment identifies and removes potential hazards (for example, clutter, poor lighting, and uneven floor surfaces) and modifies the environment to improve mobility and safety (for example, installation of grab bars and raised toilet seats and the lowering of the bed height). Specific environmental interventions should include the following: adequate lighting in all hallways and stairwells, bathroom grab bars next to the toilet and in the tubs or shower, nonskid mats in tubs or shower, raised toilet seats, handrails in the hallways, secure stairway banisters, and furniture that is easy to rise from. Of special importance is bed height. Most beds are adjustable and are often in an inappropriately raised position for the convenience of the staff. Proper bed height is such that when the patient sits on the side of the bed with feet touching the floor, the knees are bent at a 90-degree angle. Furniture can also be rearranged to support an unstable patient for ambulation to the bathroom. Box 8.2 lists the most important items to include in an environmental assessment, which are based on published safety checklists and guidelines (61).

BOX 8.2. Environmental assessment: summary of the most important items

Floor Surfaces
  Wall-to-wall, low-pile carpeting should be used
  Carpet edges should be tacked down
  Wood or vinyl floors should be kept dry and clean
  Nonskid wax should be used
  Thresholds should be removed or no higher than
    1/2" and beveled
Lighting
  Hallways and stairs should be well lit
  Reduce glare by using lamp shades and frosted
    light bulbs
  Light switches should be easily accessible
Bedroom
  Mattress should be firm
  Bed height should allow the patient's feet to touch
    the floor with knees at a 90-degree angle when
    sitting on the edge of the bed
  Bedside table should be accessible from the bed
  Call button and light should be accessible from
    the bed
  Furniture should be arranged to provide support
    for patient when walking
Bathroom
  Floors should have nonslip surface
  Grab bars should be attached to wall next to toilet
    and in bathtub or shower
  Toilet seat should be at height to allow easy
    transferring
  Shower seat and nonslip appliques should be used
    in bathtub or shower

Although not usually considered a part of the environment, proper footwear is important for safety. Ill-fitting shoes, shoes with worn soles and heels, heels that are too high or too narrow, or shoes left untied or unbuckled are unsafe. The habit of many nursing home residents of wearing slippers without soles or backs or wearing stockings without shoes is particularly hazardous. A study that examined the stability of older men when barefoot and when wearing different types of shoes showed that shoes with thin, hard soles provide the most stability (62).

Nursing Interventions

Nursing practice interventions are probably the most widely used fall prevention strategies in institutional settings. The goal of most current nursing interventions is to identify at admission residents who are at high risk for falling and to institute appropriate precautions. To assist in the identification of such high-risk residents, fall assessment tools have been developed and described in the literature

(12,63). Using these tools, the nursing staff assesses such factors as mental status, history of falls, ambulation status, medications, physical status, continence, and sensory deficits. A resident's status for risk for falling is determined by either the number of risk factors present or by a summary score (11,62). Once a resident has been identified as being at high risk for falling, a nursing care plan is usually developed that includes interventions aimed at injury prevention. Such interventions include indicating on the medical chart and the resident's door that the resident is at high risk for falls, moving high-risk residents to rooms close to the nursing station to increase observation, periodically reassessing residents after new episodes of illness or change in medication, lowering side-rails and bed heights for residents who climb out of bed, increasing the nurse-to-resident ratio, and instituting fall prevention education for residents and staff.

Few published reports have supported the validity of assessment tools or the effectiveness of these types of prevention programs. However, one recent study (63) reported high reliability and validity of a scored fall assessment tool developed to identify hospitalized patients at high risk for falling. Implementing this tool, using standardized nursing care plans for high-risk patients, and installing new safety equipment (such as safety vests and bed alarm systems) resulted in an average 20% decrease in the number of falls during the first year of the program.

Fall Prevention Devices

Until recently, the most common "devices" that were used in the nursing home to prevent falls were physical restraints such as poseys and bedrails. In U.S. nursing homes in the 1980s, the reported prevalence of restraint use ranged from 25% to 85% of residents (64). This is in marked contrast to rates in many European countries and to current recommendations that restraints be used only in relatively rare and well-documented situations in which less restrictive measures are clearly unfeasible (65). Since the new federal regulations went into effect in 1990 (65), there has been a major move away from the use of physical restraints, and research has shown that the adverse effects of physical restraints on functional status and quality of life are worse than any potential benefit in preventing falls (66). Specifically, evidence suggests that physical restraints actually contribute to falls (7), injuries (18), and death (67).

Nursing homes are now beginning to look at reducing the use of physical restraints by implementing individualized care alternatives such as alterations in nursing care (as described previously) and environmental changes. In one nursing home where care alternatives were implemented, physical restraints were successfully removed in 92% of previously restrained residents (68). One of the reasons that many nursing homes have been reluctant to discontinue the use of restraints has been the fear of potential legal liability for injuries sustained by an unrestrained patient (65). However, no nursing home has ever been held legally liable for injuries to a resident solely on the basis of failing to apply restraints. Rather, lawsuits against nursing homes have been successful on the basis of injuries associated with the use of restraints (65). Given these legal realities, clinicians should be more aggressive in finding alternatives to restraints and should help residents and their families understand that all falls may not be preventable and that the risk for a fall is often preferable to restraints.

Several devices that alert caregivers to patient movement or that protect patients from injuries from falls are currently being developed and marketed as possible alternatives to restraints for many high-risk patients. The most widely available devices are various alarm systems that are activated when patients try to get out of bed or move unassisted. One such alarm system was pilot-tested on an orthopedic and a general medicine hospital ward. Preliminary 5-month data indicated that the number of patient falls was reduced 33% and 45% on each ward, respectively (69). An infrared scanning system that activates an alarm in the nursing station when a patient sits up or gets out of bed was found to reduce the incidence of nighttime falls from 2.8 to 1.0 falls per month when installed on a psychogeriatric unit (70). Video recording systems are also being used as a means of providing closer monitoring of patient activities (71).

Injury-prevention alternatives such as hip protective pads are also being tested but are not generally available. A recent Danish study (72) tested hip protective pads in a nursing home where hip fractures had been extremely common. In wards randomly assigned to use the pads, hip fracture rates were markedly lower than those in the comparison wards, with a risk reduction of almost 60%. Even more striking was that no hip fractures occurred among patients actually wearing external hip pads.

CONCLUSION

Research in the nursing home has verified the complex multifactorial causes of falls. Many specific identifiable risk factors substantially increase the risk for falls and fall-related injuries. The clinician should focus on identifying these risk factors and intervening actively to prevent future falls. Although further research is needed, evidence suggests that a vigorous diagnostic, therapeutic, and preventive approach should be used for all nursing home residents who fall, as well as for those identified as being at high risk for falling.

REFERENCES

1. Hogue C. Injury in late life: I. Epidemiology. J Am Geriatr Soc. 1982;30:183-90.
2. Hogue C. Injury in late life: II. Prevention. J Am Geriatr Soc. 1982;30:276-80.
3. Gryfe CI, Amies A, Ashley MJ. A longitudinal study of falls in an elderly population: I. Incidence and morbidity. Age Ageing. 1977;6:201-10.
4. Pablo RY. Patient accidents in a long-term-care facility. Can J Public Health. 1977;68:237-47.
5. Feist RR. A survey of accidental falls in a small home for the aged. J Gerontol Nurs. 1978;4:15-7.
6. Cacha CA. An analysis of the 1976 incident reports of the Carillon nursing home. J Am Health Care Assoc. 1979;5:29-33.
7. Miller MB, Elliott DF. Accidents in nursing homes: Implications for patients and administrators. In: Miller MB, ed. Current Issues in Clinical Geriatrics. New York: Tiresias Press; 1979:97-137.
8. Louis M. Falls and their causes. J Gerontol Nurs. 1983;9:143-9, 156.
9. Colling J, Park D. Home, safe home. J Gerontol Nurs. 1983;9:175-9, 192.
10. Blake C, Morfitt JM. Falls and staffing in a residential home for elderly people. Public Health. 1986; 100:385-91.
11. Berry G, Fisher RH, Lang S. Detrimental incidents, including falls, in an elderly institutional population. J Am Geriatr Soc. 1981;29:322-4.
12. Berryman E, Gaskin D, Jones A, Tolley F, MacMullen J. Point by point: Predicting elders' falls. Geriatr Nurs (New York). 1989;10:199-201.
13. Gross YT, Shimamoto Y, Rose CL, Frank B. Why do they fall? Monitoring risk factors in nursing homes. J Gerontol Nurs. 1990;16:20-5.
14. Rubenstein LZ, Robbins AS, Josephson KR, Schulman BL, Osterweil D. The value of assessing falls in an elderly population. A randomized clinical trial. Ann Intern Med. 1990;113:308-16.
15. Gostynski M. Haufigkeit, Umstande und Konsequenzen von Sturzen institutionalisierter Betagter; eine Pilotstudie. Soz Praventivmed. 1991;36:341-5.

16. Neufeld RR, Tideiksaar R, Yew E, Brooks F, Young J, Browne G, et al. A multidisciplinary falls consultation service in a nursing home. Gerontologist. 1991;31:120-3.
17. Svensson ML, Rundgren A, Larsson M, Oden A, Sund V, Landahl S. Accidents in the institutionalized elderly: a risk analysis. Aging (Milano). 1991;3:181-92.
18. Tinetti ME, Liu WL, Ginter SF. Mechanical restraint use and fall-related injuries among residents of skilled nursing facilities. Ann Intern Med. 1992;116:369-74.
19. Baker SP, Harvey AH. Falls injuries in the elderly. Clin Geriatr Med. 1985;1:501-7.
20. Rhymes J, Jaeger R. Falls. Prevention and management in the institutional setting. Clin Geriatr Med. 1988;4:613-22.
21. Lipsitz LA, Jonsson PV, Kelley MM, Koestner JS. Causes and correlates of recurrent falls in ambulatory frail elderly. J Gerontol. 1991;46:M114-22.
22. Brocklehurst JC, Exton-Smith AN, Lempert-Barber SM, Hunt LP, Palmer MK. Fractures of the femur in old age: A two-centre study of associated clinical factors and the cause of the fall. Age Ageing. 1978;7:2-15.
23. Clark AN. Factors in fracture of the female femur. A clinical study of the environmental, physical, medical and preventative aspects of this injury. Geront Clin (Basel). 1968;10:257-70.
24. Exton-Smith AN. Functional consequences of aging: clinical manifestations. In: Exton-Smith AN, Evans JG, eds. Care of the Elderly: Meeting the Challenge of Dependency. London: Academic Press; 1977:41-57.
25. Lucht U. A prospective study of accidental falls and injuries in the home among elderly people. Acta Sociomed Scand. 1971;2:105-20.
26. Morfitt JM. Falls in old people at home: intrinsic versus environmental factors in causation. Public Health. 1983;97:115-20.
27. Robbins AS, Rubenstein LZ, Josephson KR, Schulman BL, Osterweil D, Fine G. Predictors of falls among elderly people. Results of two population-based studies. Arch Intern Med. 1989;149:1628-33.
28. Sheldon JH. On the natural history of falls in old age. Br Med J. 1960;2:1685-90.
29. Campbell AJ, Borrie MJ, Spears GF. Risk factors for falls in a community-based prospective study of people 70 years and older. J Gerontol. 1989;44:M112-17.
30. Tinetti ME, Williams TF, Mayewski R. Fall risk index for elderly patients based on number of chronic disabilities. Am J Med. 1986;80:429-34.
31. Sudarsky L. Geriatrics: gait disorders in the elderly. N Engl J Med. 1990;322:1441-6.
32. Hing E, Sekscenski E, Strahan G. The National Nursing Home Survey: 1985 summary for the United States. Vital and Health Statistics. Series 13, No. 97. DHHS Pub. No. (PHS) 89-1758. Public Health Service. Washington, D.C.: U.S. Government Printing Office; 1989.
33. Murray MP, Gardner GM, Mollinger LA, Sepic SB. Strength of isometric and isokinetic contractions: Knee muscles of men aged 20 to 86. Phys Ther. 1980;60:412-9.
34. Ashley MJ, Gryfe CI, Amies A. A longitudinal study of falls in an elderly population. II. Some circumstances of falling. Age Ageing. 1977;6:211-20.
35. Stewart RB, Moore MT, May FE, Marks RG, Hale WE. Nocturia: A risk factor for falls in the elderly. J Am Geriatr Soc. 1992;40:1217-20.
36. Robbins AS, Rubenstein LZ. Postural hypotension in the elderly. J Am Geriatr Soc. 1984;32:769-74.
37. Mader SL, Josephson KR, Rubenstein LZ. Low prevalence of postural hypotension among community-dwelling elderly. JAMA. 1987;258:1511-4.
38. Lipsitz LA, Fullerton KJ. Postprandial blood pressure reduction in healthy elderly. J Am Geriatr Soc. 1986;34:267-70.
39. Jonsson PV, Lipsitz LA, Kelley M, Koestner J. Hypotensive responses to common daily activities in institutionalized elderly. A potential risk for recurrent falls. Arch Intern Med. 1990;150:1518-24.
40. Tinetti ME, Liu WL, Claus EB. Predictors and prognosis of inability to get up after falls among elderly persons. JAMA. 1993;269:65-70.
41. Lipsitz LA, Wei JY, Rowe JW. Syncope in an elderly, institutionalized population: prevalence, incidence, and associated risks. Q J Med. 1985;55:45-55.
42. Granek E, Baker SP, Abbey H, Robinson E, Myers AH, Samkoff JS, et al. Medications and diagnoses in relation to falls in a long-term care facility. J Am Geriatr Soc. 1987;35:503-11.
43. Myers AH, Baker SP, Van Natta ML, Abbey H, Robinson EG. Risk factors associated with falls and injuries among elderly institutionalized persons. Am J Epidemiol. 1991;133:1179-90.
44. Wolfson L, Whipple R, Amerman P, Tobin JN. Gait assessment in the elderly: a gait abnormality rating scale and its relation to falls. J Gerontol. 1990;45:M12-9.
45. Whipple RH, Wolfson LI, Amerman PM. The relationship of knee and ankle weakness to falls in nursing home residents: an isokinetic study. J Am Geriatr Soc. 1987;35:13-20.
46. Wells BG, Middleton B, Lawrence G, Lillard D, Safarik J. Factors associated with the elderly falling in intermediate care facilities. Drug Intell Clin Pharm. 1985;19:142-5.
47. Kerman M, Mulvihill M. The role of medication in falls among the elderly in a long-term care facility. Mt Sinai J Med. 1990;57:343-7.
48. Aisen PS, Deluca T, Lawlor BA. Falls among geropsychiatry inpatients are associated with PRN medications for agitation. International Journal of Geriatric Psychiatry. 1992;7:709-12.
49. Tinetti ME. Factors associated with serious injury during falls by ambulatory nursing home residents. J Am Geriatr Soc. 1987;35:644-48.
50. Ray WA, Griffin MR, Schaffner W, Baugh DK, Melton LJ 3d. Psychotropic drug use and the risk of

hip fracture. N Engl J Med. 1987;316:363-9.

51. Tinetti ME. Performance-oriented assessment of mobility problems in elderly patients. J Am Geriatr Soc. 1986;34:119-26.

52. Rosado JA, Rubenstein LZ, Robbins AS, Heng MK, Schulman BL, Josephson KR. The value of Holter monitoring in evaluating the elderly patient who falls. J Am Geriatr Soc. 1989;37:430-4.

53. Neufeld RR, Tideiksaar R, Yew E, Brooks F, Young J, Browne G, et al. A multidisciplinary falls consultation service in a nursing home. Gerontologist. 1991;31:120-3.

54. Ory MG, Schechtman KB, Miller JP, Hadley EC, Fiatarone MA, Province MA, et al. Frailty and injuries in later life: The FICSIT trials. J Am Geriatr Soc. 1993;41:283-343.

55. Fiatarone MA, Marks EC, Ryan ND, Meredith CN, Lipsitz LA, Evans WJ. High-intensity strength training in nonagenarians. Effects of skeletal muscle. JAMA. 1990;263:3029-34.

56. Mulrow CD, Gerety MB, Kanten D, Cornell JE, DeNino LA, Chiodo L, et al. A randomized trial of physical rehabilitation for very frail nursing home residents. JAMA. 1994;271:519-24.

57. Trueblood PR, Rubenstein LZ. Assessment of instability and gait in elderly persons. Compr Ther. 1991; 17:20-9.

58. Froehling DA, Silverstein MD, Mohr DN, Beatty CW. Does this dizzy patient have a serious form of vertigo? JAMA. 1994;271:385-8.

59. Norré ME, Beckers A. Benign paroxysmal positional vertigo in the elderly. Treatment by habitual exercises. J Am Geriatr Soc. 1988;36:425-9.

60. Gurwitz JH, Soumerai SB, Avorn J. Improving medication prescribing and utilization in the nursing home. J Am Geriatr Soc. 1990;38:542-52.

61. Rubenstein LZ, Robbins AS, Schulman BL, Rosado J, Osterweil D, Josephson KR. Falls and instability in the elderly [Clinical Conference]. J Am Geriatr Soc. 1988;36:266-78.

62. Robbins S, Gouw GJ, McClaran J. Shoe sole thickness and hardness influence balance in older men. J Am Geriatr Soc. 1992;40:1089-94.

63. Schmid NA. 1989 Federal Nursing Service Award Winner. Reducing patient falls: a research-based comprehensive fall prevention program. Mil Med. 1990;155:202-7.

64. Schnelle JF, Simmons SF, Ory MG. Risk factors that predict staff failure to release nursing home residents from restraints. Gerontologist. 1992;32:767-70.

65. Kapp MB. Nursing home restraints and legal liability. Merging the standard of care and industry practice. J Leg Med. 1992;13:1-32.

66. Evans LK, Strumpf NE, Williams C. Redefining a standard of care for frail older people: Alternatives to routine physical restraint. In: Katz PR, Kane RL, Mezey MD, eds. Advances in Long-term Care. New York: Springer Publishing Company; 1991:81-101.

67. Miles SH, Irvine P. Deaths caused by physical restraints. Gerontologist. 1992;32:762-6.

68. Werner P, Koroknay V, Braun J, Cohen-Mansfield J. Individualized care alternatives used in the process of removing physical restraints in the nursing home. J Am Geriatr Soc. 1994;42:321-5.

69. Widder B. A new device to decrease falls. Geriatr Nurs (New York). 1985;6:287-8.

70. Duber NP, Creech R. Using infrared scanning to decrease nighttime falls on a psychogeriatric unit. Hosp Community Psychiatry. 1988;39:79-81.

71. Connell BR. Patterns of naturally occurring falls among frail nursing home residents. Gerontologist. 1993;33:58.

72. Lauritzen JB, Petersen MM, Lund B. Effect of external hip protectors on hip fractures. Lancet. 1993; 341:11-3.

9

Nutrition

John E. Morley, MB, BCh, and Andrew Jay Silver, MD

Malnutrition (the state produced by intake of either too few macronutrients or too many micronutrients) of many types is common in nursing home residents. Protein energy undernutrition is endemic in nursing homes, with a prevalence ranging from 17% to 65% (Table 9.1). Protein energy undernutrition has been associated with decubitus ulcers, cognitive problems, postural hypotension, infections, and anemia (1). In community nursing homes, nutritional deficiencies have been associated with increased hospitalizations (2), and, in Veterans Affairs intermediate care (Geriatric Evaluation and Management Units) and nursing homes, protein energy undernutrition has been associated with increased infections, hospitalizations, and mortality (3–5). Obesity is less common in nursing home residents, but when it occurs, it can be associated with immobility, decreased functional status, intertriginous infections, and the development of decubitus ulcers. Residents often have low blood levels of water-soluble vitamins; folate and pyridoxine deficiencies are the most common vitamin deficiencies (6). Low vitamin C levels have been associated with decubitus ulcers (7), and protein energy undernutrition and vitamin D deficiency are important factors in the pathogenesis of hip fractures, a frequent cause of morbidity and mortality in residents (8). Vitamin supplementation improves immune function and decreases infection rates in community-dwelling older persons (9). Residents are also at high risk for trace mineral deficiencies,

and both zinc and selenium deficiency can aggravate immune deficiency and delay wound healing (1). Inadequate fluid intake leads to dehydration, hypotension, and, in persons with diabetes mellitus, hyperosmolarity. Finally, food intake itself can cause postprandial hypotension (which, in turn, can precipitate falls), produce shifts in electrolytes due to insulin release, and, in persons with dysphagia or cognitive problems, result in aspiration pneumonia.

PROTEIN ENERGY UNDERNUTRITION

Causes

In nursing home residents, weight loss may occur because of any of several reasons. In some cases, the physician can do little to stop the weight loss (for example, when the cause is cancer or end-stage disease such as that seen with cardiac cachexia). However, because most causes of weight loss in elderly patients can be treated, the physician should concentrate on identifying undernutrition and on reversing the causes and risk factors of malnutrition (10) (Box 9.1). A recent study of weight loss among community nursing home residents suggested that a potential cause could be found in most cases (11).

A physiologic cause of weight loss is a decrease in the resting metabolic rate. One study reported decreases of 20% in elderly men and 13% in elderly women (12). A decrease in the resting metabolic rate

TABLE 9.1. Prevalence of protein energy undernutrition in nursing homes*

Study (Reference)	Patients, n	Age, y	Nutritional Status
Shaver et al. (77)	115	Male, 79.9 ± 9.0	<90% ABW: 42.5%; albumin <35 g/L: 32.1%
		Female, 80.9 ± 9.9	
Muncie and Carbonetto (78)	30	63.5 ± 21.0	<90% ABW: 47%; albumin <35 g/L: 60%
Pinchofsky-Devin and Kaminski (79)	232	72.9 ± 12	PEU: 59%
Siebens et al. (27)	240	81.7 ± 9.5	Dependent eaters: 32%
Sandman et al. (26)	44	76.0 ± 8.0	PEU: 50%
Rudman and Feller (80)†	176	69	<90% ABW: 60.9%; albumin <36.9 g/L: 37%
Silver et al. (36)†	88	78 ± 9	Albumin <35 g/L: 24%; <80% ABW: 23%; weight loss >20 lb: 45%; anergic: 44%
Thomas et al. (81)	50	76 ± 13	PEU: 54%
Abbasi and Rudman (82)†‡	26 institutions		80% ABW: 2% 20%; albumin >35 g/L: 5% 58%
Ferguson et al. (83)	81	83.1	99% of residents admitted to acute hospital had an albumin level >35 g/L

* The studies used differing definitions of protein energy undernutrition (PEU). Insufficient data were available to reconcile these differences, and therefore PEU is defined by the individual authors. Means are expressed ± SD. ABW = average body weight.
† Study done in Veterans Affairs nursing homes (predominantly male).
‡ No patient count or age given in study.

is accompanied by diminished food intake, which may be due to a decrease in the endogenous opioid (dynorphin) feeding drive and an increase in the satiation effect of the gut hormone cholecystokinin (13). Malnutrition, in turn, increases circulating cholecystokinin levels in older persons, which may further decrease appetite (14).

Adverse drug effects and depression are the most common reversible causes of protein energy undernutrition. Medications can induce weight loss by causing anorexia, nausea, vomiting, diarrhea, constipation, cognitive disturbance, or increased metabolism. Medications that commonly cause these side effects include digitalis, psychotropic agents, fluoxetine, sertraline, and theophylline (anorexia); erythromycin, aspirin, and nonsteroidal anti-inflammatory drugs (gastrointestinal irritation); narcotics and calcium channel antagonists (constipation); theophylline suspension (diarrhea due to sorbitol vehicle); all psychotropic agents, clonidine, and metoclopramide (cognitive disturbance); and excess dosage of l-thyroxine or theophylline (increased metabolism). Recently we noted that in some residents (after the Omnibus Budget Reconciliation Act [OBRA] 1987 mandate) who received long-term therapy with psychotropic drugs, severe weight loss developed when the therapy was discontinued (11).

Depression occurs in 8% to 38% of nursing home residents (15). Depression is more likely to be associated with anorexia and weight loss in older persons than in younger persons (15). Katz and colleagues (16) reported that, in residents, "failure to thrive" was closely correlated with depression, and an analysis of 6832 minimum data sets from 202 nursing homes in seven states showed that depression was associated with weight loss (17). Poor oral intake, eating dependency, decubiti, and chewing problems were associated with both low body mass index and weight loss. In one community nursing home study, one third of residents with weight loss had depression (11), and in another study, patients regained their weight after depression was appropriately treated (18).

Anorexia nervosa has also been reported in the geriatric population. In some patients, it may be the recurrence of a pre-existing condition, but in others, anorexia nervosa occurs for the first time in later life, in which case it is termed anorexia tardive. These patients may display certain oral control patterns, such as avoiding eating when hungry (19). Thus, one needs to consider abnormal eating attitudes when looking for causes of weight loss.

In the case of late-life paranoia, the resident may believe that she or he is being poisoned and refuse to eat. Other residents refuse to eat as a way of

BOX 9.1. Mnemonic for treatable causes of malnutrition in nursing home residents*

Medications
Emotional problems (depression)
Anorexia tardive (nervosa); alcoholism
Late-life paranoia
Swallowing disorders

Oral factors
No money (insufficient funds in Medicaid facilities for palatable, individualized diets and consultant dietitian)

Wandering and other dementia-related behavior
Hyperthyroidism, hyperparathyroidism, hypoadrenalism
Enteric problems (malabsorption)
Eating problems (inability to feed oneself)
Low-salt, low-cholesterol diets
Social problems (ethnic food preferences, isolation, "disgusting" food habits of other residents)

* The mnemonic "MEALS ON WHEELS" is adapted from our previously published mnemonic for the ambulatory elderly (12).

manipulating the staff. Older persons who see that a malnourished resident receives special attention during feeding times may stop eating to increase the time that the staff spend socializing with them.

Swallowing disorders are another cause of decreased food intake, and these may result from cerebrovascular accidents, neuromuscular disorders, generalized weakness, dementia, or Parkinson disease. Residents with Parkinson disease and Huntington chorea also lose weight because of the increased metabolism associated with their increased movements.

At least 80% of nursing home residents have some degree of tooth loss (20). Half of the residents who wear dentures need replacement or relining of their dentures, and approximately one third of residents have mucosal lesions. In another study, untreated dental decay was present in 70% of residents (21). Oral health factors such as these can result in decreased nutrient intake. Although two community-based studies failed to find a correlation between oral health and weight loss (22,23), a Veterans Affairs based study found that oral health problems were a significant predictor of weight loss (24). In addition, problems with olfaction, taste, and xerostomia may decrease the enjoyment of eating. Nursing home residents often do not receive adequate dental care. Increasing the use of dental tech-

nicians may be one solution to this problem.

Nursing homes that are funded primarily through Medicaid are limited in what they can spend on food. Thus, diets may become monotonous, and it may be impossible for the facility to meet individual dietary preferences or to cater to the preferences of separate ethnic groups. The lack of reimbursement for food supplements tends to discourage the early use of supplements to prevent the development of malnutrition. Recently, it has been demonstrated in Veterans Affairs nursing homes that the nutritional status of residents can be related to the cost of care, with better nutritional status seen in residents when more money was spent on care (25).

A large proportion of patients with cognitive impairment have protein or energy undernutrition despite adequate reported intakes (26). Many cognitively impaired residents cannot feed themselves, and a disproportionate amount of overall nursing home costs are spent on the management of "dependent eaters." In one study, the inability to feed oneself was the reason for institutionalization in 18% of patients (27). Causes of weight loss in patients with dementia include swallowing difficulties (especially in patients with multi-infarct dementia), insufficient time spent on feeding because adequate staff are not available, and infections caused by the fact that protein needs are not being met. Residents who pace all day may need greater nutritional intake to compensate for their energy expenditure. No evidence of an increased catabolic state that causes weight loss has been found in cognitively impaired persons (28).

Metabolic disorders such as hyperthyroidism and hyperparathyroidism are not uncommon causes of weight loss in older persons, but both may be overlooked because of unusual presentations in this age group. Patients may present with decreases in serum albumin, the carrier protein for calcium, which may obscure the presence of the hypercalcemia of hyperparathyroidism for the hurried physician; however, free calcium levels or simultaneous albumin levels clarify the diagnosis. Persons with hyperthyroidism may have a coexisting euthyroid sick syndrome, resulting in high normal thyroid function levels and making diagnosis extremely complicated. Pheochromocytoma should be considered in residents who are hypertensive despite weight loss.

Older persons who have tremors may spill much of their food simply in transporting it from the plate to the mouth; a heavy-handled spoon is easier for these persons to hold and helps them avoid such "spills." Persons with stroke disability may fail to eat meat because it is too difficult for them to cut. In this case, a rocker-bottom knife may enable such persons to feed themselves. Residents of nursing homes may also find it difficult to eat because of inappropriate positioning at the table and because of weakness.

Malabsorption should always be considered as a cause of malnutrition. The differential diagnosis includes late-life onset of gluten enteropathy, particularly in residents with diabetes mellitus.

Low-salt, low-cholesterol diets are unpalatable and are often associated with protein energy malnutrition and postural hypotension in older persons. Two recent studies have shown that weight loss, low albumin levels, and orthostatism are associated with therapeutic diets (29,30). In the nursing home, special diets should therefore be avoided whenever possible. Social situations may be another cause of weight loss. Institutionalization itself produces feelings of loss of control and isolation, which can lead to a refusal to eat. Some residents find it impossible to eat when they have to share dining space with residents who have catheters, ulcers, or nasogastric tubes or who are incontinent. Residents may also find it difficult to eat with cognitively impaired residents, who may have unappetizing hygiene and eating habits.

Illnesses, such as chronic infections, are another common cause of weight loss. In persons with chronic infections, weight loss is probably secondary to the release of cytokines such as interferon or interleukins, whereas in the case of local infection (for example, with *Candida* species), weight loss may result from dysphagia. Tuberculosis may present insidiously with weight loss. Residents with chronic obstructive pulmonary disease often have protein energy undernutrition related both to an increase in energy expenditure (caused by the use of accessory muscles for breathing) and to a decrease in food intake secondary to a decrease in oxygen saturation associated with feeding.

Occasionally, older persons develop early satiation and can eat only a small proportion of their meals. During the last decade, we have successfully treated several of these persons with nitrates, believing that they had ischemic bowel disease. Recently, nitric oxide has been shown to facilitate food intake by allowing adaptive relaxation of the fundus of the stomach (31). In ongoing studies, one of us (JEM) has found that in older rats, there is a decrease in messenger RNA for nitric oxide synthase and a nitric oxide synthase inhibitor induces an increased inhibition of food intake.

EVALUATION

Recognizing the many risk factors for poor nutritional status in nursing home residents is the key to a successful evaluation and treatment plan. An interdisciplinary team can be helpful in this respect. Sometimes the simplest maneuvers are the most effective; for example, the aides or volunteers who assist with feeding can provide invaluable information about total consumption, which is likely to be more useful than calorie counts. They can also provide the dietitian with information about the residents' likes and dislikes of particular foods, and they can identify which patients have swallowing problems. The dietitian can spend time with patients discussing lifelong food habits and, together with the social worker, plan meals in accordance with the cultural diversity that may exist in a particular institution. The nursing staff can help identify persons who are compatible with each other at mealtimes, and the pharmacist can identify various potential drug nutrient interactions. Nursing home personnel can assist in evaluation, through use of formal screening tests, of mental status (for example, the Folstein Mini-Mental Status Examination), affect (for example, Yesavage depression scale), and nutritional attitudes (for example, the EAT-26 questionnaire) (19). Without input from the staff, the physician is not likely to be successful in evaluation and treatment.

Although the time that the physician is available in the nursing home remains limited, obtaining a history from the resident (when possible), staff, and family members remains the cornerstone to making the correct diagnosis. In taking the history, it is important to determine if the following are present: weakness, changes in the ability to taste, olfactory changes, abdominal pain, decreased appetite, nausea, vomiting, diarrhea, constipation, dysphagia, problems with dentition, and changes in mental or functional status. Disease states associated with weight loss are numerous and may include anemia, hip fractures, depression, dementia, decubiti, hypothyroidism, and cancer. A detailed medical and medication history is also necessary because of the numerous drug–nutrient interactions (Table 9.2). On physical examination, one may find obvious signs

TABLE 9.2. Drug–nutrient interactions*

Drug[†]	Nutrient Interaction[‡]
Alcohol	Zinc, A, B_1, B_2, B_6, folate, B_{12}
Antacids	B_1, folate, total calories
Colchicine	B_{12}
Digitalis preparation	Zinc, total calories
Diuretics	Zinc, B_6, potassium
Isoniazid	Pyridoxine, niacin
Levodopa	B_6
Laxatives (including mineral oil, fiber)	Calcium, A, D, K, E, B_2, B_{12}
Metformin	Total calories and B_{12}
Phenytoin	D
Salicylates	C, folate
Serotonin uptake inhibitors	Total calories
Theophylline preparations	Total calories
Trimethoprim	Folate

* Adapted from Silver AJ. Malnutrition. In: Beck JC, ed. Geriatric Review Syllabus: A Core Curriculum in Geriatric Medicine. 1st ed. New York: American Geriatrics Society; 1989:100.
† All drugs reduce nutrient availability.
‡ Letters refer to vitamins.

of protein energy undernutrition, such as alopecia, dependent edema, glossitis, skin desquamation, and dry, depigmented hair.

A serum albumin level less than 35 g/L has been used as the gold standard for identifying patients at risk for malnutrition. The literature provides ample support to suggest that patients with low albumin levels are at increased risk for infection, decubitus ulcers, prolonged nursing home stays, and mortality. However, the albumin level may appear to be normal on admission because of its long half-life or may be artificially high because of dehydration, and therefore, although it is helpful, the albumin level may not adequately reflect the patient's true nutritional state. Also, some data indicate that patients with albumin levels between 35 and 39 g/L have the same mortality rate as those whose levels are less than 35 g/L, suggesting that the practitioner may have to institute nutritional support earlier than previously recognized. Some patients present with marasmus—that is, they are malnourished on the basis of weight loss but maintain normal serum albumin levels. Further, because serum albumin is an acute-phase reactant, low serum albumin levels may represent an inflammatory response to the release of cytokines. Thus, although it is helpful, the serum albumin level is not necessarily the most accurate indicator of nutritional status.

Weight trends, when combined with the serum albumin level, may help better identify which residents are at risk for malnutrition. Patients who have had a weight loss of 10% or more of their total body weight over 6 months, 7.5% or more over 3 months, or 5% or more over 1 month should be studied. Patients who weigh less than 90% of age-matched controls likewise need to be evaluated. We strongly recommend that residents be weighed at least biweekly during the first month of their stay in the nursing home, especially those who are either returning from or being transferred from an acute hospital stay. In our experience, many of these residents need intervention to regain weight or improve their protein status. Furthermore, although accurate weights are difficult to obtain in many nursing homes, weight accuracy is essential in quality assurance programs.

Except for Master and colleagues' table (32), weight-for-height tables for the elderly have not been standardized. Estimates of height given during the history are also frequently inadequate, and heights are difficult to measure in some residents (for example, those who are bedridden). Alternatives to height measurement have been developed, such as knee-height and armspan measurements. However, although weight-for-height is valuable in evaluating nutritional status, studying weight trends may be more useful.

Several studies suggest that a low serum cholesterol level (<4 mmol/L) may be another useful marker of inadequate nutrition. Rudman and colleagues (5) noted a tenfold increase in mortality in patients with low cholesterol levels compared with patients with cholesterol levels of 4 mmol/L or greater. Forette and colleagues (33) likewise found low cholesterol levels to be a predictor of increased mortality in older women. Cholesterol levels should be checked in residents returning to the nursing home after an acute hospital stay, because during an acute hospital stay, elderly persons may develop hypocholesterolemia. Low cholesterol levels are also associated with cognitive impairment (34) and depression (35) in older persons.

Other methods to evaluate altered nutritional status include anthropometrics other than height and weight measurements, such as measurement of skinfold thickness or mid-arm circumference, lymphocyte count, and reactivity to skin testing. Skinfold measurements (that is, triceps and subscapular) are poorly standardized in older persons, however, and are not inter-rater reliable. Also, the lymphocyte count and presence or absence of anergy can be affected by numerous other disease states and, by themselves, add little to the evaluation process. In fact, anergy and lymphocytopenia have been reported in 10% of elderly persons, with no apparent pathology. Nevertheless, anergy in nursing homes is often associated with more severe conditions; anergic residents are more likely to have low body weight and have low serum albumin levels, and a significant association between 1-year mortality rates and anergy and albumin levels less than 35 g/L has been reported (36,37). The prognosis is even worse when anergy is combined with other low nutritional variables.

MANAGEMENT

The management of nutritional problems should be interdisciplinary and individualized. Malnourished residents should be encouraged to ingest as many calories orally as possible, but most of the more frail and compromised residents will not be able to keep up with the nutritional intake necessary to reverse their deficits. Commercially available products, either single nutrients or liquid meal replacements, should be tried before invasive techniques are used. Also, undernourished residents should be asked about their favorite foods and allowed ad libitum access to these foods. Flexible mealtimes may also help encourage food intake.

When one is considering the nutritional needs of residents, the major emphasis should be placed on caloric needs. Caloric needs can be calculated from the formula

Total caloric need
  = resting metabolic rate (RMR)
  + activity-related expenditure
  + illness-related expenditure
  + diet
  = induced thermogenesis.

RMR is calculated using the Harris–Benedict equation

$$RMR_{women} = 65.5 + (9.5 \, W) + (1.8 \, H) - (4.7 \, A)$$
$$RMR_{men} = 66 + (13.7 \, W) + (5 \, H) - (6.8 \, A)$$

where W is usual weight in kilograms, H is height in centimeters, and A is age in years.

Recently, Poehlman (28) created new equations for resting metabolic rate for older persons, which in time may prove more useful than the classic Harris–Benedict equation. In these new equations, diet-induced thermogenesis is calculated as 5% of the total energy requirements. Energy estimates for activity are 400 kcal/d for bedridden individuals, 600 kcal/d for residents who are not bedridden but who are relatively inactive, and 1200 to 1800 kcal/d for "wanderers" (residents who roam the nursing home facility freely). A further 10% of the resting metabolic rate is added when a recurrent infection or chronic obstructive pulmonary disease is present. In most cases, residents tolerate the full calculated amount of calories from admission. If osmotic diarrhea develops, caloric intake should be halved and then increased at the rate of approximately 10 kcal/h daily (or 240 kcal/d) until the appropriate caloric amount is reached. One should bear in mind, however, that many residents who are assumed to have osmotic diarrhea may later be found to have diarrhea due to pathologic causes—for example, *Clostridium difficile* infection or fecal impaction with overflow diarrhea.

Caloric intake in residents can be improved by some apparently simple maneuvers. A semicircular table that allows one aide to feed as many as three to four residents at the same time is particularly recommended. As discussed earlier, use of a heavy-handled spoon may decrease food spillage in persons with tremors, and residents with stroke disability may benefit from the use of a rocker-bottom knife, which allows them to cut their own food. Residents with swallowing problems should be positioned as erectly as possible at the table and kept from leaning forward to the plate. Avoidance of special diets (for example, low-salt, low-cholesterol and diabetic diets), except when absolutely necessary, prevents protein energy undernutrition in residents.

A nasoenteric tube may be considered for alert and functional residents who require a short course (≤2 weeks) of supplementation such as those admitted for rehabilitation after hip or knee surgery, those with decubitus ulcers, and those transferred back from the acute hospital setting. One might attempt these feedings at night (with the head of the bed elevated) to avoid interference with daytime eating.

Duodenal feeding tubes are fraught with difficulty. Radiographic evidence that the tube has passed the pyloric sphincter may be difficult to obtain. Although metoclopramide (Reglan; ACh. Robins Company, Inc., Richmond, Virginia) is often used to facilitate tube placement by increasing stomach motility, studies suggest that it does not improve success with tube intubation and may, in fact, worsen the mental state of the patient.

More patients are now entering the nursing home who have already had percutaneous endoscopically placed gastrostomy or jejunostomy tubes placed. It is possible that both of these feeding tubes are associated with fewer instances of aspiration or self-extubation than nasogastric tubes, but this has not been proven. Jejunostomy tubes should be reserved for the comatose patient, who is more likely to aspirate. Feedings placed in jejunostomy tubes must be partially digested.

Although a full discussion of the many formulas currently available for enteral feeding is beyond the scope of this article, some general comments are appropriate. Lactose-free iso-osmolar products to minimize diarrhea are favored by some clinicians. Others prefer supplements with added fiber to improve bowel function. Protein (16% to 20%) should be considered in patients with increased nitrogen needs, such as those with decubiti or infection; however, the overall caloric intake must be adequate to prevent protein metabolism as the source of energy. Finally, the physician should be aware that some polymeric diets may be missing some micronutrients; residents who are to receive tube feeding long term should continue to be weighed after these diets have been instituted, because it is not uncommon for these patients to be chronically underfed.

The complications of enteral nutrition are numerous and include mechanical complications caused by tube placement, electrolyte imbalance, hyperglycemia, and diarrhea. Metabolic derangements are less likely if 18-hour infusions are provided as opposed to 24-hour infusions or bolus feedings. A hyperosmolar state can be avoided by flushing the feeding tube with 100 to 200 mL of free water every 4 to 6 hours.

Finally, it should be recognized that long-term tube feeding is not necessarily appropriate for all residents. The resident or responsible family member has the right to exert his or her autonomy and refuse tube feeding.

TUBE FEEDINGS: NEW INDICATIONS

Although physicians have traditionally reserved the use of feeding tubes for the "maintenance" of end-stage residents or for residents who are no longer able to feed themselves, the role of nutritional support may be changing, especially for those residents admitted to the nursing home for rehabilitation. Recent data suggest that the *early* use of enteral supplementation may decrease morbidity and mortality. For example, rehabilitation time was shortened and mortality decreased in a group of women with femoral neck fractures who received supplementary tube feedings of 1000 calories each night while they were asleep (38). Median rehabilitation time was significantly decreased from the time of operation to the time of independent mobility but not from the time of operation to the time of weight bearing with support. This suggests a 10- to 14-day lag time from the institution of supplementation to improvement in muscle strength and functional status. In another study, immediate and 6-month mortality rates were lower in orthopedic patients undergoing rehabilitation after hip fracture who received supplementary tube feedings of 250 calories per day (39). Finally, a group of patients with chronic obstructive pulmonary disease who received enteral supplementation of 1000 calories more than their usual intake had improved lung function, as determined by maximum expiratory pressures and mean sustained inspiratory pressures (40). Aggressive feeding of high-protein diets can also accelerate healing in persons with decubitus ulcers (41).

Another group of patients that may benefit from early intervention with enteral supplementation are those who are depressed. Identifying and treating depression is frequently delayed, with concomitant loss of weight. One may be reluctant to label a newly admitted resident as depressed, considering the numerous losses new residents tend to experience, including loss of independence. However, if this diagnosis is not considered, valuable intervention time is wasted. Furthermore, in the resident with severe cachexia and depression, it may take some time before therapy is effective. Therefore, the depressed resident is an ideal candidate for aggressive and early nutritional intervention with tube feedings. For depressed residents who do not respond to treatment with antidepressants and psychological support, electroconvulsive therapy is the treatment of choice.

Ethical issues are frequently raised regarding the level of aggressiveness in treating patients with dementia who have had weight loss, including whether or not to use tube feeding. This should be less of a problem as more residents early in the course of the disease are advised on living wills and durable power of attorney. Another concern is that the confused resident will dislodge the tube. However, in one study, 50% of severely demented residents had their tubes in place for more than 1 year (36).

A final group of residents likely to benefit from early aggressive feedings are those transferred back from the acute hospital setting. Many of these patients have had procedures for which they were to receive nothing by mouth or were too sick to feed themselves, with no one attending to their nutritional status during the hospital stay. Others may have found it difficult to eat because they were in an unfamiliar environment or because the diet was too restrictive. Because a catabolic phase generally occurs 3 to 10 days after illness or trauma and patients may be discharged from the hospital early (owing to Diagnosis Related Groups), these patients would benefit greatly from nutritional resuscitation.

APPETITE STIMULANTS

In one study in which malnourished nursing home residents received recombinant growth hormone, muscle mass improved and weight gain was noted (42). Medroxyprogesterone acetate has been reported to stimulate food intake in persons with cancer-related cachexia (43); however, in our experience, it often causes severe constipation in older persons. Serotonin antagonists have also been administered to nursing home residents with mixed results. As mentioned previously, nitrates may enhance food intake in persons with early satiation. Also, glyceryl trinitrate (2.6 mg) has been found to reduce abnormal antral filling in patients with functional dyspepsia (44), and antidepressant drugs may increase food intake in depressed residents.

VITAMINS

Low blood levels of numerous vitamins have been found in many of nursing home residents (6). These residents tend to have low caloric intakes, although drug nutrient interactions may also account for these low blood levels (Table 9.2). Illness, too, may alter the absorption, metabolism, or secretion of some vitamins. The consequences of these low vitamin levels is uncertain. Skin changes suggestive of vitamin deficiencies that are commonly found in residents include hemorrhage, cheilosis, skin dryness, and a bald tongue. Vitamin C is widely used to promote decubitus ulcer healing (1). Low

levels of vitamins B_1, B_2, and C have been correlated with cognitive dysfunction (45), and thiamine supplementation has been shown to improve cognitive function in community-dwelling older persons who have vitamin deficiencies (46). Vitamin supplementation resulted in a decrease in infections in older community dwellers (9), and vitamin C may be associated with prolongation of life in men (although not in women) (47). The few interventional studies that have been done (Table 9.3) do not clearly recommend that nursing home residents receive vitamin supplementation if caloric intake is adequate. However, large controlled trials are needed to resolve this issue.

Vitamin B_{12} deficiency is a separate case. Vitamin B_{12} deficiency may be due to an autoimmune disease process resulting in lack of intrinsic factor (that is, pernicious anemia). These persons are at increased risk for having other autoimmune endocrine disorders, such as diabetes mellitus, hypothyroidism, adrenal insufficiency, and celiac disease. Others develop vitamin B_{12} deficiency because of poor dietary intake, bacterial overgrowth, or malabsorption, which may occur because of an inability to split vitamin B_{12} from its protein complex in food. The results of the Schilling test can be normal in patients with vitamin B_{12} deficiency due to this failure to split vitamin B_{12} from its protein complex (48). Persons with Alzheimer dementia may be particularly prone to vitamin B_{12} deficiency (49). In patients with neuropsychiatric abnormalities, vitamin B_{12} deficiency can occur without anemia or macrocytosis (50). Finally, normal vitamin B_{12} levels do not necessarily rule out vitamin B_{12} deficiency: More than half of persons with vitamin B_{12} levels between 200 and 300 pg/mL may have deficiency as shown by elevated methylmalonic acid and homocysteine in the urine (51). Thus, urinary measurement of these metabolites may be necessary to make or rule out the diagnosis of vitamin B_{12} deficiency. Vitamin B_{12} can be replaced orally as well as by injection (52). A study of more than 150 patients has suggested that vitamin B_{12} therapy in deficient persons can produce significant improvement in neuropsychiatric abnormalities (48,53). However, another study has suggested that well-established B_{12} deficiency may be associated with structural brain abnormalities and masked brain atrophy (54). Clinical experience suggests that dramatic improvements after vitamin B_{12} treatment may be less common than the literature suggests.

TABLE 9.3. Vitamins in nursing homes: interventional studies*

Study (Reference)	Outcome
Multivitamin	
Brocklehurst et al. (84)	Fewer skin hemorrhages and capillary fragility
McLeod (85)	No change in tongue or in capillary fragility
Altman et al. (86)	Decrease in excitement
Vitamin B_6	
Tolonen et al. (87)	Improved clock drawing
Vitamin C	
Schorah et al. (88)	Weight gain and improved nurse assessment
Schorah et al. (89)	Weight gain, improved albumin levels, and decrease in purpura
Arthur et al. (90)	No decrease in purpura or hemorrhage

*Adapted from data in Reference 6.

HIP FRACTURE AND NUTRITION

Hip fracture is a major problem in nursing homes. These fractures usually result from falls, often in conjunction with osteopenia. Older persons develop type II osteopenia, which is due to inadequate calcium intake, protein malnutrition, and vitamin D deficiency; vitamin D deficiency is especially common in nursing home residents. Institutionalized persons often get little sunlight; the skin of older persons is less capable of synthesizing cholecalciferol in the presence of ultraviolet light; the kidneys of older persons have less of the 1 α-hydroxylase necessary to make the active form of vitamin D (that is, 1,25[OH]2 vitamin D); and vitamin D receptors in the gut are less functional with advancing age. An inadequate amount or effect of vitamin D can lead to poor calcium absorption and osteomalacia.

Calcium supplementation (an intake of at least 12.4 mmol/d) slows bone loss, although amounts as high as 24.8 to 37.2 mmol/d are classically recommended for older persons. Unfortunately, calcium supplementation often aggravates constipation in institutionalized persons. Chapuy and colleagues (55) showed that supplementation with 29.8 mmol of elemental calcium per day and 800 IU (20 µg) of vitamin D_3 per day in women who were 69 to 106 years old and living in nursing homes or apartment houses decreased the incidence of hip fractures by 43% and the incidence of nonvertebral

fractures by 32%. In our experience, nursing home residents with calcium levels less than 2.24 mmol/L and with elevated alkaline phosphatase levels are at high risk for falls and have secondary hyperparathyroidism or vitamin D deficiency. These persons appear to be ideal candidates for calcium and vitamin D supplementation.

DIABETES MELLITUS

Diabetes mellitus has many nutritional implications. Nursing home residents with diabetes mellitus tend to have more limitations than other residents (56). Residents with diabetes mellitus are often below average weight, and therefore, in most cases, calorie-restricted diets are inappropriate. Coulston and colleagues (57) showed no advantage in glycemic control in nursing home residents with diabetes who were given an American Diabetes Association diet compared with those who were given a regular diet.

There is increasing evidence that hyperglycemia causes cognitive dysfunction and that control of glucose improves mental functioning (58). Hyperglycemia can also result in increased pain perception (59). Good glycemic control can be obtained in the nursing home without excessive hypoglycemia provided that physicians and staff pay careful attention to weight loss and the eating habits of these residents.

Diabetes mellitus has been associated with multiple vitamin and trace element deficiencies (60); borderline zinc status due to decreased absorption of zinc and to hyperzincuria is especially common (61). Zinc deficiency has been linked to poor wound healing and decreased immune function (62). Residents with diabetes mellitus and decubitus ulcer or peripheral vascular disease ulcers may benefit from zinc replacement.

FLUID INTAKE AND DEHYDRATION

Dehydration is a common problem among nursing home residents that often leads to hospitalization. Even healthy older persons have decreased thirst response to dehydration owing to complex factors such as a lack of the µ-opioid drinking drive (63). In healthy older persons, this leads to slightly higher osmolality than in younger persons (64). Diseases, such as stroke, can further decrease the thirst response in older persons. Furthermore, nursing home residents who are confined in bed by bedrails or in a chair by physical restraints may not be able to reach the nearby water on the bedside table. Recently, we found that the application of a Posey restraint, even in healthy young persons, causes a marked decrease in their fluid intake (unpublished observation). Finally, the loss of the circadian rhythm of arginine vasopressin that occurs with aging leads to nocturia and increased fluid loss (65). Dehydration can result in postural hypotension, constipation, and delirium. In nursing home residents, an increase in the blood urea nitrogen:creatinine ratio of greater than 20:1 is a useful indicator of incipient free water deprivation.

Hyponatremia is also not uncommon in institutionalized persons. Both low-salt diets and inadequate salt in tube-feeding solutions are important causes of hyponatremia, as is the frequent use of diuretics. The syndrome of inappropriate antidiuretic hormone is associated with many of the diseases that result in institutionalization. Several drugs result in decreased free water clearance and hyponatremia; besides thiazides, these include chlorpropamide, carbamazepine, morphine, tricyclic antidepressants, haloperidol, and phenothiazines. Atrionatriuretic factor is elevated in older persons, particularly those with congestive cardiac failure, and may play a role in the pathogenesis of hyponatremia (66). Water retention can also lead to hyponatremia and may complicate the ability to manage diuretic-induced hyponatremia.

PHYSICAL ACTIVITY

Physical activity is an important component of nursing home care. Physical conditioning in older persons has numerous positive effects, such as slowing of the age-related changes in muscle strength, balance, aerobic conditioning, flexibility, and bone loss. In addition, Shephard (67) has suggested that many of the benefits of physical activity are nutrition-related, such as enhanced appetite, enhanced protein intake, improved bowel function (decreased constipation), and a decreased likelihood of glucose intolerance. Exercise may also enhance immune function in older persons (68).

Fiatarone and colleagues (69) studied frail nursing home residents who took part in a high-intensity exercise program over a 10-week period. Muscle strength, cross-sectional thigh muscle area, and stair-climbing ability improved in these residents. They also had an increase in total energy intake, although this was not necessarily greater than what was necessary to meet the needs of their increased energy output. Unfortunately, the exercise program had only a minimal effect on injurious falls. A meta-analysis of the FICSIT trials also failed to show that exercise affected the incidence of injurious falls (70). Exercises specifically aimed at improving balance, on the other hand, appeared to play an important part in reducing the incidence of falls. Other studies by the Roiton group have found that exercise training enhanced insulin action, increased GLUT-4 levels (71), and increased bone mineral density (72).

Sauvage and colleagues (73) found small improvements in strength (5% to 10%) as the result of a high-intensity exercise program in the nursing home. A year-long endurance exercise program in a nursing home resulted in only minimal improvements in upper body strength and in no improvements in leg strength (74). Two studies have suggested that a simple exercise program (75) and a walking program (76) may be as likely to be clinically beneficial in frail elderly persons as the more expensive, high-intensity exercise programs.

FINAL CONSIDERATIONS

Nutritional deficiencies are commonly present in nursing home residents. In some cases, disease-associated malnutrition is the major reason for institutionalization. Nutritional problems may interfere with residents' quality of life as well as with short-term rehabilitation. They may also result in readmission to the hospital either directly (for example, in the case of dehydration) or indirectly (for example, in the case of infection). Because the consultant dietitian is a key member of the interdisciplinary team, increased funding for dietitians is needed. The key to good nutritional care is early recognition of weight loss. In residents who have weight loss (or whose albumin level is less than 35 g/L), caloric supplements (200 to 600 kcal/d) should be ordered and should be carefully sought (Box 9.1). If weight loss continues, the option of tube feeding should be discussed with the resident and his or her family. Careful documentation of this discussion and the outcome is essential to protect against future litigation. This approach will result in improvement in many residents.

REFERENCES

1. Morley JE. Nutritional status of the elderly. Am J Med. 1986;81:679-95.
2. Keller HH. Malnutrition in institutionalized elderly. J Am Geriatr Soc. 1993;41:1212-8.
3. Sullivan DH, Patch GA, Walls RC, Lipschitz DA. Impact of nutrition status on morbidity and mortality in a select population of geriatric rehabilitation patients. Am J Clin Nutr. 1990;51:749-58.
4. Sullivan DH. Risk factors for early hospital readmission in a select population of geriatric rehabilitation patients: the significance of nutritional status. J Am Geriatr Soc. 1992;40:792-8.
5. Rudman D, Mattson DE, Nagraj HS, Feller AG, Jackson DL, Caindec N, et al. Prognostic significance of serum cholesterol in nursing home men. J Parenter Enteral Nutr. 1988;12:155-8.
6. Drinka PJ, Goodwin JS. Prevalence and consequences of vitamin deficiency in the nursing home: a critical review. J Am Geriatr Soc. 1991;39:1008-17.
7. Goode HF, Burns E, Walker BE. Vitamin C depletion and pressure sores in elderly patients with femoral neck fracture. Br Med J. 1992;305:925-7.
8. Pierron RL, Perry HM III, Grossberg G, Morley JE, Mahon G, Stewart T. The aging hip. J Am Geriatr Soc. 1990;38:1339-52.
9. Chandra RK. Effect of vitamin and trace-element supplementation on immune responses and infection in elderly subjects. Lancet. 1992;340:1124-7.
10. Morley JE. Why do physicians fail to recognize and treat malnutrition in older persons? J Am Geriatr Soc. 1991;39:1139-40.
11. Morley JE, Kraenzle D. Causes of weight loss in a community nursing home. J Am Geriatr Soc. 1994;42:583-5.
12. Durnin JV. Energy metabolism in the elderly. In: Munro H, Schierf G, eds. Nutrition in the Elderly. New York:Vevey/Raven; 1992:51-63.
13. Morley JE, Silver AJ. Anorexia in the elderly. Neurobiol Aging. 1988;9:9-16.
14. Berthelemy P, Bouisson M, Vellas B, Moureau J, Nicole-Vaysse M, Albarede JL, et al. Postprandial cholecystokinin secretion in elderly with protein energy undernutrition. J Am Geriatr Soc. 1992;40:365-9.
15. Fitten LJ, Morley JE, Gross PL, Petry SD, Cole KD. Depression. J Am Geriatr Soc. 1989;37:459-72.
16. Katz IR, Beaston-Wimmer P, Parmelee P, Friedman E, Lawton MP. Failure to thrive in the elderly: Exploration of the concept and delineation of psychiatric components. J Geriatr Psychiatry Neurol. 1993;6:151-69.
17. Blaum CS, Fries BE, Fiatarone MA. Factors associated with low body mass index and weight loss in nursing home residents. J Gerontol. 1995;50:M162-8.
18. Kahn R. Weight loss and depression in a community nursing home. J Am Geriatr Soc. 1995;43:83.
19. Miller DK, Morley JE, Rubenstein LZ, Pietruszka FM. Abnormal eating attitudes and body image in older undernourished individuals. J Am Geriatr Soc. 1991;39:462-86.
20. Thomson WM, Brown RH, Williams SM. Dentures, prosthetic treatment needs, and mucosal health in an institutionalised elderly population. N Z Dent J. 1992;88:51-5.
21. Vigild M. Dental caries and the need for treatment among institutionalized elderly. Community Dent Oral Epidemiol. 1989;17:102-5.
22. Horn JV, Hodge WC, Treuer JP. Dental condition and weight loss in institutionalized demented patients. Spec Care Dentist. 1994;14:108-11.
23. Bush LS, Morley JE, Martin WE. Comparison of oral health care delivery to institutionalized elderly in two settings. Nursing Home Medicine. 1995;3:3-7.
24. Sullivan DH, Martin W, Flaxman N, Hagen JE. Oral health problems and involuntary weight loss in a population of frail elderly. J Am Geriatr Soc. 1993;41:725-31.
25. Rudman D, Mattson DE, Alverno L, Richardson TJ, Rudman IW. Comparison of clinical indicators in two nursing homes. J Am Geriatr Soc. 1993;41:1317-25.
26. Sandman PO, Adolfsson R, Nygren C, Hallmans G, Winblad B. Nutritional status and dietary intake in institutionalized patients with Alzheimer's disease and multi-infarct dementia. J Am Geriatr Soc. 1987;35:31-8.
27. Siebens H, Trupe E, Siebens A, Cook F, Anshen S, Hanauer R, et al. Correlates and consequences of eating dependency in institutionalized elderly. J Am Geriatr Soc. 1986;34:192-8.
28. Poehlman ET. Regulation of energy expenditure in aging humans. J Am Geriatr Soc. 1993;41:552-9.
29. Buckler DA, Kelber ST, Goodwin JS. The use of dietary restrictions in malnourished nursing home patients. J Am Geriatr Soc. 1994;42:1100-2.
30. Morley JE, Kraenzle DK, Jensen JM, Gettman J, Tetter L. The role of a nurse practitioner in quality improvement in nursing homes. Nursing Home Medicine. 1994;2:11-19.
31. Morley JE, Flood JF. Evidence that nitric oxide modulates food intake in mice. Life Sci. 1991;49:707-11.
32. Master AH, Lasser RP, Butman G. Tables of average weight and height of American aged 65-94 years. JAMA. 1960;172:658-62.
33. Forette B, Tortrat D, Wolmark Y. Cholesterol as risk factor for mortality in elderly women. Lancet. 1989;1:868-70.
34. Swan GE, LaRue A, Carmelli D, Reed TE, Fabsitz RR. Decline in cognitive performance in aging twins. Heritability and biobehavioral predictors from the National Heart, Lung, and Blood Institute Twin Study. Arch Neurol. 1992;49:476-81.
35. Morgan RE, Palinkas LA, Barrett-Connor EL, Wingard DL. Plasma cholesterol and depressive symptoms in older men. Lancet. 1993;341:75-98.
36. Silver AJ, Morley JE, Strome LS, Jones D, Vickers L. Nutritional status in an academic nursing home. J Am Geriatr Soc. 1988;36:487-91.

37. Rudman D, Feller AG, Nagraj HS, Jackson DL, Rudman IW, Mattson DE. Relation of serum albumin concentration to death rate in nursing home men. Journal of Parenteral and Enteral Nutrition. 1987;11:360-3.
38. Bastow MD, Rajsin CH, Bengoa JM, Delmar PD, Vasey H, Bonjour JP, Rawlings J, Allison SP. Benefits of supplementary tube feeding after fractured neck of femur: a randomized controlled trial. BMJ. 1983;287:1589-92.
39. Delmi M, Rapin CH, Bengoa JM, Delmas PD, Vasey H, Bonjour JP. Dietary supplementation in elderly patients with fractured neck of femur. Lancet. 1990;335:1013-6.
40. Whittaker JS, Ryan CF, Buckley PA, Road JD. The effects of refeeding on peripheral and respiratory muscle function in malnourished chronic obstructive pulmonary disease patients. Am Rev Respir Disease. 1990;142:283-8.
41. Breslow RA, Hallfrish J, Guy DB, Crawley B, Goldberg AP. The importance of dietary protein in healing pressure ulcers. J Am Geriatr Soc. 1993; 41:357-62.
42. Kaiser FE, Silver AJ, Morley JE. The effect of recombinant human growth hormone on malnourished older individuals. J Am Geriatr Soc. 1991;39:235-40.
43. Niiranen A, Kajanti M, Tammilehto L, Mattson K. The clinical effect of medroxyprogesterone in elderly patients with lung cancer. Am J Clin Oncol. 1990;13:113-6.
44. Hausken T, Berstad A. Effects of glyceryl trinitrate on antral motility and symptoms in patients with functional dyspepsia. Scand J Gastroenterol. 1994; 29:23-8.
45. Goodwin JS, Goodwin JM, Garry PJ. Association between nutritional status and cognitive functioning in a health elderly population. JAMA. 1983;249: 2917-21.
46. Smidt LJ, Cremin FM, Grivette LE, Clifford AJ. Influence of thiamin supplementation on the health and general well-being of an elderly Irish population with marginal thiamin deficiency. J Gerontol. 1991;46:M16-22.
47. Enstrom JE, Kanim LE, Klein MA. Vitamin C intake and mortality among a sample of the United States population. Epidemiology. 1992;3:194-202.
48. Miller A, Furlong D, Burrows BA, Slingerland DW. Bound vitamin B_{12} absorption in patients with low serum B_{12} levels. Am J Hematol. 1992;40:163-6.
49. Ikeda T, Furukawa Y, Mashimoto S, Takahashi K, Yamada M. Vitamin B_{12} levels in serum and cerebrospinal fluid of people with Alzheimer's disease. Acta Psychiat Scand. 1990;82:327-9.
50. Lindenbaum J, Healton EB, Savage DG, Brust JC, Garrett TJ, Podell ER, et al. Neuropsychiatric disorders caused by cobalamin deficiency in the absence of anemia or macrocytosis. N Engl J Med. 1988; 318:1720-8.
51. Pennypacker LC, Allen RH, Kelly JP, et al. High prevalence of cobalamin deficiency in elderly outpatients. J Am Geriatr Soc. 1990;38:A9 (abstract).
52. Lederle FA. Oral cobalamin for pernicious anemia. Medicine's best kept secret? JAMA. 1991;265: 94-5.
53. Healton EB, Savage DG, Brust JC, Garrett TJ, Lindenbaum J. Neurologic aspects of cobalamin deficiency. Medicine. 1991;70:229-45.
54. Pirttila T, Salo J, Laippala P, Frey H. Effect of advanced brain atrophy and vitamin deficiency on cognitive functions in non-demented subjects. Acta Neurol Scand. 1993;87:161-6.
55. Chapuy MC, Arlot ME, Duboeuf F, Brun J, Crouzet B, Arnaud S, et al. Vitamin D_3 and calcium to prevent hip fractures in elderly women. N Engl J Med. 1991;327:1637-42.
56. Mooradian AD, Osterweil D, Petrasek D, Morley JE. Diabetes mellitus in elderly nursing home patients: A survey of clinical characteristics and management. J Am Geriatr Soc. 1988;36:391-6.
57. Coulston AM, Mandelbaum D, Reaven GM. Dietary management of nursing home residents with non-insulin dependent diabetes mellitus. Am J Clin Nutr. 1990;51:67-71.
58. Morley JE, Flood JF. Psychosocial aspects of diabetes mellitus in older persons. J Am Geriatr Soc. 1990;38:605-6.
59. Morley GK, Mooradian AD, Levine AS, Morley JE. Mechanism of pain in diabetic peripheral neuropathy. Effect of glucose on pain perception in humans. Am J Med. 1984;77:79-83.
60. Mooradian AD, Morley JE. Micronutrient status in diabetes mellitus. Am J Clin Nutr. 1987;45:877-95.
61. Kinlaw WB, Levine AS, Morley JE, Silvis SE, McClain CJ. Abnormal zinc metabolism in Type II diabetes mellitus. Am J Med. 1983;75:273-7.
62. Niewoehner CB, Allen JI, Boosalis M, Levine AS, Morley JE. Role of zinc supplementation in Type II diabetes mellitus. Am J Med. 1986;81:63-8.
63. Silver AJ, Morley JE. Role of the opioid system in the hypodipsia associated with aging. J Am Geriatr Soc. 1992;40:556-60.
64. McLean KA, O'Neill PA, Davies I, Morris J. Influence of age on plasma osmolality: A community study. Age Ageing. 1992;21:56-60.
65. Asplund R, Aberg H. Diurnal variation in the levels of antidiuretic hormone in the elderly. J Intern Med. 1991;229:131-4.
66. Davis KM, Fish LC, Elahi D, Clark BA, Minaker KL. Atrial natriuretic peptide levels in the prediction of congestive heart failure risk in frail elderly. JAMA. 1992;267:2625-9.
67. Shephard RJ. Exercise and nutrition in the elderly. In: Morley JE, Glick Z, Rubenstein LZ, eds. Geriatric Nutrition: A Comprehensive Review. 2nd ed. New York:Raven Press; 1995:303-10.
68. Fiatarone MA, Morley JE, Bloom ET, Benton D, Solomon GF, Makinodan T. The effect of exercise on natural killer cell activity in young and old subjects. J Gerontol. 1989;44:M37-45.
69. Fiatarone MA, O'Neill EF, Ryan ND, Solanes GR, Nelson ME, Roberts SB, et al. Exercise training and nutritional supplementation for physical frailty

in very elderly people. N Engl J Med. 1994;330: 1769-75.

70. Province MA, Hadley EC, Hornbrook MC, Lipsitz LA, Miller JP, Mulrow CD, et al. The effect of exercise on falls in elderly patients. A preplanned meta-analysis of the FICSIT trials. Frailty and injuries: Cooperative studies of intervention techniques. JAMA. 1995;273:1341-7.

71. Hughes VA, Fiatarone MA, Fielding RA, Kahn BB, Ferrara CM, Shepherd P, et al. Exercise increases muscle GLUT-4 levels and insulin action in subjects with impaired glucose tolerance. Am J Physiol. 1993;264:E855-62.

72. Nelson ME, Fiatarone MA, Morganti CM, Trice I, Greenberg RA, Evans WJ. Effects of high intensity strength training on multiple risk factors for osteoporotic fractures: A randomized controlled trial. JAMA. 1994;272:1909-14.

73. Sauvage LA Jr, Mykleburst BM, Crow-Pan J, Novak S, Millington P, Hoffman MD, et al. A clinical trial of strengthening and aerobic exercise to improve gait and balance in elderly male nursing home residents. Am J Phys Med Rehab. 1992;71:333-42.

74. Naso F, Carner E, Blankfort-Doyle W, Coughey K. Endurance training in the elderly nursing home patient. Arch Phys Med Rehabil. 1990; 71:241-3.

75. Jirovec MM. The impact of daily exercise on the mobility, balance, and urine control of cognitively impaired nursing home residents. Int J Nurs Stud. 1991;28:145-51.

76. Conright KC, Evans JP, Nassralla SM, Tran MV, Silver AJ, Morley JE. A walking program improves gait and balance in nursing home patients. J Am Geriatr Soc. 1990;38:1267.

77. Shaver HJ, Lopez JA, Lutes RA. Nutritional status of nursing home patients. JPEN J Parenteral Enteral Nutr. 1980;4:367-70.

78. Muncie HL Jr, Carbonetto C. Prevalence of protein calorie malnutrition in an extended care facility. J Fam Pract. 1982;14:1061-4.

79. Pinchofsky-Devin CD, Kaminski MV Jr. Correlation of pressure sores and nutritional status. J Am Geriatr Soc. 1986;34:435-40.

80. Rudman D, Feller AG. Protein-caloric undernutrition in the nursing home. J Am Geriatr Soc. 1989;37: 173-83.

81. Thomas DR, Verdery RB, Gardner L, Kant A, Lindsay J. A prospective study of outcome from protein energy malnutrition in nursing home residents. J Parenter Enteral Nutr. 1991;15:400-4.

82. Abbasi AA, Rudman D. Observations on the prevalence of protein-calorie undernutrition in VA nursing homes. J Am Geriatr Soc. 1993;41:117-21.

83. Ferguson RP, O'Connor P, Crabtree B, Batchelor A, Mitchell J, Coppola D. Serum albumin and prealbumin as prediction of clinical outcomes of hospitalized elderly nursing home residents. J Am Geriatr Soc. 1993;41:545-9.

84. Brocklehurst JC, Griffiths LL, Taylor GF, Marks J, Scott DL, Blackley J. The clinical features of chronic vitamin deficiency. A therapeutic trial in geriatric hospital patients. Gerontol Clin (Basel). 1968;10: 309-20.

85. McLeod RD. Abnormal tongue appearances and vitamin status of the elderly A double blind trial. Age Ageing. 1972;1:99-102.

86. Altman H, Mehta D, Evenson RC, Sletten IW. Behavioral effects of drug therapy on psychogeriatric inpatients. II. Multivitamin supplement. J Am Geriatr Soc. 1973;21:249-52.

87. Tolonen M, Schrijver J, Westermarck T, Halme M, Tuominen SE, Frilander A. Vitamin B_6 status of Finnish elderly. Comparison with Dutch younger adults and elderly. The effect of supplementation. Int J Vitam Nutr Res. 1988;58:73-7.

88. Schorah CJ, Newill A, Scott DL, Morgan DB. Clinical effects of vitamin C in elderly inpatients with low blood vitamin C levels. Lancet. 1979;1:403-5.

89. Schorah CJ, Tormey WP, Brooks GH, Robertwhaw AM, Young GA, Talukder R, et al. The effect of vitamin C supplements on body weight, serum proteins, and general health of an elderly population. Am J Clin Nutr. 1981;34:871-6.

90. Arthur G, Monro JA, Poore P, Rilwan WB, Murphy EL. Trial of ascorbic acid in senile purpura and sublingual haemorrhages. BMJ. 1967;1:732-3.

10

Rehabilitation

Roy V. Erickson, MD

This chapter describes the programmatic and recent clinical advances in geriatric rehabilitation that are needed to care for nursing home residents. The increasingly regulated and rapidly changing care in the nursing home requires those physicians who are primarily responsible for the care of nursing home residents to understand the principles of rehabilitation:

1. Rehabilitation services are now a required part of the plan of care of all nursing home residents. Based on the nursing home reform legislation in the Omnibus Budget Reconciliation Act (OBRA) of 1987, enacted in 1991(1), the nursing facility must make a comprehensive assessment of a resident's needs at the time of admission and after a significant change in condition or function has occurred; at the minimum, this assessment must be done annually (Reg. 483.20 (b) (ii)). The goal for each resident is to obtain or maintain the highest practicable physical, mental, and psychosocial well-being in accordance with the comprehensive assessment and plan of care (Reg. 483.25).

2. Nursing homes are expanding their ability to provide short-term rehabilitation programs under the general rubric of "subacute care." Nursing homes now provide ventilator care and wound care, as well as care for patients with postoperative and post-traumatic complications, for patients with acquired immunodeficiency syndrome, and medically and surgically complex older patients (2).

3. Because patients are being released from the acute-care setting to the nursing home "sicker and quicker" (3,4), more nursing home residents, both short-term and long-term, require rehabilitation as part of the physician-ordered plan of care and treatment.

The type and availability of rehabilitation services provided in nursing homes vary widely, ranging from per diem contracted services with physical and occupational therapists, to comprehensive, intensive rehabilitation programs with full-time therapy staff similar to those seen in hospital-based or free-standing rehabilitation facilities. The latter programs require the patient to participate in 3 to 4 hours per day of therapy and frequent medical supervision, while most rehabilitation in the nursing home requires a minimum of 1 hour of physical therapy daily, 5 days per week, for Medicare payment. Realistic goals must be set and achieved for coverage to continue.

Medically and surgically complex patients may qualify for Medicare skilled nursing facility coverage without the need for daily physical therapy. For some skilled nursing services (for example, bladder and bowel training, postoperative supervision), the criteria are less well defined or are met by a conglomerate of needed services (Box 10.1). When provided, Medicare coverage is 100% for the first 20 days and 80% for up to a maximum of 100 days. Custodial care and maintenance rehabilitation services are not covered by Medicare.

BOX 10.1. Criteria for Medicare reimbursement in a skilled nursing facility

1. A hospital stay of at least 3 consecutive days within 30 days before admission to the skilled nursing facility that provides the care required for the condition for which the patient was treated in the hospital.
2. Physician certification that the patient needs skilled service and observation on a daily basis provided by a licensed professional. These skilled services may include but are not limited to
   - Intravenous or intramuscular injection and intravenous feedings
   - Enteral tube feeds
   - Skilled ostomy care and teaching
   - Wound and pressure ulcer treatment
   - Bowel and bladder training
   - Postoperative supervision
   - Physical, occupational, and speech therapy
   - Respiratory services
3. An aggregate need of several skilled services often improves the probability of Medicare coverage.
4. Custodial and/or unskilled services are not covered.

Adapted from Ouslander JG, Osterweil D, Morley JE. Rehabilitation in the nursing home. In: Medical Care in the Nursing Home. New York: McGraw-Hill; 1991:327.

Rehabilitation services for nursing home residents include

1. *Short-term restorative services.* These are usually provided to short-stay nursing home residents who are admitted for restorative rehabilitation after onset of a new disability, and are likely to be funded by Medicare. Guidelines for this care may apply to long-term residents who have similar onset of new disabilities, but only after a required 3-day acute-care hospitalization within the preceding 30 days.

2. *Rehabilitation services for long-term nursing home residents.* These focus on change or maintenance of function in patients with chronic disease and on the prevention of further disability.

SHORT-TERM REHABILITATION PROGRAMS IN THE NURSING HOME

The most common short-term rehabilitation programs in nursing homes include *orthopedic* programs (for example, joint replacement, hip, or lower extremity fractures; vertebral compression fractures); *neurologic* programs (for example, stroke, Guillain–Barré syndrome); programs for lower extremity *amputations;* and *medical rehabilitation*

(that is, reconditioning, restoration of activities of daily living) after prolonged medical or surgical illness. Before a nursing home resident is placed in a short-term rehabilitation program, the following should be assessed:

1. *Severity of new disability.* This is assessed in terms of functional impairment and potential for improvement with rehabilitation services.

2. *Knowledge of premorbid level of function.* This is a frequent predictor of eventual outcome from rehabilitation.

3. *Coexisting medical conditions.* Cardiovascular, pulmonary, joint, and peripheral vascular disease may limit the intensity of the rehabilitation program.

4. *Cognitive status.* This involves determining whether delirium, dementia, or both are present. Impaired ability to follow two-step commands, to retain information day to day, and to use adaptive equipment limits participation in restorative rehabilitation programs. Dementia may significantly limit rehabilitation, whereas delirium may not.

5. *Depression and mood disorders.* These disorders are prevalent in older patients after the onset of new disability and may interfere with motivation to participate in a rehabilitation program.

6. *Availability, commitment, and capacity of the family or caregiver.* These often determine whether short-term rehabilitation patients will return home or remain institutionalized.

7. *Eligibility for Medicare.* This or eligibility for an alternate payment source should be determined.

Orthopedic Patients

Approximately 250,000 hip fractures occur each year in the United States. By the age of 90 years, 32% of women and 17% of men have suffered a hip fracture (5). Hip fractures often increase morbidity, mortality, and functional decline, and they frequently result in long-term institutional care (6,7).

Pre-existing comorbidities such as cognitive impairment, advanced age, limited ability to bathe and transfer independently, less family involvement, and perioperative factors of limited physical therapy, depression, longer hospital stays, and postoperative complications have been associated with increased risk for institutional placement for patients with a hip fracture (8–10). However, data suggest that of patients with hip fracture who come from the community, 70% ambulate within 1 year of fracture, 40% to 70% return home directly after hospitalization. Approximately 50% achieve prefracture functional status and at least 15% require continued long-term care 1 year later (11). The prognosis for full functional recovery for institutionalized elderly persons who have *femoral neck fractures* with coexisting neurologic or heart disease is 15% to 20% less (12).

Physical therapy within a full nursing home rehabilitation program for patients who have had hip procedures strengthens the muscles of the affected lower extremity for ambulation as well as the periarticular muscles, to prevent displacement of the hip prosthesis or to provide stability for hip fractures repaired by pinning or a compression screw. Patients progress in ambulation from a walker to a wide-base quad cane to a hand-held single point cane. Improving upper extremity strength and function is also important to aid in the use of assistive devices for ambulation as well as to ensure safe and effective bathing and dressing, both of which may be adversely affected by lower extremity disability.

Distinct from hip fractures, *elective orthopedic surgery* (that is, unilateral or bilateral total hip replacement) can be done safely and with good results in patients 80 years of age and older (13). Patient outcomes after total knee replacement are largely favorable, with up to 89% of patients reporting good-to-excellent outcomes at 4 years of follow-up (14). Elective orthopedic surgical patients, particularly those with medical comorbidities, often benefit from 2 to 4 weeks of an intensive supervised rehabilitation program before returning to community living.

COMMON MEDICAL PROBLEMS

Prophylaxis against Deep Venous Thrombophlebitis/Pulmonary Embolus. Prophylaxis against deep venous thrombophlebitis/pulmonary embolus with preoperative and postoperative anticoagulation is necessary for patients who have joint replacement or repair. Recent data suggest that enoxaparin may be more effective than standard heparin (15,16) and probably cost effective (17,18), despite data suggesting a small increased risk of bleeding (19). Data are limited in defining optimal anticoagulation after the first postoperative week. Although patients may be at risk for the development of deep venous thrombosis/pulmonary embolus for up to 2 months after surgery, there are significant variations in orthopedic and medical practice (20,21). Recommendations include 1) no further deep venous thrombophlebitis prophylaxis if the results of venous Doppler studies are negative at 7 to 10 days; 2) warfarin sodium (Coumadin), at either a fixed low dose (1 to 2 mg) (22) or dose-adjusted for 2 to 6 weeks; 3) antiplatelet therapy with Ecotrin/aspirin for 2 to 8 weeks (23). Anticoagulation with Coumadin, maintaining an international normalized ratio (IMR) between 1.5 and 2.5 (although in conflict with the American College of Chest Physicians recommendations of an IMR of 2.0 to 3.0) for 3 to 4 weeks postoperatively, has reduced the incidence of clinically apparent deep venous thrombophlebitis without significant bleeding (24). It may be appropriate to continue anticoagulation up to 8 weeks for patients at higher than usual risk for deep venous thrombophlebitis—that is, non–weight-bearing, limited mobility, previous history of deep venous thrombophlebitis, varicose veins, congestive heart failure, and other risk factors (21).

Delirium. Although more common in the acute-care hospital, delirium may either persist or subsequently develop during a short-term rehabilitation program in the nursing home. The incidence of postoperative delirium after either elective or trauma-related orthopedic surgery in older patients is reported to range from 2% to 50%. One recent study reported a 41% incidence in cognitively normal older patients who had elective bilateral knee replacements (25); and another reported an incidence of 61% in older patients who had had surgery for femoral neck fractures (26). Recent data also suggest that confusional states may persist for weeks or longer, particularly in patients with pre-existing cognitive impairment (27). Risk factors for delirium include advanced age, cognitive impairment, development of infection, and use of neuroleptic or narcotic drugs (28). In the nursing home setting, physicians need to monitor mental status and carefully evaluate patients for the onset, recurrence, or persistence of confusion. Evaluation and treatment of the underlying cause and drug therapy either with low-dose, short-acting benzodiazepines or neuroleptic drugs may be necessary if the patient's agitation enhances the risk for injury or if confusion interferes with the patient's participation in therapy.

Pain Control. Adequate pain control is essential for older postoperative patients for comfort and to maximize their ability to participate in rehabilitation. One week after surgery, aspirin or acetaminophen is rarely adequate for pain control in older patients. Nonsteroidal anti-inflammatory drugs should be used with caution in older patients because of gastrointestinal and renal toxicity. Oxycodone with aspirin or acetaminophen may often be adequate, particularly if available at appropriate time intervals, that is, every 3 to 4 hours—not every 6 hours—and given 1 hour before therapy. Propoxyphene has an analgesic effect no better than aspirin or acetaminophen and has major side effects of lethargy, impaired cognition, and renal toxicity (29). Pentazocine may cause confusion and agitation in older patients (30). Some older patients require strong opioids such as hydromorphone hydrochloride (Dilaudid) or morphine to achieve adequate pain control.

Other Medical Problems. Other common medical problems of the orthopedic rehabilitation patient in the nursing home include postoperative iron deficiency anemia; postsurgical inflammation and dependent edema in the affected extremity; urinary retention, frequently secondary to immobility or medications or both; urinary tract infections; and nutritional disturbances (31).

Patients with Stroke

Nursing homes with comprehensive therapy services may provide short-term rehabilitation for older patients with strokes. Therapy programs for these patients involve physical, occupational, and, often, speech therapy services. Physical therapists focus first on sitting and standing balance and safe transfers, and then safe ambulation, usually with graded assistive devices from most assistive (that is, use of a walker and long leg braces if needed) to least assistive (that is, a straight cane). Occupational therapists treat upper extremity deficits in strength and coordination, focus on the patient's function in activities of daily living, and address perceptual and cognitive deficits. Speech therapists assess and treat language function and address issues related to dysphasia, dysarthria, and cognitive function.

For patients who will return home, involvement and education of the family or caregivers or both are invaluable to establish appropriate goals for rehabilitation in terms of activities of daily living function once home. Evaluation of the home by physical and occupational therapists before discharge is important for assessing the safety of the home environment and determining the need for adaptive equipment.

Numerous studies defined clinical risk factors for institutionalization after stroke rehabilitation (32–37): dense hemiparesis, moderate cognitive impairment, urinary incontinence, perceptual deficits (particularly the presence of neglect or impulsivity), older age, and the nonavailability of caregiver support (38). Although outcome data vary according to site, population, and selection criteria, up to 80% of patients entering intensive stroke rehabilitation programs return home (39). Restoration of mobility in both upper and lower extremities is maximal during the first 6 weeks after stroke with mild to moderate weakness and the first 11 weeks after stroke with severe weakness (40,41).

COMMON MEDICAL PROBLEMS

Thrombotic Complication. Thrombotic complication, specifically deep venous thrombophlebitis/pulmonary embolus, is a major source of morbidity and mortality in stroke patients. Deep venous thrombophlebitis incidence rates range from 22% to 75%, and patients who survive stroke for 8 days or more have a 25-fold greater risk for dying from a pulmonary embolus than patients who survive less than 7 days (42). Unless contraindicated, patients with nonhemorrhagic stroke should begin a low dose (5000 U every 8 or 12 h) of subcutaneous heparin within the first 48 to 72 hours after stroke. Although data are limited (43,44), anticoagulant therapy should be continued with either heparin or Coumadin for a maximum of 12 weeks or until the patient is able to ambulate 50 to 100 feet, either independently or with an assistive device, several times daily. Delay in initiating prophylactic anticoagulation has been associated with an increased incidence of deep vein thrombophlebitis (42).

Coronary Artery Disease. The frequent coexistence of coronary artery disease with cerebrovascular disease may raise appropriate concerns about the intensity of rehabilitation that patients with stroke can tolerate without risk for cardiac ischemia. Limited studies have demonstrated 27% and 34% prevalence rates of cardiac complications during intensive stroke rehabilitation programs (45,46). The presence of hemiplegia may increase the energy requirement by 65% to ambulate at a normal walking speed (47). Data suggest that the cardiovascular response to exercise in patients with stroke includes increase in blood pressure, pulse rate, and rate-pressure product (48). In a nursing home rehabilitation program, the blood pressure and heart rate should be monitored during and after therapy in patients with stroke who have known or suspected cardiovascular disease. Therapy activities should be modified if they induce pain, dyspnea, lightheadedness, fatigue, or other symptoms suggestive of cardiac ischemia. In some nursing homes, ambulatory Holter monitoring may be of benefit to document ST-T wave changes of ischemia or arrhythmias related to therapy. Rest periods, modification of cardiac drug regimes, and appropriate cardiac consultation may allow the patient to continue therapy (48,49).

Dysphagia. Dysphagia is a frequent but often under-recognized complication of stroke in older patients, with prevalence rates of 25% to 35% (50). Aspiration pneumonia is a frequent complication of dysphagia and a source of significant morbidity and mortality in these patients. Bedside evaluation of swallowing function by speech or occupational therapists or both should be done routinely for elderly patients who have had a stroke. In patients in whom dysphagia is suspected by bedside evaluation, or in those in whom aspiration is suspected on clinical grounds (for example, unexplained recurrent fever, cough, choking while eating or drinking), a modified barium swallow may be of benefit to diagnose dysphagia accurately and to help in determining plan of treatment (51).

Oral dysphagia treatment programs include modifying the consistency of diet by thickening liquids, puréeing, chopping, or grinding foods, paying careful attention to patient positioning and posture during feeding, as well as engaging the patient in strengthening exercises, thermal stimulation, and biofeedback to improve swallowing muscle function. The availability and sophistication of speech therapy for swallowing disorders vary widely in nursing homes. Although data on the overall effectiveness of specific therapy techniques on the improvement of swallowing function per se are ambiguous (52), recognition of probable dysphagia and modification of diet or feeding techniques or both may help avoid aspiration.

Arthritis. Arthritis can complicate stroke rehabilitation. Patients with osteoarthritis or rheumatoid arthritis may experience exacerbations during rehabilitation due to an intense physical and occupational therapy program. Treatment with rest, splinting with orthotics, ultrasonography, acetaminophen, and thermal modalities (heat or cold) usually provides symptom relief. A limited and carefully monitored trial of anti-inflammatory agents may be necessary if patients do not benefit from these measures.

Moderately severe pulmonary disease (chronic obstructive pulmonary disease) may also be exacerbated by the increased energy requirements brought about by physical and occupational therapy. Re-evaluation of previous medication regimens may be in order; simple pulse oximetry, if available, can detect significant desaturation with exercise and the need for supplemental oxygen.

Hypertension. Like cardiovascular disease, hypertension should be monitored during both physical and occupational therapy. As already noted, fluctuations with exercise are common, and drug regimens may need to be modified. If present, orthostatic hypotension may limit the patient's ability to perform certain transfers and may adversely effect standing balance and limit gait training and ambulation.

Delirium. Delirium is well documented as a complication in older patients with stroke (53,54). In the nursing home rehabilitation setting, such patients with either persistent or new onset of delirium should be evaluated for treatable causes, such as infection, medications, environmental change, dehydration, and nutritional and metabolic disorders, and should receive treatment with low-dose psychotropic medications if symptoms persist despite treatment of the cause (55).

Depression. Depression is common after stroke, both in reaction to functional losses caused by the stroke and correlated with the anatomic site of infarction (56); in both cases, the depression may be alleviated by the restoration of function through rehabilitation. Supportive counseling may be sufficient, but often for both the patient and family members and caregivers, antidepressant medication (for example, tricyclics, selective serotonin re-uptake inhibitors, psychostimulants) should be initiated if the symptoms of depression interfere with the patient's ability to participate in therapy. Although nortriptyline has been found to be of benefit for depression in patients with stroke, the anticholinergic, hypotensive, orthostatic, and cardiovascular side effects of the tricyclic antidepressants should be monitored carefully (57–59). While the benefit of antidepressants such as the selective serotonin reuptake inhibitors or butyrophenone has not been well documented in controlled studies, their more tolerable side effect profile may provide an advantage to older patients with stroke. Psychostimulants have the added advantage of few side effects and rapid onset of action.

Patients with an Amputation

Nursing homes are often the site for rehabilitation of an older patient with an amputation. Postoperative needs to be met in the nursing home include proper care of the amputed limb to promote healing, continuing exercise to strengthen muscles proximal to the amputation, and maintenance of proper positioning, as well as exercise to prevent flexion contractures of the knee or hip or both. Shrinking of the amputed limb to accommodate the socket of a temporary prosthesis can be accomplished with either stump shrinkers (tight elastic cuffs) or frequent tight ace wraps. Patients can usually be fitted for a temporary prosthesis 4 to 8 weeks after surgery and for a permanent prosthesis 8 to 12 weeks after surgery (60,61).

Advanced age should not be considered a contraindication to the institution of a prosthetic training program. However, an amputed limb that has healed poorly, threatened gangrene of the opposite extremity, poor motivation, and irreducible flexion contractures of the knee or hip are relative contraindications. A prosthetic training program emphasizes techniques of transfer from bed to wheelchair and from wheelchair to toilet. When feasible, gait training begins with weight bearing on a temporary prosthesis, first in the parallel bars and then on a walker, on crutches, and on a cane. Occupational therapy to strengthen upper extremities to enable the use of assistive devices, as well as to teach compensatory techniques for activities of daily living function, is also an integral part of prosthetic training.

Severe cardiovascular disease or pulmonary disease may limit tolerance of, or participation in, an intense physical therapy training program because of increased energy expenditure requirements for ambulation (61). However, even patients with severe chronic obstructive pulmonary disease (forced expiratory volume <1 L) have been reported to complete prosthetic training programs successfully (62). Peri-pheral vascular disease, arthritis, and motor, sensory, or other neurologic impairment in the opposite extremity may also limit the patient's ability to ambulate independently and safely.

Postamputation depression may interfere with prosthetic training. Emotional support for the patient, treatment of severe depression with antidepressant medication, if necessary, and involvement, support and education for the caregiver and family are critical. Of older patients with an amputation, 75% to 80% ambulate with a prosthesis, and most ambulate independently without an assistive device (63,64).

Rehabilitation of Older Medical/Surgical Patients

Many older persons can benefit from a short nursing home rehabilitation program after a prolonged medical or surgical illness. The physiologic complications of bed rest have been well described (65): decreased cardiac output, muscle atrophy and loss of strength, loss of bone mass, impaired ambulation, atelectasis, orthostatic intolerance, and pressure ulcers. Continued skilled nursing care and daily physical and occupational therapy may help reverse deconditioning and restore older residents to their previous level of function. The medical issues addressed earlier in this chapter for other short-term nursing home rehabilitation patients are similar. Patients need to meet criteria for placement in a skilled nursing facility as shown in Box 10.1.

REHABILITATION SERVICES FOR LONG-TERM NURSING HOME RESIDENTS

Although long-term nursing home residents may require short-term restorative rehabilitation programs after the onset of a new disability (for example, hip fracture or stroke), rehabilitation evaluation is often required for activities of daily living impairment secondary to progressive chronic disease and/or superimposed medical or surgical illness. The improvement in or restoration of function through rehabilitation can improve quality of life for residents by fostering continued independence and minimizing dependency. To refer patients for therapy evaluation and potential treatment, the attending physician should refer patients based on impairment of function rather than on the specific disease process.

Ambulation

Gait impairments in nursing home residents result from many causes, including stroke, Parkinson disease, primary motor disorders, peripheral neuropathies, entrapment syndromes, arthritis, contractures, hip fracture, or amputation. Deconditioning resulting from illness and prolonged bed rest or limited mobility secondary to pain is a frequent cause of impaired ambulation in older patients.

Table 10.1 lists the assistive devices for ambulation commonly used by nursing home residents. Patients should be evaluated by the physical therapists who will prescribe these assistive devices. Both walkers and canes can be modified to accommodate upper extremity deformity or weakness. Patients usually prefer the assistive device that is the least cumbersome and conspicuous (for example, a single-point cane instead of a wide-based quad cane). Visual, perceptual, and cognitive deficits may affect the resident's ability to use these devices properly.

Mobility

Rehabilitation services can also benefit nursing home residents by teaching the proper use of wheelchairs to move from place to place, to transfer, and to move from one surface to another safely and independently.

WHEELCHAIRS

For many nursing home residents, wheelchairs become an over-used aid for mobility; there is the risk that wheelchairs may be used for staff convenience rather than for helping residents with their disability. Residents should be properly assessed and fitted for a wheelchair, usually by a physical therapist or physical therapy assistant. The resident's range of motion, weight, height, muscle strength, skin condition, cardiac function, cognitive function, and visual capacity should be evaluated so that the most appropriate wheelchair can be prescribed. For example, a wheelchair seat that is too narrow can hinder transfers and enhance the risk of pressure sores; if the seat is too wide, sitting balance may be impaired as well as the resident's ability to propel the wheelchair. If the arms of the chair are too high, the shoulder muscles can fatigue; if they are too low, the patient may aggravate and foster kyphosis and have an impaired sitting balance. Wheelchair propulsion requires increased work of the upper extremities, with increased (up to 12%) oxygen consumption (47).

Wheelchairs can be modified and individualized: A reclining back can accommodate spinal deformity; low-pressure cushions (for example, foam, gel) can reduce both pressure and shearing force in residents at risk for pressure ulcers; a one-arm drive wheelchair can allow residents with hemiplegia wheelchair mobility, and adjustable arms can facilitate safe transfers.

TRANSFERRING

Transfers are a routine part of daily life for nursing home residents and staff. Safe and efficient transfers require a combination of physical and percep-

TABLE 10.1. Assistive devices for ambulation

Device	Indicators	Considerations
Cane	Unilateral lower extremity weakness or pain	May displace up to 25% of body weight Must be held in hand of unaffected side Progress from wide-base quad cane to single-point cane
Walker	Bilateral lower extremity weakness— need upper extremity strength/ standing balance to use effectively	May be modified to accommodate upper extremity weakness/deformity Standard two-wheeled or four-wheeled May displace up to 50% of body weight
Lower extremity orthotics: ankle-foot orthotic (AFO), knee-ankle-foot orthotic (KAFO)	Painful, weak, or healing lower extremity	Plastic AFO commonly used for patients with improving lower extremity weakness Monitor for skin breakdown, especially if sensory impairment is present

tual capacities, proper equipment, and training in techniques for staff and resident appropriate for each resident's functional abilities.

An independent bed-to-wheelchair transfer requires the resident to have adequate sitting and standing balance, upper extremity function to lock the wheelchair brakes and grasp the siderail of the bed, and the ability to pivot from the standing position and sit down in the wheelchair (stand-pivot transfer). Cognitive impairment, hemiplegia with neglect of the affected side, upper or lower extremity weakness, depression, obesity, deconditioning, and orthostatic hypotension are all factors that may adversely affect the patient's ability to perform this transfer independently.

Wheelchair-to-toilet transfer requires that the resident rise from the wheelchair and stand-pivot onto the toilet. If the ability to make this transfer independently is impaired, adaptive equipment may be used to facilitate this transfer: Raised toilet seats and handrails on either or both sides of the toilet can assist patients with upper extremity weakness and hemiplegic residents in safe transfer on and off the toilet.

Feeding, Bathing, and Dressing

Independence in feeding, bathing, and dressing not only enhances self-esteem but allows residents to receive a less intensive level of care within nursing facilities (that is, intermediate care instead of skilled care). Loss of independence in bathing, feeding, or dressing may be caused by weakness, limited range of motion, difficulty with coordination, deficits in perception or safety awareness, or depression. Residents with Parkinson disease, stroke, muscle weakness or spasticity, deformity secondary to arthritis, generalized weakness, or impaired upper extremity function may benefit from the assistive devices listed in Box 10.2. Evaluation by an occupational therapist is needed to ensure that the appropriate assistive device is prescribed and that the resident is physically capable of using the device effectively. Perceptual deficits, upper extremity weakness, spasticity, or deformity must be evaluated to ensure that the assistive device will be effective. In general, the less cumbersome, complex, or conspicuous the aid, the greater the chance that it will be used. Assistive devices for feeding, bathing, or dressing may be expensive, and their costs are frequently not covered by Medicare or Medicaid.

In evaluating residents for assistive devices for

BOX 10.2. Assistive devices for feeding, bathing, and dressing

Feeding:	Rocker knife, enlarged silverware handles, weighted utensils, plate guards, high-rimmed dishes
Bathing:	Long-handled bath sponge, wash mitts, enlarged handles and length of combs and brushes
Dressing:	Button hook and zipper pulls, Velcro attachments to clothing/shoes, long-handled reachers, stocking-donning device

feeding, evaluation of swallowing function is frequently indicated. Dysphagia is a common problem among long-term nursing home residents. Dysphagia is usually acquired (for example, stroke), or the result of degenerative neurologic disorders (for example, Parkinson disease) or primary progressive dementias. Workup of dysphagia is similar to that described for patients with stroke-related dysphagia and may include a neurologic evaluation and a modified barium swallow, if necessary (51). Treatment of dysphagia in long-term residents may include several options: modification of diet to provide the safest consistencies of food and liquid (for example, diced or chopped food, thinned or thickened liquids); proper positioning of the resident (that is, having the resident sit as vertically as possible to best facilitate swallowing); speech therapy for oral motor and bolus control exercises or thermal stimulation, particularly for those patients with delayed triggering of the swallowing reflex (66,67).

CHALLENGES IN THE PROVISION OF REHABILITATION SERVICES FOR NURSING HOME RESIDENTS

1. *Does the site of provision of rehabilitation services for older patients affect outcome?* Will the provision of subacute care services in skilled nursing facilities provide rehabilitation services and outcomes comparable to the level of care that a hospital provides, and will this be an improvement over present skilled nursing facility–based rehabilitation services? Do the short-term rehabilitation programs that are provided in nursing homes for older persons with the new onset of disability (for example, stroke, hip fracture) provide

the same outcome that hospital-based rehabilitation programs provide? To date, most data on outcomes of stroke rehabilitation come from hospital-based rehabilitation programs of patients of similar disability and morbidity (68). A recent study comparing subacute rehabilitation in a skilled nursing facility with comprehensive inpatient rehabilitation found that inpatients received twice the rehabilitation services at twice the average charge and had greater gains in functional impairment measures (69). However, the proportion of patients discharged to the community varied little and the cost per point of functional impairment measure gain was substantially higher in the inpatient group, suggesting that subacute rehabilitation may be more cost effective (69). Similar data are needed to determine if patients with nontraditional rehabilitation diagnoses benefit from a short-term stay in a skilled nursing facility rehabilitation unit. For example, are patients who are discharged from acute hospital care for recurrent episodes of congestive heart failure or exacerbations of chronic obstructive pulmonary disease less likely to be readmitted to the acute-care setting if they receive posthospital rehabilitation services?

2. *If Medicare funded maintenance or preventative rehabilitation services, could the need for costly restorative rehabilitation services be reduced?* Patients with Parkinson disease, for example, often receive their first comprehensive physical therapy evaluation and treatment after incurring a broken hip, rather than participate in an exercise and gait training program designed to prevent fall and fracture. To date, limited data have demonstrated the benefit of maintenance rehabilitation services for long-term nursing home residents (70). Mulrow and colleagues (71) evaluated a 4-month period of thrice-weekly physical therapy for very frail long-term nursing home residents and found modest improvements in mobility (that is, patients were less likely to use assistive devices and wheelchairs), but these were accompanied by substantial financial costs and an increased rate of falls. Other studies involving healthier, more ambulatory nursing home residents have demonstrated that strengthening exercises and intensive weight and resistance training of the lower extremities can improve muscle function and strength (72–77). Relatively simple interventions, such as seated exercise, have demonstrated improved functional status and well-being of nursing home residents (78). Does earlier intervention with less frail individuals reduce longer-term risks of more significant disability, and hence reduce cost? Can lower-cost, less intensive rehabilitation resources (that is, use of physical therapy assistants, group therapy) be of benefit to select populations of nursing home residents with significant maintenance of function and with decreased disability and dependency, thus reducing the cost and perhaps the (later) need of institutional care?

3. *Are rehabilitation resources equitably distributed among nursing home residents?* The selection of patients for short-term rehabilitation services is often based on age, payment source, perception of family and patient motivation, and bed availability (79). A nursing home resident who suffers a stroke may be less likely to be accepted into a restorative intense rehabilitation program than a community-dwelling patient with stroke. A study of rehabilitation services of 8500 patients in 65 nursing homes found that the use of short-term rehabilitation services was correlated with neurologic and orthopedic diagnoses, partial dependence in activities of daily living, clear mental status, improvement in medical status, and having Medicare as a primary payment source (80). Has diagnosis-based reimbursement for rehabilitation created a system in which rehabilitation resources are over-utilized for short-term patients and under-utilized for long-term residents? If reimbursement were based on functional impairment rather than diagnosis, could rehabilitation resources be more appropriately allocated among both short-term and long-term nursing home residents?

4. *Will earlier physician referral of nursing home residents for rehabilitation evaluation result in better functional outcomes?* One of the most common reasons rehabilitation services are not included in the plan of care is the failure of physicians to refer patients. A recent study documented the impact of not referring patients for rehabilitation services on subsequent hospitalization and mortality (81). Earlier referral and intervention by rehabilitation for patients with stroke may also improve outcome (82). Rehabilitation evaluations should be prescribed as part

of the care plan for many nursing home residents who develop gait impairment or who are deconditioned by acute illness, to help reduce further morbidity and mortality.

In the role as advocates, physicians must recognize that for nursing home residents, quality of life is often equated with preservation of function and maintenance of some, albeit limited, independence. The effective prescription of rehabilitation services by physicians can play an important role in obtaining this goal.

Acknowledgments. The author gratefully acknowledges the thoughtful and critical review of this manuscript by Richard W. Besdine, MD, Laurence Z. Rubenstein, and Robert U. Massey, MD, and the technical support provided by Rosemary Brener, Sandy Blake, and Frances Finn.

REFERENCES

1. State Operations Manual. Provider Certification, Transmittal 250. Department of Health and Human Service, Health Care Financial Administration; April 1992.
2. Zimmer JG, Eggert GM, Treat A, Browdows B. Nursing homes as acute care providers. J Am Geriatr Soc. 1988;36:124-9.
3. Shaughnessy SW, Kramer AM. The increased needs of patients in nursing homes and patients receiving home health care. N Engl J Med. 1990;322:21-7.
4. Tresch DD, Duthie EH, Gruchow HW. Coping with DRGs—a nursing home experience. Am J Med Sci. 1989;298:309-13.
5. Marottoli RA, Berkman LF, Cooney LM, Jr. Decline in physical function following hip fracture. J Am Geriatr Soc. 1992;40:861-6.
6. Alberts KA, Nilsson MH. Consumption versus need of institutional care after femoral neck fracture. Scand J Rehabil Med. 1989;21:159-64.
7. Broos PL, Stappaerts KH, Luiten EJ, Gruwez JA. Home-going prognostic factors concerning the major goal in treatment of elderly hip fracture patients. Int Surg. 1988;73:148-50.
8. Bonar SK, Tinetti ME, Speechley M, Cooney LM. Factors associated with short-versus long-term skilled nursing placement among community living hip fracture patients. J Am Geriatr Soc. 1990;38:1139-44.
9. Magaziner J, Simonsick EM, Kashner TM, Hebel JR, Kenzora JE. Predictors of functional recovery one year following hospital discharge for hip fracture: a prospective study. J Gerontol. 1990;45:M101-7.
10. Ensberg MD, Paletta MJ, Galecki AT, Dacko CL, Fires BE. Identifying elderly patients for early discharge after hospitalization for hip fracture. J Gerontol. 1993;48:M187-95.
11. Perez ED. Hip fracture: physicians take more active role in patient care. Geriatrics. 1994;49:31-7.
12. Folman Y, Geptstein R, Assaraf A, Liberty S. Functional recovery after operative treatment of femoral neck fracture in an institutionalized elderly population. Arch Phys Med Rehabil. 1994;75:454-7.
13. Petersen VS, Solgaard S, Simonsen B. Total hip replacement in patients aged 80 years and older. J Am Geriatr Soc. 1989;37:219-22.
14. Callahan CM, Drake BG, Heck DA, Dittus RS. Patient outcomes following tricompartmental total knee replacement. JAMA. 1994;271:1349-57.
15. Colewell CW Jr, Spiro TE, Trowbridge AA, Morris BA, Kwaan HC, Blaha JD, et al. Use of enoxaparin, a low molecular weight heparin for the prevention of deep vein thrombosis after elective hip replacement. J Bone Joint Surg. 1994;76:3-14.
16. Turpie AG, Gent M, Cote R, Levine MM, Ginsberg JS, Powers PJ, et al. A low-molecular-weight heparinoid compared with unfractionated heparin in the prevention of deep vein thrombosis in patients with acute ischemic stroke. Ann Intern Med. 1992;117:353-7.
17. O'Brien BJ, Anderson DR, Goerci R. Cost-effectiveness of enoxaparin versus warfarin prophylaxis against deep vein thrombosis after total hip replacement. Can Med Assoc J. 1994:150:1083-90.
18. Spiro TE, Johnson GJ, Christie MJ, Lyons RM, MacFarlane DE, Blasier RB, et al. Efficacy and safety of enoxaparin to prevent deep venous thrombosis after hip replacement surgery. Ann Intern Med. 1994;121:81-9.
19. Imperiale TF, Speroff T. A meta-analysis of methods to prevent venous thromboembolism following total hip replacement. JAMA. 1994;271:1780-5.
20. Trowbridge A, Boese CK, Woodruff B, Brundly HH Sr, Lowry WE, Spiro TE. Incidence of posthospitalization proximal deep vein thrombosis after total hip arthroplasty. A pilot study. Clin Orthop. 194; 299:203-8.
21. Paiement GD, Bersaw NE, Harris WH, Wessinger SJ, Wyman EM. Advances in prevention of venous thromboembolic disease after elective hip surgery. Instr Course Lect. 1990;39:413-21.
22. Wilson MG, Pei LF, Malone KM, Polck JF, Creager MA, Goldhaber SZ. Fixed low-dose versus adjusted higher-dose warfarin following orthopedic surgery. A randomized prospective trial. J Arthroplasty. 1994;9:127-30.
23. Antiplatelet Trialists Collaboration. Collaborative overview of randomised trials of antiplatelet therapy-III. Reduction in venous thrombosis and pulmonary embolism by antiplatelet prophylaxis among surgical and medical patients. BMJ. 1994; 308:235-46.
24. Reis SE, Hirsch DR, Wilson MG, Donovan BC, Goldhaber SZ.. A program for the prevention of venous thromboembolism in high-risk orthopedic patients. J Arthroplasty. 1991;6 Suppl:S11-6.

25. Williams-Russo P, Urquhart BL, Sharrock NE, Charlson ME. Post-operative delirium: Predictors and prognosis in elderly orthopedic patients. J Am Geriatr Soc. 1992;40:759-67.
26. Gustafson Y, Berggren MD, Brännström B, Bucht G, Norberg A, Hansson LI, et al. Acute confusional states in elderly patients treated for femoral neck fractures. J Am Geriatr Soc. 1988;36:525-30.
27. Murray AM, Levkoff E, Wetle TT, Beckett L, Cleary PD, Schor JD, et al. Acute delirium and functional decline in the hospitalized elderly patient. J Gerontol. 1993;48: M181-6.
28. Schor JD, Levkoff SE, Lipsitz, LA, Reilly CH, Cleary PD, Rowe JW, et al. Risk factors for delirium in hospitalized elderly. JAMA. 1992;267:827-31.
29. Beaver WT. Impact of non-narcotic oral analgesics in pain management. Am J Med. 1988;84::3-15.
30. Hanks GW. The clinical usefulness of agonist-antagonist opioid analgesics in chronic pain. Drug Alcohol Depend. 1987;20:338-46.
31. Newington DP, Bannister GC, Fordyce M. Primary total hip replacement in patients over 80 years of age. J Bone Joint Surg [Br]. 1990;72:450-2.
32. Kotila M, Waltimo O, Niemi ML, Laaksonen R, Lempinen M. The profile of recovery from stroke and factors influencing outcome. Stroke. 1984;15: 1039-44.
33. Thorngren M, Westling B, Norrving B. Outcome after stroke in patients discharged to independent living. Stroke. 1990;21:236-40.
34. Wade DT, Skilbeck CE, Hewer R. Predicting Barthel ADL score at 6 months after an acute stroke. Arch Phys Med Rehabil. 1983;64:24-8.
35. Heinemann AW, Roth EJ, Cichowski K, Betts HB. Multivariate analysis of improvement and outcome following stroke rehabilitation. Arch Neurol. 1987;44:1167-72.
36. Jongbloed L. Prediction of function after stroke: a critical review. Stroke. 1986;17:765-76.
37. Granger CV, Hamilton BB. Measurement of stroke rehabilitation outcome in the 1980s. Stroke. 1990;21:46-7.
38. Evans RL, Bishop DS, Matlock AL, Stranahan S, Halar EM, Noonan W. Prestroke family interaction as a predictor of stroke outcome. Arch Phys Med Rehabil. 1987;68:508-12.
39. Granger CV, Hamilton BB, Fiedler RC. Discharge outcome after stroke rehabilitation. Stroke. 1992; 23:978-82.
40. Nakayama H, Jorgensen HS, Rauaschou HO, Olsen TS. Recovery of upper extremity function in stroke patients. The Copenhagen Stroke Group, Arch Phys Med and Rehabil. 1994;75:394-8.
41. Jorgensen HS, Nakayama H, Raaschou HO, Olsen TS. Recovery of walking function in stroke patients. The Copenhagen Stroke Group. Arch Phys Med Rehabil. 1995;75:27-32.
42. Pambianco G, Orchard T, Landau P. Deep vein thrombosis: prevention in stroke patients during rehabilitation. Arch Phys Med Rehabil. 1995;76: 324-30.
43. Brandstater ME, Roth EJ, Siebens HC. Venous thromboebolism in stroke: literature review and implications for clinical process. Arch Phys Med Rehabil. 1992;73(5-S):379-91.
44. McCarthy ST, Turner J. Low-dose subcutaneous heparin in the prevention of deep-vein thrombosis and pulmonary emboli following acute stroke. Age Aging. 1986;15:84-8.
45. Roth EJ, Mueller K, Green D. Stroke rehabilitation outcome: impact of coronary artery disease. Stroke. 1988;19:42-7.
46. Roth EJ, Green D. Cardiac complications in stroke rehabilitation [abstract]. Arch Phys Med Rehabil. 1990;71:776.
47. Corcoran PJ, Peszayenshi M. Gait and gait retraining. In: Basmajian JV, ed. Therapeutic Exercise. Baltimore:Williams & Williams;1984:285-302.
48. Roth EJ. Heart disease in patients with stroke. Arch Phys Med Rehabil. 1994;75:94-101.
49. Leach CM, Leach JA. Stroke rehabilitation in elderly patients with coronary artery disease. In: Erickson RV, ed. Medical Management of the Elderly Stroke Patient. Physical Medicine and Rehabilitation: State of the Art Review. Philadelphia: Hanley and Belfus; 1989: 3:611-8.
50. Horner J, Masseu EW. Silent aspiration following stroke. Neurology. 1988;38:317-19.
51. Splaingard ML, Hutchins B, Sulton LD, Chaudhuri G. Aspiration in rehabilitation patients: video fluoroscopy vs. bedside clinical assessment. Arch Phys Med Rehabil. 1988;69:637-40.
52. Miller RM, Langmore SE. Treatment efficacy for adults with oropharyngeal dysphagia. Arch Phys Med Rehabil. 1994;75:1256-62.
53. Dunne JW, Leedman PJ, Edis RH. Inobvious stroke: a cause of delirium and dementia. Aust N Z J Med. 1986;16:771-8.
54. Schmidley AW. Agitated confusional states in patients with right hemisphere infarctions. Stroke. 1984;15:883-5.
55. Dicks RS, Erickson RV. Evaluation of altered mental status: delirium. In: Erickson RV, ed. Medical Management of the Elderly Stroke Patient. Physical Medicine and Rehabilitation: State of the Art Review. Philadelphia: Hanley and Belfus; 1989:3: 629-44.
56. House A. Mood disorders after stroke: a review of the evidence. Int J Geriatric Psychiatry. 1987;2:211-21.
57. Reding MJ, Orto LA, Winter SW, Fortuna IM, Di Ponte P, McDowell FH. Antidepressant therapy after stroke: a double-blind trial. Arch Neurol. 1986;43: 763-5.
58. Lipsey JR, Robinson RG, Pearlson GD, Rao K, Price TR. Nortriptyline treatment of post-stroke depression: a double-blind study. Lancet. 1984; 297-300.
59. Sinyor D, Amato P, Kaloupek DG, Becker R, Goldenberg M, Coopersmith H, et al. Post-stroke depression: relationships to functional impairment, coping strategies, and rehabilitation outcome. Stroke. 1986;17:1102-7.

60. Sakuma J, Hinterbuchner C, Green R, Silber M. Rehabilitation of geriatric patients having bilateral lower extremity amputations. Arch Phys Med Rehabil. 1985;55:101-11.

61. Malone JM, Moore W, Leal JM, Childers SJ. Rehabilitation for lower extremity amputation. Arch Surg. 1981;116:93-8.

62. Sioson ER. The elderly amputee with severe chronic obstructive pulmonary disease. J Am Geriatr Soc. 1990;38:51-2.

63. Reyes RL, Leahey EB, Leahy EB Jr. Elderly patients with lower extremity amputations: three-year study in a rehabilitation setting. Arch Phys Med Rehabil. 1977;58:115-23.

64. Steinberg FU, Sunwoo I, Roettger RF. Prosthetic rehabilitation of geriatric amputee patients: a follow-up study. Arch Phys Med Rehabil. 1985;66:742-5.

65. Harper CM, Lyles YM. Physiology and complications of bed rest. J Am Geriatr Soc. 1988;36:1047-54.

66. Veis SL, Logemann JA. Swallowing disorders in persons with cerebrovascular accidents. Arch Phys Med Rehabil. 1985;66:372-75.

67. Lazzara G, Lazarus C, Logemann J. Impact of thermal stimulation on the triggering of the swallow reflex. Dysphagia. 1986;1:73-7.

68. Granger CV, Hamilton BB, Gresham GE. The stroke rehabilitation outcome study. Part I: General Description. Part II: Relative merits of the total Barthel index score and a four-item subscore in predicting patient outcomes. Arch Phys Med Rehabil. 1988;69:506-9;70:100-4.

69. Keith RA, Wilson DB, Gutierrez P. Acute and subacute rehabilitation for stroke: a comparison. Arch Phys Med Rehabil. 1995;76:495-500.

70. Smith ME. The organization, delivery, utilization and financing of rehabilitation care for the elderly. DRG 1990;7:1-11.

71. Mulrow CD, Gereth MD, Kanten D, Cornell JE, DeNino LA, Chiodo L, et al. A randomized trial of physical rehabilitation for very frail nursing home residents. JAMA 1994;271:519-24.

72. Sauvage LR, Mykelbust BM, Crow-Pan J, Novak S, Millington P, Hoffman MD, et al. A clinical trial of strengthening and aerobic exercise to improve gait and balance in elderly male nursing home residents. Am J Phys Med Rehabil. 1992;71:333-42.

73. Fisher NM, Pendergast DR, Calkins E. Muscle rehabilitation in impaired elderly nursing home residents. Arch Phys Med Rehabil. 1991;72:181-5.

74. Jirovec MM. The impact of daily exercise on the mobility, balance, and urine control of cognitively impaired nursing home residents. Int J Nurs Stud. 1991;281:145-51.

75. Fiatarone MA, Marks EC, Ryan ND, Meredith CN, Lipsitz LA, Evans WJ. High-intensity strength training in nonagenarians. JAMA. 1990;263:3029-84

76. Li L. A nursing home strength training and exercise program [abstract]. J Am Geriatr Soc. 1993;41: SA29.

77. Hadley EC. The research findings of FICSIT trials. Gerontologist. 1993;33:204.

78. McMurdo ME, Rennie LA. A controlled trial of exercise by residents of old peoples' homes. Age Ageing. 1993;22:11-5.

79. Caplan AL, Callahan D, Haas J. Ethical and policy issues in rehabilitation medicine. A Hastings Center Report.1987;17:1-20.

80. Murtaugh CM, Cooney LM, DerSimonian RR, Smits HL, Fetter RB. Nursing home reimbursement and the allocation of rehabilitation therapy resources. Health Serv Res. 1988;23:467-93.

81. Evan RL, Haselkorn JK, Bishop DS, Hendricks RV. Characteristics of hospital patients receiving medical rehabilitation: an exploratory outcome comparison. Arch Phys Med Rehabil. 1991;72:685-9.

82. Ottenbacher KJ, Jamell S. The results of clinical trials in stroke rehabilitation research. Arch Neurol. 1993;50:37-44.

— 11 —

Ethical and Legal Issues

Deon Cox Hayley, DO, Christine K. Cassel, MD, FACP,
Lois Snyder, JD, and Mark A. Rudberg, MD, MPH

The withholding or withdrawal of life-sustaining treatment. The capacity to give informed consent. Surrogate decision making. Advance directives. Ethics committees. These have become familiar terms in hospitals throughout the country, but what happens to these and other ethical and legal concepts when the scene shifts from the hospital to the nursing home? Although ethical and legal issues abound in medicine, these dilemmas are even more frequent and complicated for practitioners who care for nursing home residents, because of both the nursing home environment and the underlying medical and social conditions of the residents. This chapter gives an understanding of why ethical issues in the nursing home are different from those in the hospital setting and of how the environment and residents make these situations unique. Although we are unable to analyze the ethical and legal issues in depth in this chapter, this can be a starting point for physicians to think about the ethical and legal dilemmas that might arise in the nursing home and how to deal with them.

THE NURSING HOME ENVIRONMENT

The ethical situations that arise in the nursing home have no exact parallels in any other health care setting. The environment and process of care are therefore unique.

Who Is in the Nursing Home?

The nursing home population consists predominately of poor, elderly, and physically or mentally disabled persons. Most individuals probably would not choose to live in an institution, but because of lack of financial resources to get nursing care at home or in another setting, many arrive impoverished. Approximately 63% of nursing home residents have some type of cognitive impairment that may affect their ability to participate fully in decisions about their care (1,2).

Becoming a Resident

Becoming a nursing home resident means leaving at the door a certain amount of autonomy, often beginning with the process for admission. Many times the resident has not chosen the facility—a family member or someone else decides. A Federal Trade Commission draft report found that the nursing home resident (whom the report referred to as "the ultimate consumer") "frequently has the least to say during the critical selection process" (3). The selection of a facility is often made under crisis circumstances, such as the rapid deterioration of health, or because of caregiver stress or the death of a caregiver. In addition, a shortage of beds or geographic considerations may severely limit choice. For many, the choice is a final one; one third of new admissions stay for more than a year, and these residents are likely to die in the nursing home (4).

The selection and admissions processes often foster an atmosphere that from the start diminishes the role of the individual. Some institutions disregard the legal requirement that competent individuals sign admissions contracts; they frequently presume the individual lacks the capacity to sign (or accept another's pronouncement that the prospective resident is incompetent) and insist on dealing with a family member or other responsible party to sign the contract. The print in admissions contracts is often too small for the prospective resident to read, and the facility may see the signing of the agreement as perfunctory, 3 hours or less being the standard amount of time for the admissions process.

Vulnerability

Autonomy, or self-determination, is fundamental in medical ethics, the law, and the daily lives of most Americans (5). We accept that individuals should be able to make their own decisions regarding personal and medical care. The physician caring for nursing home residents should acknowledge the lessened emphasis of the values of choice, control, dignity, and privacy in the nursing home.

Elderly persons face many physical and cognitive losses, and these losses are often the reason for nursing home admission. Many residents experience changes in their social support system as the result of loss of family members, friends, home, and finances. Although values such as security and companionship may be considered important in the nursing home setting (6), moving from a familiar setting of former independence to the nursing home confirms and adds a new dimension to the loss of autonomy and self-determination.

In the institutional context, "deliberate efforts [may be required] to help residents feel more powerful, such as providing appropriate emotional support, effective counseling, adequate information, optimal medication regimen, and involvement opportunities for family and friends" (7).

Most decisions in the nursing home are made by someone other than the resident. Physicians write orders for medications, treatment, and therapies; prescribe recreation, activities, and diet; and give instructions for other aspects of daily life. Nursing home life is also controlled by nursing home policies; local, state, and federal laws and regulations; and accreditation standards; thus, the nursing home

has been described as "a total institution" (8). The many rules and regulations have improved the quality of care, but they are often imposed on inadequate numbers of nursing staff for residents who need close supervision. Thus, unfortunately, it is very difficult to provide personalized care and autonomy. Furthermore, autonomy may be restricted by well-meaning staff members and regulators who "protect" physically or mentally dependent residents. Protection is sometimes necessary, other times overdone.

Privacy is closely linked to autonomy and is likewise difficult to protect in the nursing home. Bedrooms are usually shared, common rooms are often noisy and crowded, and staff members may walk in on residents without permission. Because of limited privacy, the sexuality of residents is constrained. It may be acceptable to restrict sexual relations in a short hospital stay, but less so in a place substituting for home.

In addition it is difficult to maintain confidentiality of personal information in the nursing home. Current and previous medical, psychiatric, and social problems are recorded in such a way that all caregivers have access to these records. This open distribution of information further diminishes the resident's sense of privacy and autonomy.

Regulations to address residents' rights and welfare were passed in 1987 in the Nursing Home Quality Reform Act of the Omnibus Budget Reconciliation Act of 1987 (OBRA 1987, Pub L No. 100-203). These regulations in OBRA 1987 include

- Assuring resident rights to privacy and decision making regarding accommodations, medical treatment, personal care, visits, written and telephone communications, and meetings with others.

- Maintaining confidentiality of personal and clinical records.

- Requiring comprehensive resident assessments and individualized care plans in accordance with those assessments.

- Ensuring proper use of physical restraints and psychoactive drugs.

- Requiring a minimum amount of nursing and social work coverage.

- Requiring that notice of rights be provided at the time of admission. Implementing admissions policy requirements.

- Ensuring transfer and discharge rights (9).

Along with developments in the law, the literature in medical ethics has indicated ways in which individualized care in the nursing home can be promoted (10), beginning with concrete aspects of the structure of the institution and the behavior of staff. Although it may be difficult to personalize care schedules, attention to small details may make a big difference in residents' satisfaction and sense of autonomy. For instance, a resident's long-cherished routine of reading the morning paper with a cup of coffee or coming to breakfast in robe and slippers may not fit with the schedule of the staff but would be relatively easy to accommodate. Nursing home residents have also strongly suggested that "permeability" between the nursing home and the outside world be encouraged through excursions, telephone calls, and mail to help increase feelings of independence and integrity (11).

Whether it is the right to have visitors or the right to privacy in using the bathroom when feasible or the right to decide whether to undergo a medical test or procedure, the physician is often in the best position to help enhance resident autonomy and set a tone that respects resident dignity, privacy, choice, and control.

ETHICAL PRINCIPLES

Issues of confidentiality, consent, and assessment of decision-making capacity all are part of a practitioner's average day. These issues also have legal implications. Often, there is no conflict, and the situation is handled without incident. However, sometimes these issues are not easily resolved.

Clinical medical ethics attempts to address "the identification, analysis, and resolution of moral problems that arise in the care of a particular patient. These moral concerns are inseparable from the concerns surrounding the correct diagnosis and treatment of the patient" (12).

Although principle-based medical ethics has been critiqued, the principles of beneficence, respect for persons, fidelity, and justice can be used as a framework to approach an ethical issue and parcel out the different values (13). It may be helpful to consider the implications of each principle for the issue at hand; however, doing so may not lead to clear conclusions, because each principle may lead to different plans of action, or the principles may conflict.

The principle of beneficence refers to the obligation of doing what is best for the patient. Benefi-cent care of the patient encompasses attention to both scientific expertise and compassionate, low-tech care. Included in the consideration of what is best is nonmaleficence, or doing no harm. However, occasionally, what will not cause harm and what is best for the patient may come in conflict; for instance, a proposed treatment that would help the patient may be painful. Beneficence should be distinguished from paternalism, in which the physician's determination of what is best for the patient is considered more important than the patient's determination of what is best.

The next principle, respect for persons, encompasses a basic respect for human life and centers around the concept of autonomy. Autonomy is one of the most important aspects in considerations of informed consent, disclosure of information, making health care decisions in advance (including advance directives), and the right to refuse treatment. The autonomous wishes of an individual may occasionally come in conflict with the medical plan that is considered beneficent, for example, when a resident refuses the proposed therapy despite the physician's recommendation that it would restore the resident's health.

Another aspect of respect for persons is constituted by respectful action, which becomes critical with loss of cognitive capacity. If residents cannot engage in meaningful dialogue, then many of the usual components of interaction that normally elicit respect are absent. Because the majority of nursing home residents have some degree of cognitive impairment, caregivers must exercise special attention to the fundamental humanity of the most unresponsive or demented persons. This includes a whole range of concerns with how patients are addressed, handled, clothed, and treated during the course of an interaction.

The principle of fidelity embraces the all-important doctor–patient relationship on which the clinical practice of medicine is based. It implies trust and confidentiality. This principle addresses the balance needed between the autonomous decisions of patients and the beneficent recommendations made by physicians. Fidelity holds particular responsibilities for the nursing home physician because the doctor–patient relationship is particularly asymmetric; the physician is both more knowledgeable and more powerful, whereas the patient is extremely vulnerable. Patients have certain rights regarding confidentiality of information, truthfulness, and availability that physicians must acknowledge and address.

Last, the principle of justice may be easy to identify but harder to resolve. Justice addresses equitable treatment and distribution of resources. This principle can be considered at a variety of levels: the levels of equity for the patient, for an institution, and even for society at large. Justice poses special difficulties because it can conflict with fidelity or beneficent treatment. For example, the treatment that is thought best for the patient may result in an unequal distribution of resources. In this case, the welfare of the patient should be considered above societal justice.

SELECTED ISSUES

A multitude of issues that arise in the nursing home can be considered ethical or moral dilemmas. As already mentioned, the most difficult balance to attain is between autonomy (or extended autonomy) and protection. Thus, we might categorize the issues based on those concerned with decision making and those focused on the protection of residents.

Decision Making

The practice of medicine is filled with decisions to be made jointly by physicians and patients. In the nursing home, the types of decisions and approaches to them may differ from those in the hospital or outpatient setting.

DECISION-MAKING CAPACITY, COMPETENCE, AND CONSENT

Many nursing home residents have limited ability to make personal and medical decisions because of cognitive impairment or difficulties with communication. However, limited decision-making capacity does not mean that residents are completely unable to make decisions. Most residents with dementia are able to make some decisions for themselves. Even so, residents may defer decision making to trusted family members even when they retain the capacity to make decisions themselves. Additionally, in decisions of great importance, it is often practical to include close family members or friends in discussions so that they can support the resident and help clarify issues, if necessary.

When determining whether a resident is able to participate in decision making, the health care provider must consider and evaluate competence and decision-making capacity separately. Determination of incompetence is de jure and implies an absolute and unchanging condition (14). In reality, many residents with cognitive impairment have variable abilities to make decisions. This variability is expressed as *decision-making capacity,* which may be partial and may vary over time or with the situation (15).

In cases of limited decision-making capacity, the concept of a sliding scale may be helpful to determine acceptance or refusal of proposed treatment. A sliding scale implies that to consent, a resident must have a higher level of understanding of a treatment with potentially more risk and less benefit (16). For instance, the level of understanding required for consent to have blood drawn is considerably less than that required for elective surgery because of the higher relative risks.

An example of a situation in which altered decision-making capacity must be considered is the resident with moderate dementia who presents with iron-deficiency anemia and hemepositive stools. When presented with the situation and possible diagnostic approaches, the nursing home resident may be unable to make complicated decisions about a colonoscopy that might find a curable lesion, but the resident may be able to strongly express that he does not want to go through painful and disruptive procedures. The resident may also be able to express general values, for example, by saying he is old and knows he will not live much longer and would not want his life to be artificially prolonged. The clinician must weigh the benefit-burden ratio of possible life prolongation and possible prevention of a painful obstruction against invasive testing and the associated discomfort and disruption of the resident's life. The resident should participate as much as possible in decision making, but assistance from others who know the person well can aid the physician in coming to a treatment plan that reflects both what the resident would want if he were able to make the decision himself and what is in his best interest.

The assessment of whether residents understand the risks and benefits of any proposed intervention and of their ability to make a choice based on personal values is not always easy, but it is a necessary clinical skill for all physicians who see nursing home residents. The determination of decision-making capacity should not automatically fall to psychiatrists, because knowledge of the patient and surrounding circumstances give the primary care physician particular strength in making these determinations (17). However, if decision-making capacity is unclear, an expert second opinion is recommended.

A resident's ability to give informed consent is closely linked to decision-making capacity. Informed consent is more than a completed form for diagnostic and therapeutic procedures; it is a concept that expresses the resident's ability to communicate and understand the information that is needed for reasoning and deliberating about choices (18). Consent should extend beyond the usual invasive procedures for which forms are usually signed and should be an ongoing process for the use of medications, restraints, and other components of nursing home life in which physicians give orders.

Many nursing home residents are completely unable to make decisions. However, most of these residents have not been legally declared incompetent. For some, this is not necessary from a practical standpoint because the residents have concerned family members who will make decisions. In the case of an elderly woman with end-stage dementia, her husband and children are assumed to have the moral authority to act as surrogate decision makers. In some states, surrogacy laws authorize family members and friends to make decisions for those who do not have advance directives and are unable to make decisions themselves (19).

Some of the most difficult situations in nursing home care surround life-and-death decisions for individuals who are functionally incompetent and have no family or friends to share the resident's views or make decisions for the resident. In this case, autonomy and extended autonomy through a surrogate decision maker are moot. Beneficence is often unclear in this situation, so nonmaleficence and respect for the person may predominate in the decision making. Legal guardianship and/or consultation by an ethics committee may help the physician determine appropriate actions.

SURROGATE DECISION MAKING

Physicians must commonly turn to surrogates to assist in medical decision making when residents cannot make decisions alone. Ideally, the person who serves as a surrogate should agree to do so and should know the resident well enough to be able to bring his or her goals and values to the discussion (20). Unfortunately, many decisions, particularly in day-to-day care, must be made without knowledge of what the resident would have wanted.

In the absence of an advance directive, surrogates should consider the resident's previous statements and known values to make decisions for the resident. This standard is referred to as *substituted judgment,* and although critics are concerned with the accuracy of these decisions (21,22), there is evidence that, in most situations, the elderly's trust in family outweighs the need for accurate decisions (23). If no previous stated preferences can be determined, physicians and surrogates should agree on the resident's best interest. Some experts raise concerns that conflicts of interest (for example, an inheritance) invariably complicate the role of family members as surrogates (24). If the physician suspects that the family is not acting in the resident's best interests or if the family members disagree, a mechanism to resolve conflict, such as an ethics committee, is advisable.

Surrogacy acts, recently passed by several states, list persons who may legally make medical decisions for those individuals without advance directives who are unable to make decisions themselves (25). Unfortunately, these acts tend to apply to end-of-life situations and are less helpful in many day-to-day decisions that do not involve terminating medical treatment.

Often, physicians caring for nursing home residents struggle to find appropriate surrogates when the choice is not clear. Many people are in the nursing home because they do not have any close friends or relatives. The friends and relatives they do have may not be able to help with decision making because of emotional or geographic distance.

ADVANCE DIRECTIVES

Advance directives (living wills and durable powers of attorney for health care or health care proxies) are formal, written documents designed to guide medical care when an individual becomes unable to make medical decisions, particularly in end-of-life situations (26). All states now have living will laws, and most recognize durable powers of attorney for health care (27). Advance care planning also includes the informal expression of desires to guide medical treatment. This informal directive is important, because most individuals have not completed the formal documents (28).

If advance directives are to extend medical self-determination in the nursing home, the nursing staff, administration, and physicians must understand both the utility of the documents and the institution's policy. Because most elderly persons who live in nursing homes will die there, it is especially pertinent that both formal advance directives and informal decisions regarding end-of-life care be addressed with the nursing home resident. If the resident is unable to make these decisions, similar discussions should be held with appropriate surrogates.

If a prospective nursing home resident has completed an advance directive document, it is important that this be recognized on admission. The Patient Self-determination Act requires all medical facilities receiving federal funds (nearly all nursing homes) to ask on admission if the prospective resident has previously completed advance directive documents (29). This should be used as a starting point for further discussion between the resident, physician, and other health care providers. Addressing the topic of advance directives provides a perfect opportunity to encourage residents to discuss wishes for future medical care. Although residents who are incapable of participation in these discussions cannot have new documents completed, the physician should try to discern previously expressed goals or preferences (either written or spoken) and should make note of these on the medical record (30).

When individuals are instructed about the usefulness of advance directives, they do not always complete a form. Discussion of advance directives should not be confused with coercion to fill out documents, especially if the goals of the document do not coincide with the goals of the resident. Nevertheless, even if documents are not completed, the discussion can produce useful information. In fact, advance planning for medical care should be considered a process in which it is appropriate that decisions of such gravity be undertaken thoughtfully. If a resident is not ready to make decisions at the time of admission, the topic of advance directives and advance care planning should be raised at a later date. Even decisions that sound definitive should be reviewed over time because changes in circumstances may precipitate changes in residents' desires. Although the legal standing and familiarity of formal documents is preferable, documentation of oral communications with residents regarding their desires for future medical care also can serve as a reliable guide for decision making (31).

DECIDING ABOUT LIFE-SUSTAINING TREATMENT

Conversations regarding advance medical care planning should specifically address desires for life-sustaining treatment. There are times when further use of life-prolonging medical technology may no longer be beneficial or desired. Nursing home residents may have strong feelings about this. If the topic has not been broached, the resident or family may appropriately initiate discussion of withholding or withdrawing treatment (32). Autonomy dictates that competent individuals "choose among medically indicated treatments and refuse any unwanted treatments" (33). However, before honoring such wishes, physicians should ensure that the individual truly desires the treatment limitations and understands the consequences. In fact, although physicians should always discuss and thoughtfully evaluate these decisions, they are morally obligated to respect the wishes of a competent resident who has made a choice. If a physician has a moral objection to these requests, another physician should be found who will honor them. Legal support for refusing treatment has been upheld in numerous court decisions (34), including the U.S. Supreme Court decision in *Cruzan* (1990), in which the court found that a competent patient's liberty interest protects his or her right to refuse life-sustaining nutrition or hydration (35). If the resident is no longer able to make decisions, formal surrogates designated by advance directives or informal surrogates, such as close family members who know the resident well, ethically may make the same decisions to withhold or withdraw treatment (36).

Limitation of treatment does not imply all or nothing. Decisions regarding treatment plans should make clinical sense but may be specific and may range from refusal of resuscitation to do-not-hospitalize orders to stopping nutrition and hydration. For instance, a treatment plan may consist of do-not-resuscitate orders and not hospitalizing a resident if he or she becomes ill but using antibiotics and intravenous therapy for infections treatable in the nursing home. However, it would not make sense clinically to have a treatment plan to withhold hospitalization yet perform resuscitation should the resident undergo cardiac arrest. Although it may seem more difficult to withdraw treatment than to withhold it, there is no difference from an ethical perspective (34). For example, it may seem easier to not begin dialysis treatment for a resident with profound dementia and progressive renal failure than to withdraw dialysis from a similar resident who has been receiving the treatment for years and has developed a profound dementia; nevertheless, ethically and legally, these situations are the same.

The decision not to use cardiopulmonary resuscitation in the event of cardiac arrest in the nursing home is a medical decision as well as a practical one. Nursing home staff vary in their ability to perform cardiopulmonary resuscitation, and since most cardiac arrests are not witnessed, chances of success, even by experienced personnel, are dismal. In fact, numerous studies have documented nearly universally fatal outcomes of resuscitation efforts in the nursing home (37). Despite these data, the policy at most nursing homes directs staff to initiate cardiopulmonary resuscitation unless there is a documented do-not-resuscitate order in the record. This discrepancy between statistics and policy emphasizes how important it is that health care providers educate residents and families beforehand about the utility of resuscitation efforts.

Clinicians may be frustrated both by the lack of transportability and by the refusal to recognize orders limiting treatment, especially do-not-resuscitate orders, between nursing homes and hospitals. This varies between states, and regulations may limit emergency medical services in accepting advance directives (such as do-not-resuscitate orders) from nursing homes. With the leadership of physicians, however, some cities have established networks for such directives that are accepted by all providers, regardless of location (38).

The issue of nutrition and hydration may be considered separately because of the strong emotions associated with eating and drinking and providing for those who are unable to do so themselves (39). Tube feeding for those with advanced dementia or terminal conditions is particularly sensitive. Some family members and staff in nursing homes have strong feelings regarding the necessity of food and water for providing comfort care and who believe that no one should be deprived of them; it is difficult to watch residents die without food or fluids (40,41). It has also been questioned whether tube feedings constitute medical treatment. Tube feeding may be recommended or used when the resident is able to take in some food and fluids. In these cases, staff and family members should continue to attempt to provide as much oral intake as the resident can handle or wants. Complicating these decisions, many nursing homes have regulations prohibiting the withdrawal of feeding tubes and requiring the use of feeding tubes for residents who are not eating well. From an ethical perspective, food and nutrition may be refused by a competent individual, and the same power extends to appropriate surrogates (42).

Protection

Although the issues of decision making addressed above focus particularly on autonomy, several issues in nursing home care emphasize protection of residents. Nursing home care is structured and regulated to address the fact that all nursing home residents need to be protected to varying degrees. Health care providers, families, and friends must appropriately balance the resident's right to act autonomously in a manner that may be harmful and moral responsibilities to protect the vulnerable.

RESTRAINTS

Mechanical restraints, which include cloth and leather restraints as well as other devices that limit movement, have been commonly used in the nursing home. Restraints are used both to protect the resident from harm and to minimize risk for the institution and other residents. Harmful behaviors that may be considered by well-meaning physicians and nursing staff to require the use of restraints are unsteadiness, disruptiveness, agitation, and wandering (43). However, there is evidence that restraints do not minimize risk to the institution and can actually cause harm to those who are restrained (44). Restraints may be misused as a form of convenience or discipline by staff members unable to give sufficient attention to residents (45).

Restraints can cause physical harm, such as ischemic limbs, contractures, skin trauma, and deconditioning, and they have even been associated with death by asphyxiation (46). Additionally, the use of restraints can result in substantial psychological morbidity, including demoralization, humiliation, fear, and stress (47).

There is a trend to decrease the use of restraints and re-evaluate their usefulness, partly because of ethical considerations and partly because of newer regulations. The enactment of OBRA 1987 has significantly reduced the numbers of nursing home residents who are restrained. Before enactment, as many as 59% of residents in some facilities were restrained (48), whereas in September 1992, according to the Health Care Financing Administration, approximately 22% of residents were restrained (49). The OBRA regulation on physical restraints emphasizes rehabilitation (50) and states that "the decision . . . should be based on the assessment of each resident's capabilities, an evaluation of less restrictive alternatives, and the ruling out of their use. A plan of care should also contain a schedule or plan of rehabilitative training to enable the progressive removal of restraints or the progressive use of less restrictive means, as appropriate."

Alternate therapies are preferable to restraints: prompt treatment of medical problems, attention to environmental safety concerns, such as nonslip floors, and behavior-modification techniques (51). For instance, some dementia units that have problems with confused residents wandering out exit doors have disguised functional doors by painting them to look like bookcases. This simple but innovative technique may keep residents from unsafely wandering out of the building without physically restraining them. Unfortunately, staff members who are overextended may feel that alternatives to physical restraints are time-consuming and difficult to implement. In fact, studies have shown the reverse to be true; it takes staff members more time to deal with the physical and behavioral consequences of restraint use (52). New strategies and approaches are being implemented, and nursing home staff need support for education and communication with other institutions to enhance their skills in this area.

Nonmaleficence and autonomy both need to be addressed when the use of restraints is being considered. In our opinion, there are very few times when the resident cannot be adequately protected without the use of potentially harmful restraints. However, there are times when using restraints would be the most nonmaleficent option, as in the resident with dementia who has had a recent amputation and does not yet recognize the loss of a leg or have the skills to get out of bed independently. Physicians should thoughtfully evaluate the need for restraints with all the caretakers involved and should discuss the use of restraints with involved family members and friends, obtaining informed consent.

PSYCHOTROPIC MEDICATION

Like mechanical restraints, psychotropic drugs have commonly been used in the nursing home to protect residents by controlling a variety of symptoms and behaviors. These drugs include major tranquilizers, sedatives, and anxiolytic agents. Although selected behaviors may respond to the judicious use of psychotropic agents, overuse is well documented.

Before the enactment of OBRA 1987, 21% to 44% of nursing home residents were being given psychotropic agents (53). Significant side effects include sedation, which can lead to falls and consequent fractures, and extrapyramidal side effects, such as tardive dyskinesia, which may be persistent. In addition, anticholinergic effects may worsen cognitive, behavioral, and medical conditions, and cardiovascular effects may be life-threatening (54).

A study following OBRA guidelines that evaluated treatment with psychotropic agents found that only half of neuroleptic drug use was appropriate (55). In response to overuse, misuse, and abuse, guidelines were set by OBRA 1987 for appropriate use of psychotropic agents in the long-term care setting:

1. A specific condition, including a psychiatric diagnosis, that warrants neuroleptic use must be documented.

2. Neuroleptic therapy is prohibited if certain behaviors are the only justification.

3. Neuroleptic use on an as-needed basis is prohibited.

4. Gradual reductions in dose should be coupled with attempts at behavioral programming, including environmental modification. A study conducted after the implementation of these regulations has shown that an educational program can reduce the amount of psychotropic agents used in the nursing home without adversely affecting care (56).

Although treatment with psychotropic agents can sometimes be helpful to control behaviors in residents with dementia, their use calls for thoughtful evaluation.

ABUSE OF RESIDENTS

Physicians have an ethical responsibility to uncover, report, and address abuse of residents in the nursing home. The definition of abuse includes willful neglect as well as physical, financial, psychological, and sexual abuse (57). Abuse can be inflicted by nursing home staff, visitors, or even other residents. Nursing home residents are particularly vulnerable to abuse not only because of physical and mental dependencies but also because they may fear that reporting abuse may adversely affect their care. If caretakers are the abusers, reporting the abuse may either increase the abuse or leave the residents without care. Many dependent residents also see that those who are perceived as complainers get lower-quality care and less time of care.

When physicians suspect abuse, their primary responsibility is to ensure the safety of the resident. They should conduct a thorough physical examination and historical review with the resident and should extensively document their findings in the medical record (with photographs, if pertinent). Next, they should report the abuse to the appropriate authorities. Forty-two states have mandatory reporting laws for even suspected abuse, and all states have some system for reporting abuse either through adult protective services or through a state long-term care ombudsman program (58).

RISK MANAGEMENT

The principle of beneficence dictates that physicians should be aware of and, when possible, should participate in the development of policies that directly improve residents' care while at the same time vigilantly preventing harm and minimizing risk to residents. As in other health care settings, a good relationship marked by frequent communication among physician, nursing home resident, and family combined with thorough documentation go a long way in preventing misunderstandings and claims.

Risk management, the reduction of preventable injuries and malpractice claims (59), has a place in the nursing home and in the consciousness of the physician who practices there. Overall, the frequency of claims against nursing homes is low. Of claims filed, approximately 25% involve injuries sustained in falls or because of wandering (60). Sources of lawsuits in the nursing home because of professional negligence include medication errors, dietary mistakes, allergic reactions, infections, improper physical and/or mental assessments, improper transfers or discharges, pressure sores and resulting conditions, lack of informed consent for

treatment or compelled participation in research, and the withholding or withdrawal of life-prolonging treatment or the refusal of such a request (60).

Incident reports can be useful to identify adverse occurrences when an unexpected poor outcome or unexpected death occurs. Incident reports and resulting consequent action can be valuable in an individual case to identify, investigate, and correct adverse trends.

RESIDENT PARTICIPATION IN RESEARCH

The topic of research in nursing homes has been debated with fervor by those who are concerned about the protection of the vulnerable as well as by those who advocate the necessity of research to define, analyze, and ameliorate problems in the nursing home. Research promises progress in the understanding and treatment of many terrible problems that nursing home residents may face, such as Alzheimer disease, urinary incontinence, falls, and decubitus ulcers.

A major concern about conducting research in the nursing home arises because residents are vulnerable to exploitation. Many residents are unable to give informed consent because of cognitive disabilities, and even residents who are able to give informed consent may feel coerced into participation because they fear their care would be jeopardized if they refused. Another concern expressed frequently by nursing directors is the precious time required of their staff in most research endeavors, which may detract from the time available to attend to residents' needs.

The physician may be asked to give permission for residents to participate in research trials. In these situations, physicians should ascertain the purpose of the research, its technical soundness, and the potential risks and benefits for the subject and should discuss the issue with the resident and any interested others (62–65). If residents have strong desires to participate in research for altruistic reasons, there are those who argue that they should not be denied that right.

ETHICS COMMITTEES AND CONSULTATIONS

Nursing home care is constrained in many ways by laws and regulations, yet most ethical issues in the nursing home are best resolved in an open and thoughtful discussion with the resident (when possible), relevant family members, and the physician and specific nursing home staff members involved in the care of the resident. The physician can positively shape the environment of care and guide treatment decisions.

Often, unfortunately, the physician may not know the resident well, or conflicting values may pose a decision-making dilemma. In these situations, many hospitals are turning to the use of ethics committees. This practice is growing, especially in large institutions and those with religious affiliations (66). Even when formal ethics committees do not exist, many nursing homes have some mechanism to evaluate and help find solutions to difficult cases. Such mechanisms will become increasingly useful because legal and regulatory guidelines can never cover the full range of complexity occurring in these cases.

CONCLUSIONS

Life in the nursing home is much different than life in the community, and medical care in the nursing home is much different than medical care in the hospital or outpatient clinic. Physicians have an ethical obligation to consider that residents are in special circumstances. Although, in general, the elderly are often at risk for having their autonomy compromised, residents in the nursing home are at even greater risk. Balancing the principles of beneficence and nonmaleficence against the autonomy and freedom of nursing home residents is an extremely delicate process, and the issues of each case must be considered individually.

Respect for individual persons is the ethical thread that runs through the care of nursing home residents. Any event in the daily life of a nursing home may bring up the issue of honoring privacy, making medical decisions, planning for future care, or protecting the resident from undue harm. Although the issues are complex, physicians who care for nursing home residents can provide a high standard of care by applying the ethical and legal precedents outlined in this chapter.

REFERENCES

1. Hing E. Use of nursing homes by the elderly: preliminary data from the 1985 National Nursing Home Survey. Vital Health Statistics. 1987;135:1-12.
2. Van Nostrand JF, Miller B. Selected issues in long term care: profile of cognitive disability. In: Heath Data on Older Americans. Hyattsville, MD: National Center for Health Statistics; 1992;21-30. Publication PHS 98-141.
3. Taylor EA. Cited by: Ambrogi DM. Legal issues in nursing home admissions. Law Med Health Care. 1990;18:254-62.
4. Kemper P, Murtaugh CM. Lifetime use of nursing home care. N Engl J Med. 1991;324:595-600.
5. Agich GJ. Reassessing autonomy in long-term care. Hastings Center Report. November-December 1990;20: 12-17.
6. Moody HR. Ethics in an Aging Society. Baltimore, MD: The Johns Hopkins University Press; 1992.
7. Lynn J. Ethical issues in caring for elderly residents of nursing homes. Prim Care. 1986;13:295-306.
8. Foldes SS. Life in an institution: a sociological and anthropological view. In: Kane RA, Caplan AL, eds. Everyday Ethics: Resolving Dilemmas in Nursing Home Life. New York: Springer Publishing Co.; 1990;21-36.
9. Kapp MB. Medicolegal problems in caring for nursing home residents. In: Kapp MB, ed. Geriatrics and the Law. 2nd ed. New York: Springer Publishing Co.; 1992;143-68.
10. Hofland BF, Callopy BJ, Jameton A, et al. Autonomy and long term care. Gerontologist. 1988;28 (Suppl):3-9.
11. Kane RA. Everyday life in nursing homes: "The way things are." In: Kane RA, Caplan AL, eds. Everyday Ethics. Resolving Dilemmas in Nursing Home Life. New York: Springer Publishing Co.; 1990; 1-20.
12. Jonsen AR, Siegler M, Winslade WJ. Clinical Ethics: A Practical Approach to Ethical Decisions in Clinical Medicine. 3rd ed. New York: MacMillan Publishing Co.; 1992.
13. Cassel CK. Ethical problems in geriatric medicine. In: Cassel CK, Riesenberg DE, Sorenson LD, Walsh JR, eds. Geriatric Medicine. 2nd ed. New York: Springer Publishing Co.; 1990;38-40.
14. Kapp MB. Informed consent and truth telling. In: Kapp MB, ed. Genetics and the Law. 2nd ed. New York: Springer Publishing Co.; 1992:15-43.
15. High DM. Planning for decisional incapacity: a neglected area in ethics and aging. J Am Geriatr Soc. 1987;35:814-20.
16. Drane JF. The many faces of competency. Hastings Center Report. April 1985;17-21.
17. Markson LJ, Kern DC, Annas GJ, Glantz LH. Physician assessment of patient competence. J Am Geriatr Soc. 1994;42:1074-80.
18. Appelbaum PS, Grisso T. Assessing patients capacities to consent to treatment. N Engl J Med. 1988; 319:1635-8.
19. Areen J. The legal status of consent obtained from families of adult patients to withhold or withdraw treatment. JAMA. 1987;258:229-35.
20. President's Commission for the Study of Ethical Problems in Medicine and Biomedical and Behavioral Research. Deciding to Forego Life Sustaining Treatment. Washington, D.C.: U.S. Government Printing Office: 1983:32-3.
21. Seckler AB, Meier DE, Mulvihill M, Paris BE. Sub-

stituted judgment: how accurate are proxy predictions? Ann Intern Med. 1991;115:92-8.

22. Tomlinson T, Howe K, Notman M, Rossmiller D. An empirical study of proxy consent for elderly persons. Gerontologist. 1990;30:54-61.

23. High DM, Turner HB. Surrogate decision making: the elderly's familial expectations. Theor Med 1987; 8:303-20.

24. Emanuel EJ, Emanuel LL. Proxy decision making for incompetent patients: an ethical and empirical analysis. JAMA. 1992;267:2067-71.

25. Menikoff JA, Sachs GA, Siegler M. Beyond advance directives: health care surrogate laws. N Engl J Med. 1992;327:1165-69.

26. Annas GJ. The health care proxy and the living will. N Engl J Med. l991;324:1210-3.

27. Choice in Dying Inc. State Law Governing Durable Power of Attorney, Health Care Agents, Proxy Appointments. New York: Choice in Dying, Inc; 1992.

28. Gallup News Service. January 6, 1991;55:1-6.

29. Cate FH, Gill BA. The Patient Self-determination Act Implementation Issues and Opportunities: A White Paper of the Annenberg Washington Program. Evanston, IL: Northwestern University Press; 1991.

30. Kapp MB. Family decision-making for nursing home residents: legal mechanisms and ethical underpinnings. Theor Med. 1987;8:259-73.

31. High DM. Planning for decisional incapacity: a neglected area in ethics and aging. J Am Geriatr Soc. 1987;35:814-20.

32. Weir RF, Gostin L. Decisions to abate life-sustaining treatment f or nonautonomous patients: ethical standards and legal liability for physicians after *Cruzan* JAMA. 1990;264:1846-53.

33. Council on Ethical and Judicial Affairs, American Medical Association. Decisions near the end of life. JAMA. 1992;267:2229-33.

34. Guidelines on the Termination of Life-sustaining Treatment and the Care of the Dying: A Report by the Hastings Center. Briarcliff Manor, NY: The Center; 1987;4-38.

35. *Cruzan v Director* Missouri Department of Health, 110 SCt 2840 (1990).

36. American Medical Association. Current Opinions of the Council on Ethical and Judicial Affairs of the AMA Withholding or Withdrawing Life Prolonging Treatment. Chicago, IL: American Medical Association; 1992;14-19. Opinions 2.20, 2.21.

37. Applebaum GE, Kino JE, Finucane TE. The outcome of CPR initiated in nursing homes. J Am Geriatr Soc. 1990;38:197-200.

38. Sachs GA, Miles SH, Levin RA. Limiting resuscitation: emerging policy In the emergency medical system. Ann Intern Med 1991;114:151-4.

39. Hodges MO, Tolle SW, Stocking C, Cassel CK. Tube feeding: internists' attitudes regarding ethical obligations. Ann Intern Med. 1994;154:1013-20.

40. Kyser Jones J.The use of nasogastric feeding tubes in nursing homes: patient, family and health care

provider perspectives. Gerontologist. 1990;30: 469-79.

41. Callahan D. On feeding the dying. Hasting Center Report. October 22–27,1983;13:22.

42. Meyers RM, Grodin MA. Decision making regarding the initiation of tube feedings in the severely demented elderly. J Am Geriatr Soc. 1991;39:526-31.

43. Evans LK, Stnumpf NE. Tying down the elderly: a review of the literature on physical restraint. J Am Geriatr Soc. 1989;37:36-65.

44. Tinetti ME, Liu W-L, Ginter SF. Mechanical restraint use and fall-related injuries among residents of skilled nursing facilities. Ann Intern Med. 1992;116:369-74.

45. Moss RJ, LaPuma J. The ethics of mechanical restraints. Hastings Center Report. January-February 1991;21:22-5.

46. Miles SH, Irvine P. Deaths caused by physical restraints. Gerontologist. 1992;32:762-66.

47. Berland B, Wachtel TJ, Kiel DP, O'Sullivan PS, Phillips E. Patient characteristics associated with the use of mechanical restraints. J Gen Intern Med. 1990;5:480-5.

48. Tinetti ME, Liu W-L, Marottoli RA, Ginter SF. Mechanical restraint use among residents of skilled nursing facilities: prevalence, patterns and predictors. JAMA. 1991;265:468-71.

49. Skolnick AA. After long delay, federal regulations for enforcing nursing home standards may be issued this year. JAMA 1993;269:2348-53.

50. Health Care Financing Administration. Survey Procedures, Forms and Interpretive Guidelines for the Long-Term Care Survey Process. Springfield, VA: Health Care Financing Administration; 1992. Report PB-92-950003.

51. Sloane PD, Mathew LJ, Scarborough M, Desai JR, Koch GG, Tangen C. Physical and pharmacologic restraint of nursing home patients with dementia: impact of specialized units. JAMA. 1991;265: 1278-82.

52. Phillips CA, Hawes C, Fries BE. Reducing the use of physical restraints in nursing homes: will it increased costs? Am J Public Health.1993;83:342-48.

53. Committee on Nursing Home Regulation. Improving the Quality of Care in Nursing Homes. Washington, DC: National Academy of Sciences and Institute of Medicine; 1986.

54. Phillipson M, Moranville JT, Jeste DV, Harris MJ. Antipsychotics. Clin Geriatr Med. 1990;6:411-22.

55. Garrard J, Makris L, Dunham T, Heston, LL, Cooper S, Ratner ER, et al. Evaluation of neuroleptic drug use by nursing home elderly under proposed Medicare and Medicaid regulations. JAMA. 1991; 265:463-67.

56. Avorn J, Soumerai SB, Everitt DE, Ross-Degnan D, Beers MH, Sherman D, et al. A randomized trial of a program to reduce the use of psychoactive drugs in nursing homes. N Engl J Med. 1992;327:168-73.

57. Lachs MS, Fulmer T. Recognizing elder abuse and neglect. Clin Geriatr Med. 1993;9:665-81.

58. Arvanis SC, Adelman RD, Breckman R, Fulmer TT,

Holder E, Lachs M, et al. Diagnostic and treatment guidelines on elder abuse and neglect. Arch Fam Med. 1993;2:371-88.

59. Showalter J. Quality assurance and risk management: a joinder to two important movements. J Leg Med. 1984;5:4497-4502.

60. Johnson SH. The fear of liability and the use of restraints in nursing homes. Law Med Health Care. 1990;18:263-73.

61. Kapp MB. Preventing malpractice suits in long-term care facilities. QRB Qual Rev Bull. 1986;12:109-13

62. Annas GJ, Glantz LH. Rules for research in nursing homes. N Engl J Med. 1986;315:1157-8.

63. Sachs G, Rhymes J, Cassel C. Biomedical and behavioral research in nursing homes: guidelines for ethical investigations. J Am Geriatr Soc. 1993; 41:771-7.

64. Markson L Snyder L, Steel RK. Cognitively impaired subjects: position paper of the American College of Physicians. Ann Intern Med. 1989;111: 843-8.

65. Cassel CK. Ethical issues in the conduct of research in long-term care. Gerontologist. 1988;28(suppl): 90-6.

66. Libow LS, Storer P. Care of the nursing home patient. N Engl J Med. 1989;321:93-6.

12

Evaluation and Management of Dementia and Delirium

Cathy A. Alessi, MD

The National Nursing Home Survey of 1985 estimated the prevalence of mental disorders in nursing homes to be 64%. Dementia was most common, with a prevalence of 47% (1). Other studies have reported the prevalence of mental disorders at 60% to 94% (2–6). The most common diagnoses are Alzheimer disease (56% of residents), multi-infarct dementia (18%), delirium (6%), and depression (6%). The prevalence of dementia is even higher in residents who have been in a nursing home for 1 year or more (2). Dementia is also a well-recognized risk factor for nursing home placement. Identifying dementia and determining the underlying cause(s) and appropriate long-term management are important to prevent further mental and functional decline, to decrease inappropriate use of psychotropic drugs and physical restraints, to prevent unnecessary hospitalizations, and to avoid further morbidity and mortality from unrecognized conditions (2).

Careful mental status testing is the most efficient and only reliable method to identify dementia and delirium. Mental status testing should be done on admission and repeated annually. In addition, a brief assessment of mental status should be included in every routine visit and during evaluation of residents with acute problems. Further, ongoing nursing staff assessment of residents' mental status is crucial. In fact, most personal care is provided by nurses' aides, who usually have little training in patient assessment but who may be the first to recognize a change in mental status.

DEMENTIA

Dementia has been defined as a syndrome of acquired persistent impairment of mental function with involvement in at least three areas of neuro-psychological activity, including language, memory, visuospatial skills, emotion or personality, and cognition (abstraction and calculation) (7). Dementia usually involves loss of intellectual function in some areas and relative maintenance of function in others (7). The most common causes of dementia in nursing home residents are Alzheimer disease (at least 50% of the cases) and vascular dementia (up to 25% of the cases) (5,8,9). Long-term management of dementia is important because the average survival of persons with dementia has been reported to be 2.5 years after admission to a nursing home (10).

Screening

The presence of dementia is usually known before admission or is detected by mental status testing administered at admission. Several screening tests have been suggested, which, if the results are normal, greatly reduce the probability of dementia. They include normal serial 7s, 7-digit span, 3-item recall, and correct clock drawing (11). However, because of the high prevalence of dementia in nursing homes and the need for ongoing monitoring, more elaborate formal testing is usually warranted. One commonly used test is the Mini-Mental Status Examination

(MMSE) (12), although many other tests are available. A common problem with most screening tests is a failure, without knowledge of previous performance, to distinguish dementia from delirium or to identify delirium superimposed on dementia. These distinctions require careful clinical evaluation.

The Omnibus Budget Reconciliation Act (OBRA) of 1987, which became effective in 1991, contains rules for nursing home care, including the requirement for a comprehensive assessment of all residents within 14 days of admission (13). This assessment includes completion of the Minimum Data Set. Two of the 16 sections of the Minimum Data Set address cognitive patterns and mood and behavior; both must be updated quarterly (14). "Triggers" in these specific areas lead to Resident Assessment Protocols for delirium, cognitive loss, or dementia, mood, or behavior problems. The disciplines usually responsible for completing the Minimum Data Set items and Resident Assessment Protocols are nursing, social work, or psychology, or a combination of the three. The data set and protocols are usually completed in the context of quarterly interdisciplinary meetings. Physicians generally do not attend these meetings and therefore need to discuss the findings during routine visits with their patients.

Evaluation

Often, the clinician is aware of the presence of dementia in an individual resident and has information on the course and cause. However, when this information is not available and the clinician is evaluating a resident with mild-to-moderate dementia for the first time, a diagnostic evaluation is indicated, especially to look for disorders in which treatment may reverse or ameliorate symptoms. Although only about 15% of patients with dementia have a potentially reversible or treatable cause, and an even smaller number actually improve after appropriate intervention (15), failure to recognize and treat these patients may be devastating. In patients with stable end-stage dementia (that is, mute and bed-bound) in which a reversible cause is extremely unlikely, extensive testing for cause is probably not warranted. However, even persons with the most severe dementia may benefit from careful evaluation for treatable conditions causing excessive disability, such as medical illness, toxic effects of drugs, and functional impairment (16).

Several laboratory tests that may be useful in identifying clinically important problems that contribute to or cause dementia include chemistry panel, complete blood count, and thyroid function tests (17). Other tests commonly ordered, but that may not be routinely warranted, include VDRL, HIV, and Lyme serology, cerebral imaging studies, and serum cobalamin (B_{12}) and folate levels (11). When a diagnostic evaluation has already been done, repeat testing is probably indicated only if the resident has a new, unexpected decline or the progression of disease differs from what is expected. Expected progression of Alzheimer disease is one of a slow but inexorable downward decline. Multiinfarct dementia is described as having a step-wise progression, but this pattern may be difficult to identify. In either disorder, the resident typically has mild day-to-day fluctuations, but major decline (usually identified by nursing staff) is not expected and, if it occurs, should be evaluated because the cause is commonly an unrecognized acute problem causing superimposed delirium. A flow chart of the general approach to evaluation of abnormal mental status is shown in Figure 12.1.

Management

Chronic management of residents with dementia includes palliation, rehabilitation, and control of coexisting illness. Palliative care includes treating pain and psychological distress, providing a safe environment that is as unrestricted as possible, and providing adequate staffing with personnel who have the skill and time to maximize resident comfort and freedom. Decline in functional status can occur with social isolation, withdrawal, loss of independence, and restriction of activity as well as iatrogenic illness from medications and forced immobility and injury from chemical or physical restraints (18,19). Rehabilitative care involves providing an appropriate environment and any necessary prosthetic devices to maximize function. The control of coexisting illnesses requires recognition and treatment of chronic comorbid conditions (18) and recognition of worsened mental status caused by a superimposed, usually medical illness (16).

Treatment goals in the care of residents with dementia should reflect the progressive course of most dementing processes. Resident comfort and well-being are the primary goals. Treatments should focus on helping the resident derive as much quality

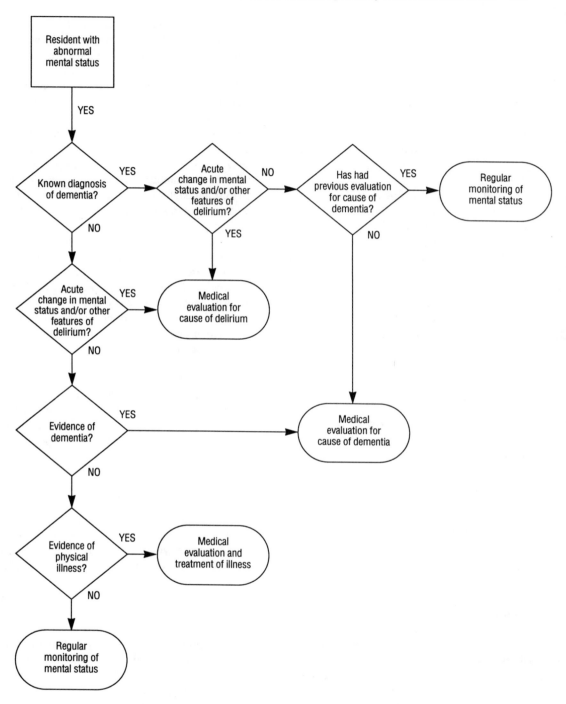

FIGURE 12.1. Simple flow chart for the evaluation of abnormal mental status in nursing home residents.

and pleasure from life as possible by maximizing participation in life, promoting physical and emotional comfort, providing safety and feelings of security, and maintaining dignity and human contact (20).

Treatment should also include management of conditions commonly associated with dementia, including urinary and fecal incontinence, sleep disorders, decubitus ulcers, infections, malnutrition, immobility, and deconditioning (20). Nursing staff play a key role in the monitoring and management of these conditions.

Ethical issues are also important. Advance directives should be sought for all residents. Residents with mild cognitive impairment may be able to participate in decision making, but when dementia prohibits participation, decisions should be made based not only on sustaining life but on sustaining quality of life. Families can play a major role in decision making for cognitively impaired residents. When the previous wishes of a resident are unknown and family members are not available, decisions can be difficult, and the clinician should above all do no harm.

Behavioral Symptoms

Studies suggest that 38% to 90% of residents have problematic behavioral symptoms (1,21,22). These symptoms are often caused by clinical conditions or precipitating events, which, when addressed, may resolve or ameliorate the symptoms. In addition, behavioral symptoms often lead to nursing home placement. In one prospective study of community-dwelling elderly persons with dementia, those placed in a nursing home did not have worse cognition but did have more behavioral symptoms and more psychiatric abnormalities than those remaining at home (23).

Most studies of behavioral symptoms have focused on Alzheimer disease; it is not clear if these findings are applicable to other causes of dementia. The most common behavioral abnormalities include memory disturbance (such as losing things, disorientation, and repetitive questions); general restlessness and agitation; day and night reversal in sleep; wandering; verbal agitation; catastrophic reactions (episodes in which the person with dementia overreacts to a situation or task that is overwhelming or difficult); delusions; physical violence; and resistance to necessary care (24,25). Difficult behaviors may be most prominent during personal care activities such as bathing (26,27). In fact, cognitive impairment has been documented to increase the amount of effort and time staff must use to provide resident care (28).

Suggested predictors of behavioral symptoms include dementia severity, age at onset, and the presence of extrapyramidal symptoms (29–31). However, other evidence suggests that certain behavioral disturbances actually decrease with increasing dementia severity (32). Psychotic symptoms appear to be more common in the middle stages of dementia (33), although the appearance of these symptoms predicts a more rapid cognitive decline (34). Premorbid personality traits may also be related to behavioral symptoms. For example, premorbid hostility is associated with paranoid symptoms (35). Finally, there is evidence that behavioral symptoms in patients with dementia may be more prominent when caregivers are stressed (25).

Clinicians should query nursing staff about the presence of behavioral symptoms. If any are present, it is helpful to determine which are the most worrisome and address these first. Have caregivers document the frequency and severity of these symptoms to help determine if they are serious enough to warrant intervention. Several scales are available to document behavioral symptoms of dementia on the basis of either direct observations or reports from informants (for example, nursing staff) (21,36–39).

NONPHARMACOLOGIC MANAGEMENT

It is important to address behavioral symptoms of dementia because these symptoms may indicate important underlying illness, cause patient distress, interfere with necessary care, and negatively affect caregivers. Physicians should evaluate residents with dementia for a causative underlying physical condition and then consider various nonpharmacologic measures as the first approach for treatment of most symptoms. General stressors that may precipitate or worsen behavioral symptoms include fatigue, change of routine, excess demands, overwhelming stimuli, and physical stressors such as acute illness or pain (40).

One behavioral approach to managing these symptoms involves 1) identifying the problem behavior (including its timing and frequency); 2) determining its antecedents (that is, the events that occur immediately before the behavior); and 3) identifying the consequences (that is, the events that occur immediately after the behavior) (41). This method relies heavily on nursing staff to observe and document the behavior and to help plan and implement management techniques. Specific non-pharmacologic measures for managing common behavioral symptoms are listed in Table 12.1. The clinician should discuss these measures with nursing staff; written orders may be necessary for some interventions to improve compliance. Follow-up discussions with nursing staff are necessary to monitor response to the intervention.

Most recommendations for nonpharmacologic management are based on experience rather than on clinical trials (20,24,42,43). A notable exception is the use of bright-light therapy. Nighttime exposure to bright light has been suggested as a treatment for sleep maintenance insomnia in older persons without dementia (44). Subsequently, Mishima and colleagues (45) exposed residents with dementia who had sleep and behavior problems to 2 hours of a light therapy device (3000 to 5000 lux) in the morning (45). Treatment was associated with increased nighttime sleep, decreased daytime sleep, and decreased behavioral symptoms. Specific guidelines for the use of bright-light therapy are lacking, but the intensity of illumination needed to affect the endogenous circadian timing system is more than that found in normal indoor lighting (46), and therefore outdoor light or a light therapy device is recommended.

PHARMACOLOGIC MANAGEMENT

In general, the effectiveness of psychotropic medications for behavioral symptoms in dementia has been disappointing (47). However, 25% to 65% of residents receive these agents, most commonly neuroleptics (48–50), and inappropriate use may be frequent. In one study, over 20% of nursing home residents who were prescribed psychotropic medications did not have a documented mental disorder (51). Another study found that 19% of all elderly residents in seven nursing homes were exposed to excessive use of tranquilizers (antipsychotics and antianxiety agents), including long duration of treatment, concurrent use of three or more psychotropic medications, or duplication of medications. In addition, residents in nursing homes with less adequate staffing and fewer resources are more likely to receive a tranquilizer and to experience deviations from established drug use criteria (52).

Key issues in the use of psychotropic medications are to avoid polypharmacy, use small doses, increase doses slowly, monitor for side effects and efficacy, and frequently re-evaluate the need for the drug. Although neuroleptics are most commonly used, alternatives to neuroleptics that have been suggested include serotoninergic agents, benzodiazepines, beta-blockers, carbamazepine, and lithium (Table 12.2).

Trials on the effectiveness of neuroleptics for managing behavioral symptoms of dementia have had mixed results. Most authors agree that low doses of neuroleptics can be useful in residents with dementia who have severe behavioral symptoms that do not respond to nonpharmacologic measures (53), but dramatic improvement is uncommon and side effects are frequent. Behavioral symptoms that respond to neuroleptic agents include psychotic behavior and severe agitation. Many other symptoms—for example, memory loss, disorientation, apathy, withdrawal, and wandering—do not respond to these agents. A meta-analysis of controlled trials of neuroleptic treatment in dementia found these agents more effective than placebo, but efficacy was modest (54). Most studies comparing various neuroleptics do not show significant differences in efficacy among agents, so choice of a particular neuroleptic is usually made on the basis of its side-effect profile.

In general, low-potency neuroleptics are more sedating and therefore may be helpful in residents with marked agitation. High-potency agents are less sedating and may be helpful in residents with severe daytime agitation, but extrapyramidal symptoms (such as akathisia, parkinsonism, dystonia, and tardive dyskinesia) can be limiting. Whichever agent is chosen, the dosing plan should be to "start low and go slow." The continued use of neuroleptics should be reviewed at each drug renewal and whenever the resident develops side effects. Residents should not be given these agents indefinitely unless symptoms repeatedly recur off of the medication.

OBRA specifically addressed the use of neuroleptics in nursing homes. The regulations state that residents have the right to be free from any psychoactive drug administered for purposes of discipline or convenience and not required to treat their medical symptoms. Interpretive guidelines for implementation of OBRA regulations are used by the Health Care Financing Administration to help surveyors inspect nursing homes (Box 12.1) (13).

TABLE 12.1. Nonpharmacologic measures for selected behavioral problems

Behavior	Examples	Estimated Prevalence (%)	Suggested Nonpharmacologic Measures*

Memory disturbance	Asking repetitive questions
	Losing things
	Accusations by the person
	  with dementia
		Almost 100	Caregiver education on behaviors related
			  to memory loss
			Memory aids, for example, word or
			  picture labels on bathroom, bedroom,
			  closets, drawers
			Regular daily routine with posted
			  daily activities
			Clocks, calendars
			Familiar objects left in their usual places
			Maintain an uncluttered environment
			Family photographs in the room

General restlessness
  and agitation
	Pacing
	Fidgeting
	Resisting care
	Uncooperative with care
	Irritable behavior
		40 to 50	Caregiver should approach resident in a
			  relaxed, friendly manner
			Simplify the environment
			Avoid environmental and sensory overload
			Limit demands made on residents
			Soft music
			Exercise, outdoors if possible
			Divert resident's attention

Day-night reversal
  in sleep
	Daytime sleepiness
	Night-time restlessness
	Frequent night-time awakenings
		40 to 70	Give required medications with sedating
			  side effects at night
			Expose residents to bright light during
			  the day
			Label bathroom clearly (and visibly at night)
			Treat painful conditions
			Daytime exercise, outdoors if possible
			Decrease daytime napping
			Keep residents dressed during the daytime
			Small snack at night
			Avoid night-time fluids and diuretics
			Soft nightlight to help orientation at night
			Minimize night-time disruption of sleep

Wandering	Leaving ward or nursing home
	Getting lost
	Can be precipitated by a move
	  to a new nursing home or
	  new room
		30 to 60	Regular daytime exercise
			Fenced yards
			Rooms that allow a safe area for residents
			  to wander
			Exit alarms triggered by door opening or
			  resident-worn device
			Door and window locks that are difficult to
			  operate or located in an unusual place
			Disguise exit (e.g., cover up doorknob or
			  place chair in front of door)
			Identification bracelet
			Inform other ward personnel and neighbors
			  of residents who wander
			Remove environmental hazards, for
			  example, loose cords, throw rugs
			Use measures suggested above for day or
			  night disturbance
			Frequent snacks if wandering seems
			  precipitated by hunger

TABLE 12.1. Nonpharmacologic measures for selected behavioral problems (continued)

Behavior	Examples	Estimated Prevalence (%)	Suggested Nonpharmacologic Measures*
Verbal agitation	Screaming Shouting Constant requests for attention Complaining Negativism	20 to 50	Patience and gentle redirection Evaluate residents for pain, hunger, thirst, other care needs (e.g., bed is wet) Limit demands of residents Simplify tasks to one step at a time Approach residents in a relaxed, friendly manner Increase personal contact; touch if appropriate
Catastrophic reactions	Substantial emotional reaction (e.g., screaming, angry outburst, physical blow) to a situation or task (e.g., bathing, grooming)	10 to 70	Caregiver education that the episode is caused by dementia Use measures suggested above for general restlessness and agitation Follow familiar routines Rely on over-learned behaviors to accomplish tasks Simplify tasks (e.g., bathing) to individual steps Avoid events known to precipitate an outburst
Delusions	"People are stealing things" "Spouse is an impostor" Abandonment by family and friends	10 to 50	Educate caregivers that these delusions are caused by dementia Patience and gentle redirection Ignore delusions that are not harmful or do not interfere with care
Physical violence	Hitting, slapping Pushing Scratching Grabbing	10 to 50	Use measures suggested above for restlessness and agitation Limit demands and stress Simplify tasks to one step at a time Do not force residents to do things they clearly do not want to do Distract their attention during necessary activities Structured ward milieu Show of force, that is, the arrival of multiple staff members Avoid physical restraints Remove potential weapons

*With all behavioral problems, residents should be evaluated for an underlying illness or condition precipitating the problem.

Alternatives to neuroleptics are increasingly being used, for example, the serotoninergic agents trazodone and buspirone. Trazodone, given at low doses at night (25 to 50 mg), has been used for agitated patients with dementia who are refractory to other medications (55 56). Trazodone has low anticholinergic activity and may be effective because of sedative and serotoninergic properties (56). Buspirone is an anxiolytic with serotoninergic properties and has been suggested for the management of agitation with overt anxiety as the major symptom. Literature on the use of selective serotonin reuptake inhibitor antidepressants (for example, fluoxetine and sertraline) for behavioral symptoms is limited, and therefore specific recommendations are not available.

TABLE 12.2. Medications suggested for managing behavioral symptoms of dementia*

Drug Class	Example(s)	Indications	Usual Starting Dose in Elderly	Side Effects	Comments
Neuroleptics*†	Haloperidol (high potency) Thioridazine (low potency)	Psychotic symptoms (e.g., delusions, hallucinations) and nonpsychotic disruptive symptoms (e.g., severe agitation, hostility)	Haloperidol: 0.5 mg (0.25 if very frail) Thioridazine: 25 mg (10 mg if very frail)	High potency: extrapyramidal effects Low potency: sedation, anticholinergic effects, orthostasis Both: falls, confusion, neuroleptic malignant syndrome	Most commonly used agents. OBRA 1987 provides guidelines for use of these agents. Most agents available as tablet, solution or elixir, and injection. Do not use prophylactic anticholinergic agent.
Serotoninergic agents	Trazodone (antidepressant) Buspirone (anxiolytic)	Trazodone suggested for agitation (especially at night) and hostility Buspirone suggested for agitation associated with anxiety	Trazodone: 25–50 mg at HS Buspirone: 5 mg tid	Trazodone: sedation, hypotension, gastro-intestinal upset (little or no anticholinergic effects) Buspirone: dizziness, headache	Trazodone is increasingly being used in this setting. Buspirone may take weeks for an effect. Patients may often be prescribed a dose that is too low (may require 15 mg tid). No euphoric effect.
Benzodiazepines	Oxazepam Lorazepam Alprazolam	Severe agitation, anxiety and restlessness, insomnia	Oxazepam: 10–15 mg Lorazepam: 0.5 mg Alprazolam: 0.25 mg (depending on symptoms, one-time dosing at night, or bid/tid daytime dosing)	Worsened confusion, sedation, paradoxical excitation, ataxia, falls	Caution is warranted in this population. Duration of action often longer than expected in older patients. Long-acting agents (e.g., diazepam, chlordiazepoxide, flurazepam) should not be used.
β-blockers	Propranolol Pindolol	Agitation or hostility	Propranolol: 40 mg/d in divided doses Pindolol: 60 mg/d in divided doses	Confusion; depression; exacerbations of other medical illness (heart failure, COPD, asthma, diabetes); increased drug levels (anticonvulsants, neuroleptics)	Most experience is with younger populations and other brain disease. Response time may be days to months. Very high doses may be required (i.e., 300–600 mg/d). Not first-line therapy; may be considered if symptoms are severe and patient fails other therapies.
Anticonvulsants	Carbamazepine	Aggression, impulsivity	50 mg bid	Leukopenia, hepatotoxicity, thyroid abnormalities, ataxia, dizziness, cardiac problems, rashes (also fatal agranulocytosis and Stevens-Johnson syndrome has been reported)	Used in a wide variety of psychiatric illnesses, but primarily studied in younger patients. May take 1 to 7 weeks to see effect. Carbamazepine levels must be monitored. Side effects may be limiting factor, not a first-line therapy.

*OBRA = Omnibus Budget Reconciliation Act; COPD = chronic obstructive pulmonary disease.
†Many neuroleptics have been used in this setting, including high potency (haloperidol, thiothixene, trifluoperazine); intermediate potency (perphenazine, loxapine, molindone); and low-potency (thioridazine, mesoridazine) agents.

BOX 12.1. Interpretive guidelines of OBRA 1987 regulations

Conditions that justify the use of antipsychotic agents: Organic mental syndromes (including dementia and delirium) if associated with

- Psychotic features (hallucinations, paranoia, delusions) that impair functional capacity; and/or
- Agitated features that present a danger to self or others, interfere with care, or impair functional capacity

Symptoms that do not justify the use of antipsychotic agents:

Wandering	Unsociability
Poor self-care	Indifference to
Restlessness	surroundings
Impaired memory	Fidgeting
Anxiety	Nervousness
Depression	Uncooperativeness
Insomnia	Unspecified agitation

Adapted from Elon R, Pawlson LG. The impact of OBRA on medical practice within nursing facilities. J Am Geriatr Soc. 1992;40:958-63.

Benzodiazepines have been used for managing severe agitation, anxiety, and restlessness with dementia, but caution is warranted. Short- or intermediate-acting agents may be useful for the short-term management of agitated patients in whom anxiety or sleep disturbance is a prominent symptom, but there is a risk for producing confusion even at low doses. Long-acting agents should not be used.

The anticonvulsant carbamazepine may be useful in agitated, violent patients with dementia who show temporal lobe abnormalities on an electroencephalogram, but the drug can have serious side effects, including clumsiness, ataxia, confusion, and sedation (57). Although valproate is also suggested, there is little data on its use for behavioral symptoms of dementia.

Several other classes of agents have been used, including beta-blockers, lithium, and estrogen. In general, these agents should be limited to residents without complicating medical illnesses who do not respond to more conventional therapies. Beta-blockers have been used for aggressive behavior with other organic brain disease. Unfortunately, extremely high doses may be required for therapeutic effect, and these doses certainly carry a major risk for side effects in the elderly. Lithium has also been suggested for agitated patients with dementia who have manic-like symptoms such as hyperactivity,

grandiosity, rapid speech, decreased sleep, and elevated mood; but risks for toxicity and the potential to worsen cognitive impairment severely limit its usefulness for these residents (56,57). Finally, there have been case reports on the use of estrogen for aggressive behavior in men with dementia. Further study is needed before any recommendations can be made about this agent.

DELIRIUM

Delirium is a syndrome of acute change in mental status that has the major neuropsychologic features of an alteration of attention and disturbance of consciousness (58,59). Delirium develops over a short period of time (usually hours to days) and tends to fluctuate (8). There is little literature on the prevalence of delirium in nursing homes. Reported point prevalence of delirium among nursing home residents was 6% in a small, random sample of current residents (5) and was 7% in a sample of consecutive admissions to eight nursing homes (60). In another study of 157 residents with cognitive impairment, 6% to 12% had improvement in their cognitive testing over time; Katz and colleagues (61) suggest that this improvement reflects delirium.

Much of our information on delirium comes from studies of hospitalized elderly persons. Some of the reported risk factors for delirium in hospital studies include preexisting cognitive impairment or dementia; age over 80 years; fracture on admission; symptomatic infection or fever during hospitalization; hypothermia; male gender; abnormal serum sodium levels or azotemia; severe illness; and hospital use of neuroleptic, narcotic, or sedative drugs (62,63).

Screening

Screening tests for delirium have been suggested, for example, the Confusion Assessment Method, which has been shown to be reliable and valid in hospitalized older patients (64). Other screening tests are available (65–67). Distinguishing between dementia and delirium can be difficult, particularly in residents who are newly admitted from the acute-care hospital. Delirium in hospitalized elderly persons is associated with an increased risk for nursing home placement (63). The tendency is for the clinician to assume that the newly admitted resident with mental status impairment has dementia. This assumption may be incorrect in the case of residents transferred from the hospital, based on recent evidence that symptoms of delirium can persist indefinitely in older patients (68). These findings stress the importance of careful monitoring of mental status in residents, particularly those recently admitted from the hospital, to identify slowly resolving delirium. If the resident's mental status improves, the clinician should reconsider decisions made earlier (for example, decisions about limited treatment plans, failure of rehabilitation, and ability of the resident to return home) when the cognitive impairment was believed to be permanent.

At least one recent study (68) suggests that partial delirium may be at least as common as the DSM-IV diagnosis; a subset of elderly patients hospitalized for major illness has an incomplete presentation of delirium. This subset may also occur in nursing homes; accordingly, clinicians must not disregard reports of a change in mental status in a resident simply because all criteria of delirium are not present. This is particularly true of residents with dementia, in whom worsening of mental status provoked by superimposed delirium is often the initial clue to an underlying acute illness. Key elements in the recognition of delirium include careful mental status evaluation, knowledge of baseline mental status, interview of caregivers and family, and review of current physical problems and medications (68).

Diagnostic Evaluation

Common causes of delirium in hospitalized older people include infection, drug effects, fluid or electrolyte disturbances, metabolic abnormalities, hypoxia, and hypotension. Causes in nursing homes have not been well documented. Clinical experience suggests that causes of delirium in nursing homes parallel those in the acute-care hospital; infection is probably most common. Other less obvious causes to consider include sensory deprivation, fecal impaction, and urinary retention.

The evaluation of residents with delirium should include a careful medical evaluation and selected laboratory testing. Data are not available on the yield of specific laboratory tests, but screening for infection, metabolic abnormalities, and drug toxicity is warranted. Commonly recommended tests include a chemistry panel (including electrolytes and renal and liver function), thyroid function tests, complete

blood count, urinalysis, and chest roentgenography (58,59,69). The latter test should be done if any evidence exists of respiratory difficulty because pneumonia can be occult in frail, elderly patients. Drug levels of potentially toxic medications should be obtained. Medications with central nervous system and anticholinergic effects are commonly implicated (59,61). Because delirium can have several causes in older residents, clinicians should not discontinue evaluation when one potential cause is identified. All laboratory abnormalities should be pursued, and all unnecessary medications should be discontinued. When delirium is suspected, evaluation should proceed rapidly, from in-expensive, common, noninvasive tests to more expensive invasive tests, until the diagnosis is made. Although electroencephalography may help establish the diagnosis of delirium in hospitalized patients (typical electroencephalographic findings include diffuse slowing or low voltage fast activity), the electroencephalogram is usually neither readily available nor necessary in the nursing home setting.

Management

In residents who have delirium or a change in mental status that does not meet all criteria for delirium, the two major aspects of management are recognition and specific treatment of the cause(s) and management of the behavioral symptoms of abnormal mental status that place elderly patients at risk for injury or further decline. Evaluation for cause(s) is discussed above. Management of behavioral symptoms includes providing a safe environment, preventing complications of immobility such as decubitus ulcers and contractures, and ensuring that the resident receives adequate nutrition and hydration. When severely agitated residents with delirium require sedation, treatment with low doses of a neuroleptic, with increasing doses as needed, may be helpful. Benzodiazepines are recommended for delirium caused by alcohol or drug withdrawal (58,59,69). Acutely ill residents with delirium are usually best evaluated and managed in the hospital. However, in residents for whom treatment plans are limited or for whom a decision has been made not to transfer the resident to the hospital for acute illnesses, the major issue in management is providing for resident comfort and safety. In addition, it appears that the hospital itself may be a risk factor for delirium.

DISTINGUISHING DELIRIUM
FROM DEMENTIA

The distinction between dementia and delirium usually cannot be made with simple mental status testing; careful clinical evaluation is also required. The most important element is knowledge of the resident's previous cognitive status. In addition, key features of delirium that help distinguish this disorder from dementia include abrupt onset, a rapid course (hours to days), fluctuating mental status, altered attention, perceptual abnormalities (such as hallucinations), impaired consciousness, rambling speech, and motor system abnormalities (such as tremor or asterixis) (58). Patients with delirium may be hypoactive, hyperactive, or show features of both. Hypoactive delirium is thought to be more common in elderly persons (59). Therefore, clinicians should aggressively pursue an acute change in mental status in older residents, whether the resident is aroused and hyperactive or hypoactive and "quietly confused."

Common features of dementia, in contrast to features of delirium, include gradual or vague onset (months to years), slow progression, intact attention and consciousness except late in the disease, less common perceptual abnormalities, and often paucity of speech and word-finding difficulties (58). The presence or absence of motor abnormalities (such as gait disturbance) depends on the cause and stage of dementia.

When a resident with unknown previous mental status presents with abnormal attention or altered consciousness, or both, raising suspicion for delirium, it is not possible to establish whether an underlying dementia is present because delirium can produce features of dementia such as memory impairment and disorientation. In these cases, an evaluation for delirium is essential because many causative disorders can be life threatening; documentation of the presence or absence of dementia must wait until the delirium resolves.

DELIRIUM SUPERIMPOSED
ON DEMENTIA

Because of the high prevalence of dementia among nursing home residents, a more common diagnostic challenge than distinguishing dementia from delirium is identifying delirium superimposed on preexisting dementia. This clinical problem is important because studies in hospitalized elderly patients have identified previous cognitive impairment as an important risk factor for delirium (62,63). Unfortunately, there are few data to help clinicians with this diagnostic dilemma. The identification of superimposed delirium may be relatively simple in residents with mild dementia who develop a marked change in mental status. However, the distinction is much more difficult in residents with severe dementia who may have day-to-day fluctuations without the presence of a coexisting delirium. Features that should raise suspicion for superimposed delirium include a sudden deterioration in cognition, increased agitation, increased lethargy and somnolence, new hallucinations, new behavioral problems, or a decrease in the resident's ability to participate in daily care activities. Any of these clues should prompt clinical evaluation. Because of more frequent interaction, nursing staff can play a key role in identifying mental status changes in residents with dementia.

OTHER MENTAL DISORDERS IN THE
NURSING HOME

Mental disorders other than dementia and delirium are also quite common. Depression is present in 10% to 30% of residents, but most depression is unrecognized and untreated (70–72). Most residents with depression have abnormal mental status; 55% to 70% of depressed nursing home residents are rated as demented or "not alert" by their clinicians (70,71). The mental status abnormality may be caused by depression presenting as cognitive impairment or by coexisting dementia and depression. Clues to depression presenting as cognitive impairment include cognitive symptoms that are mild and fluctuating, that have rapid onset and relatively short duration, and that occur with or after the onset of depression (73,74). Treatment of depression can lead to a dramatic improvement in mental status in these residents. However, coexisting depression and dementia are probably more common in this setting. In residents with coexisting depression and dementia, the dementia usually predates the depression, and dementia symptoms are of long duration and are relatively stable (73). The depression still should be treated and some improvement in cognition is common, but cognitive impairment usually remains in the demented range (75,76).

Another important group of residents with abnormal mental status are those with chronic mental illness such as schizophrenia. Unfortunately, nursing home staff are not well trained to work with these patients. In fact, one study of chronic psychiatric patients randomly assigned to nursing homes versus continued chronic psychiatric hospital care found that the nursing home group had worse self-care abilities, more behavioral deterioration, more mental confusion and depression, and less satisfaction with care (77). OBRA mandates that persons with severe nonorganic mental disorders such as schizophrenia and major affective disorders not be placed in nursing homes unless they also require basic nursing care. Even if OBRA guidelines are fully implemented, there will likely be a large remaining burden of mental illness in nursing homes (78).

CONCLUSIONS

Disorders of mental status are extremely common in nursing home residents. Regular mental status testing is essential to the recognition and appropriate management of these conditions. The most common and best-studied disorder is dementia. Clinicians must consider special care issues for residents with dementia and be alert to changes in mental status that herald a superimposed delirium. When problematic behavioral symptoms occur in residents with dementia, management with nonpharmacologic methods should be the first step; all psychoactive medications have side effects, including the potential for worsening cognitive function. When drug therapy is needed, most clinicians use neuroleptics first; however, alternatives to neuroleptic therapy are available. The key to successful drug therapy is "start low and go slow."

Delirium is a disorder of altered attention with other features variably present that typically indicates underlying acute illness. Delirium may be difficult to distinguish from dementia, particularly if the delirium occurs in a patient with preexisting dementia. Most studies of delirium in the elderly have focused on the hospital setting, but evidence suggests that the common causes of delirium are similar in nursing home and hospitals. Finally, clinicians should be aware of depression presenting as dementia, coexisting depression and dementia, and other chronic mental illnesses. Attention to detail and a focus on the overall well-being of residents are essential in the evaluation and management of these important problems in the nursing home.

REFERENCES

1. Hing E, Sekscenski E, Strahan GW, for the National Center for Health Statistics. The National Nursing Home Survey: 1985 Summary for the United States. Hyattsville, Maryland: U.S. Department of Health and Human Services; 1989:45. In: Vital and Health Statistics, Series 13, No. 97, DHHS publication no. 89-1758.
2. German PS, Rovner BW, Burton LC, Brant LJ, Clark R. The role of mental morbidity in the nursing home experience. Gerontologist. 1992;32:152-8.
3. Rovner BW, Rabins PV. Mental illness among nursing home patients. Hosp Community Psychiatry. 1985;36:119-20, 128.
4. Phillips CD, Hawes C. Nursing home case-mix classification and residents suffering from cognitive impairment: RUG-II and cognition in the Texas case-mix data base. Med Care. 1992;30:105-16.
5. Rovner BW, Kafonek S, Filipp L, Lucas MJ, Folstein MF. Prevalence of mental illness in a community nursing home. Am J Psychiatry. 1986;143:1446-9.
6. Parmelee PA, Katz IR, Lawton MP. Depression among institutionalized aged: assessment and prevalence estimation. J Gerontol. 1989;44:M22-9.
7. Cummings JL, Benson DF. Dementia: A Clinical Approach. 2d ed. Boston: Butterworth-Heinemann; 1992.
8. American Psychiatric Association: Draft Criteria for the Diagnostic and Statistical Manual of Mental Disorders. 4th ed. Washington, DC: American Psychiatric Association: 1994.
9. Barnes RF, Raskind MA. DSM-III criteria and the clinical diagnosis of dementia: a nursing home study. J Gerontol. 1981;36:20-7.
10. Diesfeldt HF, van Houte LR, Moerkens RM. Duration of survival in senile dementia. Acta Psychiatr Scand. 1986;73:366-71.
11. Siu AL. Screening for dementia and investigating its causes. Ann Intern Med. 1991;115:122-32.
12. Zillmer EA, Fowler PC, Gutnick HN, Becker E. Comparison of two cognitive bedside screening instruments in nursing home residents: a factor analytic study. J Gerontol. 1990;45:P69-74.
13. Elon R, Pawlson LG. The impact of OBRA on medical practice within nursing facilities. J Am Geriatr Soc. 1992;40:958-63.
14. Ouslander JG, Osterweil D. Physician evaluation and management of nursing home residents. Ann Intern Med. 1994;120:584-92.
15. Clarfield AM. The reversible dementias: do they reverse? Ann Intern Med. 1988;109:476-86.
16. Barry PP, Moskowitz MA. The diagnosis of reversible dementia in the elderly. A critical review. Arch Intern Med. 1988;148:1914-8.
17. Larson EB, Reifler BV, Sumi SM, Canfield CG, Chinn NM. Diagnostic tests in the evaluation of dementia. A prospective study of 200 elderly outpatients. Arch Intern Med. 1986;146:1917-22.
18. Rango N. The nursing home resident with dementia.

Clinical care, ethics, and policy implications. Ann Intern Med. 1985;102:835-41.

19. Curlik SM, Frazier D, Katz IR. Psychiatric aspects of long-term care. In: Sadavoy J, Lazarus LW, Jarvik LF, eds. Comprehensive Review of Geriatric Psychiatry. Washington, D.C.: American Psychiatric Press; 1991:547-564.

20. Fabiszewski KJ. Caring for the Alzheimer's patient. Gerontology. 1987;6:53-8.

21. Cohen-Mansfield J, Marx MS, Rosenthal AS. A description of agitation in a nursing home. J Gerontol. 1989; 44:M77-84.

22. Cohen-Mansfield J, Marx MS, Rosenthal AS. Dementia and agitation in nursing home residents: how are they related? Psychol Aging. 1990;5:3-8.

23. Steele C, Rovner B, Chase GA, Folstein M. Psychiatric symptoms and nursing home placement of patients with Alzheimer's disease. Am J Psychiatry. 1990;147:1049-51.

24. Alessi CA. Managing the behavioral problems of dementia in the home. Clin Geriatr Med. 1991;7: 787-801.

25. Rabins PV, Mace NL, Lucas MJ. The impact of dementia on the family. JAMA. 1982;248:333-5.

26. Everitt DE, Fields DR, Soumerai SS, Avorn J. Resident behavior and staff distress in the nursing home. J Am Geriatr Soc. 1991;39:792-8.

27. Burgener SC, Jirovec M, Murrell L, Barton D. Caregiver and environmental variables related to difficult behaviors in institutionalized, demented elderly persons. J Gerontol 1992;47:P242-9.

28. Aronson MK, Cox D, Guastadisegni P, Frazier C, Sherlock L, Grower R, et al. Dementia and the nursing home: association with care needs. J Am Geriatr Soc. 1992;40:27-33.

29. Gilley DW, Wilson RS, Bennett DA, Bernard BA, Fox JH. Predictors of behavioral disturbance in Alzheimers's disease. J Gerontol. 1991;46:P362-71.

30. Drachman DA, Swearer JM, O'Donnell BF, Mitchell AL, Maloon A. The Caretaker Obstreperous-Behavior Rating Assessment (COBRA) Scale. J Am Geriatr Soc. 1992;40:463-70.

31. Ray WA, Taylor JA, Lichtenstein MJ, Meador KG. The Nursing Home Behavior Problem Scale. J Gerontol. 1992;47:M9-16.

32. Lukovits TG, McDaniel KD. Behavioral disturbance in severe Alzheimer's disease: a comparison of family member and nursing staff reporting. J Am Geriatr Soc. 1992;40:891-5.

33. Cummings JL, Miller B, Hill MA, Neshkes R. Neuropsychiatric aspects of multi-infarct dementia and dementia of the Alzheimer type. Arch Neurol. 1987;44:389-93.

34. Stern Y, Mayeux R, Sano M, Hauser WA, Bush T. Predictors of disease course in patients with probable Alzheimer's disease. Neurology. 1987;37: 1649-53.

35. Chatterjee A, Strauss ME, Smyth KA, Whitehouse PJ. Personality changes in Alzheimer's disease. Arch Neurol. 1992;49:486-91.

36. Reisberg B, Borenstein J, Salob SP, Ferris SH, Franssen E, Georgotas A. Behavioral symptoms in Alzheimer's disease: phenomenology and treatment. J Clin Psychiatry. 1987;48(Suppl):9-15.

37. Teri L, Truax P, Logsdon R, Uomoto J, Zarit S, Vitaliano PP. Assessment of behavioral problems in dementia: the revised memory and behavior problems checklist. Psychol Aging. 1992;7:622-31.

38. Tariot PN. CERAD behavior rating scale for dementia (BSRD) [Abstract]. Gerontologist. 1992;32:160.

39. Devanand DP, Brockington CD, Moody BJ, Brown RP, Mayeux R, Endicott J, et al. Behavioral syndromes in Alzheimer's disease. Int Psychogeriatr. 1992;4:161-84.

40. Hall GR. Care of the patient with Alzheimer's disease living at home. Nurs Clin North Am. 1988;23: 31-46.

41. Proulx GB. Management of disruptive behaviors in the cognitively impaired elderly. Integrating neuropsychological and behavioral approaches. In: Conn DK, Greg A, Sadavoy J, eds. Psychiatric Consequences of Brain Disease in the Elderly: A Focus on Management. New York: Plenum Pr; 1989:147.

42. Winograd CH, Jarvik LF. Physician management of the demented patient. J Am Geriatr Soc. 1986;34: 295-308.

43. Mace NL, Rabins PV. The 36-Hour Day. New York: Warner Books; 1991.

44. Campbell SS, Dawson D, Anderson MW. Alleviation of sleep maintenance insomnia with timed exposure to bright light. J Am Geriatr Soc. 1993;41: 829-36.

45. Mishima K, Okawa M, Hishikawa Y, Hozumi S, Hori H, Takahashi K. Morning bright light therapy for sleep and behavior disorders in elderly pateints with dementia. Acta Psychiatr Scand. 1994;89:1-7.

46. Lewy AJ. Effects of light on human melatonin production and the human circadian system. Prog Neuropsychopharmacol Biol Psychiatry. 1983;7:551-6.

47. Avorn J, Dreyer P, Connelly K, Soumerai SB. Use of psychoactive medication and the quality of care in rest homes. Findings and policy implications of a statewide study. N Engl J Med. 1989;320:227-32.

48. Beers M, Avorn J, Soumerai SB, Everitt DE, Sherman DS, Salem S. Psychoactive medication use in intermediate-care facility residents. JAMA. 1988; 260:3016-20.

49. Buck JA. Psychotropic drug practice in nursing homes. J Am Geriatr Soc. 1988;36:409-18.

50. Lantz MS, Louis A, Lowenstein G, Kennedy GJ. A longitudinal study of psychotropic prescriptions in a teaching nursing home. Am J Psychiatry. 1990; 147:1637-9.

51. Beardsley RS, Larson DB, Burns BJ, Thompson JW, Kamerow DB. Prescribing of psychotropics in elderly nursing home patients. J Am Geriatr Soc. 1989;37: 327-30.

52. Svarstad BL, Mount JK. Nursing home resources and tranquilizer use among the institutionalized elderly. J Am Geriatr Soc. 1991;39:869-75.

53. Psychotherapeutic medications in the nursing home. Board of Directors of the American Association for

Geriatric Psychiatry, Clinical Practice Committee of the American Geriatrics Society, and Committee on Long-Term Care and Treatment for the Elderly, American Psychiatric Association. J Am Geriatr Soc. 1992;40:946-9.

54. Schneider LS, Pollock VE, Lyness SA. A meta-analysis of controlled trials of neruoleptic treatment in dementia. J Am Geriatr Soc. 1990;38:553-63.

55. Salzman C. Treatment of the elderly agitated patient. J Clin Psychiatry. 1987;48 (Suppl):19-22.

56. Mahler ME. Aggression in Alzheimer's disease. Bull Clin Neurosciences. 1989;54:43-50.

57. Risse SC, Barnes R. Pharmacologic treatment of agitation associated with dementia. J Am Geriatr Soc. 1986;34:368-76.

58. Cummings JL. Clinical Neuropsychiatry. Orlando, Florida: Grune and Stratton; 1985:68-74.

59. Lipowski ZJ. Delirium in the elderly patient. N Engl J Med. 1989;320:578-82.

60. Rovner BW, German PS, Broadhead J, Morriss RK, Brant LJ, Blaustein J, et al. The prevalence and management of dementia and other psychiatric disorders in nursing homes. Int Psychogeriatr. 1990;2:13-24.

61. Katz IR, Parmelee P, Brubaker K. Toxic and metabolic encephalopathies in long-term care patients. Int Psychogeriatr. 1991;3:337-47.

62. Schor JD, Levkoff SE, Lipsitz LA, Reilly CH, Cleary PD, Rowe JW, et al. Risk factors for delirium in hospitalized elderly. JAMA. 1992;267:827-31.

63. Francis J, Martin D, Kapoor WN. A prospective study of delirium in hospitalized elderly. JAMA. 1990;263:1097-101.

64. Inouye SK, van Dyck C, Alessi CA, Balkin S, Siegal AP, Horwitz RI. Clarifying confusion: the confusion assessment method. A new method for detection of delirium. Ann Intern Med. 1990;113:941-8.

65. Albert MS, Levkoff SE, Reilly C, Liptzin B, Pilgrim D, Cleary PD, et al. The delirium symptom interview: an interview for the detection of delirium symptoms in hospitalized patients. J Geriatr Psychiatry Neurol. 1992;5:14-21.

66. Vermeersch PE. The clinical assessment of confu-sion-A. Appl Nurs Res. 1990;3:128-33.

67. Pompei P, Foreman M, Cassel CK, Alessi C, Cox D. Detecting delirium among hospitalized older patients. Arch Intern Med. 1995;155:301-7.

68. Levkoff SE, Evans DA, Liptzin B, Cleary PD, Lipsitz LA, Wetle TT, et al. Delirium. The occurrence and persistence of symptoms among elderly hospitalized patients. Arch Intern Med. 1992;152:334-40.

69. Francis J, Kapoor WN. Delirium in hospitalized elderly. J Gen Intern Med. 1990;5:65-79.

70. Rovner BW, German PS, Brant LJ, Clark R, Burton L, Folstein MF. Depression and mortality in nursing homes. JAMA. 1991;265:993-6.

71. Heston LL, Garrard J, Makris L, Kane RL, Cooper S, Dunham T, et al. Inadequate treatment of depressed nursing home elderly. J Am Geriatr Soc. 1992;40:1117-22.

72. Parmelee PA, Katz IR, Lawton MP. Depression and mortality among institutionalized aged. J Gerontol. 1992;47:P3-10.

73. Allen A, Blazer DG. Mood disorders. In: Sadavoy J, Lazarus LW, Jarvik LF, eds. Comprehensive Review of Geriatric Psychiatry. Washington, D.C.: American Psychiatric Pr; 1991:337-51.

74. Yesavage J. Differential diagnosis between depression and dementia. Am J Med. 1993;94(Suppl 5A):23s-28s.

75. Greenwald BS, Kramer-Ginsberg E, Marin DB, Laitman LB, Hermann CK, Mohs RC, et al. Dementia with coexistent major depression. Am J Psychiatry. 1989;146:1472-8.

76. Yesavage JA. Depression in the elderly. How to recognize masked symptoms and choose appropriate therapy. Postgrad Med. 1992;91:255-8, 261.

77. Linn MW, Gurel L, Williford WO, Overall J, Gurland B, Laughlin P, et al. Nursing home care as an alternative to psychiatric hospitalization. A Veterans Administration cooperative study. Arch Gen Psychiatry. 1985;42:544-51.

78. Drinka PJ, Howell T. The burden of mental disorders in the nursing home [Letter]. J Am Geriatr Soc. 1991;39:730-1.

INDEX

Note: An "f" following page numbers indicates figures; "t" indicates tables.

A

Abuse, of residents, 150-151
Accidents, 105; *see also* Falls
Acetaminophen, 84-85, 94, 134
Acetophenazine, side effects, 82t
Activities of daily living
  assessment, 19
  rehabilitation services, 138
Acute illness
  evaluation, 20-21
  management, 6-7
Acyclovir, 55
Admission evaluation, 18-19
Advance directives, 147-148
Agitation, 160t
  verbal, 161t
Akathisia, 82
Albumin
  in nutrition evaluation, 121
  pressure ulcers and, 64-65
Alprazolam, 162t
Alzheimer disease, 92, 124; *see also* Dementia
Ambulation, rehabilitation services and devices, 136-137
Amitriptyline, 83, 95
Amputees, rehabilitation for, 136
Anal incontinence, 42-43, 65
Analgesics, 84-85, 94-96, 134
Anergy, in nutrition evaluation, 121-122
Annual review, 22-24
Anorexia nervosa, 118
Anthropometrics, in nutrition evaluation, 121-122
Antibiotics, 50-51, 52, 54
Anticholinergics, 39, 40
Anticonvulsants, 162t
Antidepressants, 83-84, 95
Antiemetics, 95
Antimicrobial therapy, 50-51, 52, 54
Antipsychotic drugs; *see* Psychoactive drugs
Appetite stimulants, 124
Arthritis
  drug treatment of osteoarthritis, 84-85
  stroke rehabilitation and, 135
Aspirin, 134

Assistive devices
  for ambulation, 137
  for feeding, bathing, and dressing, 137
Autonomy of residents, 143-144; *see also* Decision making;
  Protection

B

Bacteremia, 47, 48t, 52
Bacteriuria, 33-34, 36, 51-52
Bacteroides fragilis, 70
Balance impairment, falls and, 106, 108-109, 110-111
Bathing, rehabilitation services, 138
Bed-bound patients, positions of, 64f, 66
Bed sores; *see* Pressure ulcers
Beds
  for pressure ulcers, 68-69
  transfer to wheelchairs from, 138
Beneficence, 145, 151
Benzodiazepines, 79, 81, 83
  for delirium, 164
  for dementia, 162t, 163
  elimination half-lives, 83
Beta-blockers, 79, 162t, 163
Bethanechol, 40
Biofeedback, for pain management, 97
Bladder function, record-keeping, 32, 33f
Bladder-neck suspension and pelvic prolapse repair, 40
Bladder relaxant medications, 39, 40
Bladder retraining protocols, 36-38
Bowel function
  laxatives and stool softeners and, 85
  record-keeping, 32, 33f
Bowel-training programs, 42-43
Braden Scale, 65
Breast cancer screening, 22
Buspirone, 161, 162t

C

Caffeine, 82
Calcium
  in hip fracture prevention, 86
  supplementation, 125

Caloric needs, determining, 122
Cancer screening, 22
Canes, 137t
Capsaicin, 96
Carbamazepine, 96, 162t, 163
Cardiopulmonary resuscitation, 149
Cardiovascular disease prevention, 86
Catastrophic reactions, 161t
Cathartic syndrome, 85
Catheters, in urinary incontinence, 41-42
Cellulitis, 52
Cervical cancer screening, 22
Chlorpromazine, side effects, 82t
Chlorprothixene, side effects, 82t
Cholesterol, in nutrition evaluation, 121
Chronic obstructive pulmonary disease, 120, 123
   rehabilitation and, 135, 136
Clonazepam, 96
Clostridium difficile colonization and colitis, 54-55
Cognitive impairment
   assessment, 19
   falls and, 105, 106
   nutrition and, 119
   pain and, 92-93
Colitis, from *Clostridium difficile,* 54-55
Collagen, periurethral injections, 40
Communication, 8-9
Consent, informed, 147
Constipation, 42, 85, 95
Continuing care
   acute and subacute problems, 20-21
   annual review, 22-24
   periodic monitoring practices, 21t
   periodic visits, 20
COPD, 120, 123
   rehabilitation and, 135, 136
Coronary artery disease, stroke rehabilitation and, 134-135
Costs; *see* Economics
Coumadin, 133, 134
CPR, 149
Cruzan, 148
Cushions, for chair-bound patients, 67
Cutaneous infections, 52

D
Debridement, for pressure ulcers, 68
Decision making
   advance directives, 147-148
   capacity, competence, and consent, 146-147
   about life-sustaining treatment, 148-149
   pharmacotherapeutic, 87
   surrogate, 147
Decubitus ulcers; *see* Pressure ulcers
Deep venous thrombophlebitis, 133, 134
Dehydration, 125-126
Delirium, 163
   dementia vs., 165
   diagnostic evaluation, 164
   management, 164
   rehabilitation and, 133, 135
   screening, 163-164

   superimposed on dementia, 165
Delusions, 161t
Dementia, 155
   behavioral symptoms, 158
   delirium superimposed on, 165
   delirium vs., 165
   evaluation, 156
   falls and, 105, 106
   management, 156, 158
      nonpharmacologic, 158-159, 160-161t
      pharmacologic, 159, 161, 162t, 163
   pain and, 92-93
   screening, 155-156
   sedation in, 81-82
   tube feedings and, 123-124
Demographic trends, 4
Depression, 165
   antidepressant drugs, 83-84, 95
   assessment, 19
   protein energy undernutrition from, 118
   rehabilitation and, 135-136
   tube feedings and, 123
Desipramine, 83, 95-96
Detrusor hyperactivity, 31-32, 39
Diabetes mellitus, nutrition in, 125
Diarrhea, 54-55, 122
Diet; *see also* Nutrition
   low-salt, low-cholesterol, 120
Digoxin, 78
Diphenhydramine, 83
Dizziness, falls and, 105, 111
Dressing, rehabilitation services, 138
Dressings for pressure ulcers, 66, 67, 68
Drop attacks, 106
Drug use, 77-90
   analgesics, 94-96, 97
   antibiotics, 50-51, 52, 54
   commonly prescribed drugs, 78t
   decision making, 87
   for delirium, 164
   for dementia, 159, 161, 162t, 163
   drug-nutrient interactions, 121t
   falls and, 106, 107, 111
   histamine-2 blockers, 86
   inappropriate prescriptions, 77, 79
   laxatives and stool softeners, 85
   in long-term care, 77
   for mild to moderate pain, 84-85
   preventive care and, 85-86
   protein energy undernutrition from, 118
   psychoactive drugs, 10, 80-84, 95, 150
   regimen accretions and holidays, 77-79
   rehabilitation and, 133-134
   research recommendations, 87-88
   unique aspects of nursing home setting and, 79-80
Duodenal feeding tubes, 122-123
Durable power of attorney, 147
Dysphagia
   nutrition and, 119
   stroke rehabilitation and, 135
   workup and treatment, 138

E

Economics
of drug use, 80
of histamine-2 blockers, 86
of pressure ulcer treatment, 70
reimbursement of physicians, 10
Edema, incontinence and, 36
Education of physicians, 11-12
Electrical nerve stimulation, transcutaneous, 96-97
Elimite, 53
Enoxaparin, 133
Enteral nutrition, 122-124
Enterobacter, 51
Enterococcus, 51
Environmental assessment, in falls, 111-112
Erythema, nonblanchable, 67
Escherichia coli, 51
Estrogen therapy, 36, 39, 163
Ethical and legal issues, 143-154
decision making, 146-149
ethical principles, 145-146
nursing home environment, 143-145
protection, 149-152
Ethics committees and consultations, 151-152
Evaluation of nursing home residents, 15-26
for admission, 18-19
for continuing care
acute and subacute problems, 20-21
annual review, 22-24
periodic monitoring practices, 21t
periodic visits, 20
for falls, 107-109
federal rules and role of interdisciplinary team, 16-18
for incontinence, 32-35
for infection, 49-50
for mental status, 155
cognitive impairment, 19
delirium, 164-165
dementia, 156, 165
flow chart, 157f
for nutrition, 120-122
for pain, 92-93
points of emphasis by type of resident, 16t
for rehabilitation, 132, 136
Exercise
in falls prevention, 110
nutrition and, 126

F

Falls, 103-115
causes, 104-106
diagnostic approach, 107-109
epidemiology, 103-104
risk factors, 106-107
therapy and prevention, 109-110
devices for fall prevention, 112-113
dizziness syndromes, 111
environmental assessment, 111-112
exercise training, 126
gait and balance impairments, 110-111
nursing interventions, 112

polypharmacy and inappropriate medications, 111
postural hypotension, 111
weakness and impaired function, 110
Famciclovir, 55
Fecal impaction, 36, 42
Fecal incontinence, 42-43, 65
Federal regulation of nursing home care, 3, 9-10, 16-18, 80;
see also Omnibus Budget Reconciliation Act
Feeding, rehabilitation services, 138
Feeding tubes, 122-124
withdrawal of, 149
Fentanyl citrate, transdermal, 95
Fever, 48-49, 50; *see also* Infections
Fidelity, 145-146
Fludrocortisone acetate, 111
Fluid intake, 125-126
Fluoxetine, 84, 95
Fluphenazine, side effects, 82t
Flurazepam, 83
Fractures
hip
nutrition and, 125
prevention, 86
rehabilitation, 132-133
tube feedings and, 123
Functional assessment, for falls, 108-109
Functional incontinence, 31t

G

Gait disorders
falls and, 104-105, 106, 108-109, 110-111
rehabilitation and, 136-137
Gastrostomy tubes, 123
Gylceryl trinitrate, 124
Goals of nursing home care, 15
Gram-negative bacilli, 50-51, 52
Gram stain, in urinary tract infections, 52

H

Haemophilus influenzae, 50, 51
Haloperidol, 81, 82
for dementia, 162t
side effects, 82t
Hearing assessment, 19
Heels, pressure ulcer prevention for, 66-67
Heparin, 134
Herpes zoster, 55
Hip fractures
nutrition and, 125
prevention, 86
rehabilitation, 132-133
Hip protective pads, 113
Histamine-2 blockers, 86
History (medical)
for falls, 108
for incontinence, 33
for nutrition, 120
Holter monitoring, in falls evaluation, 109
Hospitalization, for infection, 50
H_2-receptor antagonists, 86
Huntington chorea, 119

Hydrocolloid dressings, for pressure ulcers, 68
Hyperglycemia, 125
Hyperlipidemia, 86
Hyperparathyroidism, 119
Hypertension, 86, 135
Hyperthyroidism, 119
Hypnosis, for pain management, 97
Hypnotics, 82-83
Hyponatremia, 126
Hypotension, postural, falls and, 105-106, 111

I
Ibuprofen, 84-85
Imipramine, 39, 40, 95
Immobility, pressure ulcers and, 64, 66
Immunizations, 56-57, 85
Incompetence, decision making and, 147
Incontinence; *see* Fecal incontinence; Urinary incontinence
Infections, 47-60
  clinical manifestations, 48-49
  Clostridium difficile, 54-55
  diagnostic approach, 49-50
  epidemiology in nursing homes, 47-48
  herpes zoster, 55
  hospitalization for, 50
  immunizations, 56-57, 85
  methicillin-resistant *Staphylococcus aureus,* 53-54
  pneumonia, 50-51
  prevention, 85
  skin, 52-53; *see also* Pressure ulcers
  supportive management, 50
  tuberculosis, 54
  urinary tract, 33-34, 36, 51-52
Influenza vaccine, 56, 85
Informed consent, 147
Institute of Medicine, 3
Interdisciplinary team, 7-8, 17t, 18
  for pressure ulcers, 70-71
Isoniazid, 55, 85

J
Jejunostomy tubes, 123
Joint replacement, rehabilitation, 133
Justice, 146

K
Klebsiella, 51
Kwell, 53

L
Laboratory tests
  in delirium, 164
  in dementia, 156
  in falls evaluation, 109
Lactulose, 85
Lawsuits, 91, 113, 151; *see also* Ethical and legal issues
Laxatives, 42, 43, 85
Legal issues; *see* Ethical and legal issues
Legionella, 50
Legislation for nursing home care, 3, 9-10, 16-18, 80;
  see also Omnibus Budget Reconciliation Act

Life-sustaining treatment, deciding about, 148-149
Light therapy, in dementia, 159
Lipid-lowering drugs, 86
Lithium, 163
Living wills, 147
Lorazepam, 162t
Lower extremity orthotics, 137t
Loxapine, side effects, 82t
Lymphocytes, in nutrition evaluation, 122

M
Malabsorption, 120
Malnutrition, 117-120; *see also* Nutrition
  pressure ulcers and, 64-65
Mattresses, for pressure ulcers, 66
Medical directors, 10-11
Medical evaluation; *see* Evaluation of nursing home residents
Medical records, for incontinence, 32, 33f
Medicare, 10
  coverage for rehabilitation services, 131-132
Medications; *see* Drug use
Medroxyprogesterone acetate, 124
Memory disturbance, 160t
Mental abilities, assessment, 19
Mental disorders; *see also* Cognitive impairment; Delirium;
  Dementia
    delirium, 163-165
    dementia, 155-163, 165
    depression, 165
    evaluation and management, 155-168
    flow chart, 157f
    schizophrenia, 166
Meperidine, 95
Metabolic rate, resting, calculating, 122
Metabolism, weight loss and, 117-118, 119
Metaclopramide, 40
Methadone, 95
Methicillin-resistant *Staphylococcus aureus,* 53-54
Metronidazole, 55, 69
Mexiletine, 96
Minerals, 117
Mini-Mental State Examination, 19
Minimum Data Set, 9, 17-18, 19
  areas covered by, 17t
  incontinence and, 29
  mental disorders and, 156
  pressure ulcers and, 65
Mobility
  impairment assessment, 19
  rehabilitation services, 137-138
Molindone, side effects, 82t
Monitoring, periodic, 21t
Morphine, 91, 94-95, 97
Multidisciplinary team, 7-8, 17t, 18
  for pressure ulcers, 70-71
Muscle weakness, falls and, 104, 110
Mycobacterium tuberculosis, 54

N
Nasoenteric tubes, 122
Nausea, opiate-induced, 95

Neuroleptics, 159, 162t, 164
Nitric oxide, 120
Nonmaleficence, 150
Nonsteroidal anti-inflammatory drugs, 84-85, 94, 134
Norton Scale, 65
Nortriptyline, 83, 135
NSAIDs, 84-85, 94, 134
Nurse practitioners, 8
Nurses, 5-6
Nursing Home Quality Reform Act regulations, 144
Nursing home residents; *see* Residents of nursing homes
Nursing homes
  as setting for care, 4-6
  communication with physicians, 8-9
  environment, ethics and, 143-145
  historical perspective, 3
  visit codes, 11t
Nursing interventions, in falls, 112
Nutrition, 117-129
  appetite stimulants, 124
  decision making and, 149
  drug-nutrient interactions, 121t
  evaluation, 120-122
  fluid intake and dehydration, 125-126
  hip fracture and, 125
  in diabetes mellitus, 125
  management, 122-123
  physical activity and, 126
  pressure ulcers and, 64-65
  protein energy undernutrition, 117-120
  tube feedings, new indications, 123-124
  vitamins, 124, 125t

O

Obesity, 117
OBRA; *see* Omnibus Budget Reconciliation Act
Omnibus Budget Reconciliation Act, 9, 16-17, 166
  incontinence and, 16-17
  Nursing Home Quality Reform Act regulations, 144
  psychotropic drugs and, 150, 159, 163
  rehabilitation and, 131
  restraints and, 149-150
Opiates, 91, 94-95, 97, 134
Oral health, nutrition and, 119
Orthopedic rehabilitation, 132-134
Orthostatic hypotension
  falls and, 105-106, 111
  rehabilitation and, 135
Orthotics, lower extremity, 137t
Osteoarthritis
  drug treatment, 84-85
  stroke rehabilitation and, 135
Osteomyelitis, 53, 70
Overflow incontinence, 31t, 40
Oxazepam, 83, 162t
Oxybutynin, 39
Oxycodone, 134

P

Pads for incontinence, 40-41
Pain, 91-99

assessment, 92-93
epidemiology, 92
management, 91, 92, 93-94
  future directions, 97
  "high-tech" strategies, 97
  nonpharmacologic strategies, 96-97
  prescribing analgesic drugs, 94-96
  rehabilitation and, 133-134
  sensitivity, 91-92
Paranoia, nutrition and, 118-119
Parkinson disease, 119, 139
Paroxetine, 95
Pentacozine, 95, 134
Peptic ulcers, from NSAIDs, 94
Perphenazine, side effects, 82t
Phenylpropanolamine, 39-40
Pheochromocytomas, 119
Physical activity, nutrition and, 126
Physical examination
  for falls, 108
  for incontinence, 33
Physical restraints, 149-150
  falls and, 112-113
Physical therapy; *see also* Rehabilitation
  for pain management, 96
Physician assistants, 8
Physicians
  evaluation by; *see* Evaluation of nursing home residents
  in nursing homes, 6
  roles of, 3-13
    clinical skills, 6-7
    communication, 8-9
    education, 11-12
    medical director, 10-11
    patient advocate, 8
    quality improvement, 9-10
    team approach to care, 7-8
    visits and reimbursement, 10, 11t
Pindolol, 162t
Pneumococcal vaccine, 56, 85
Pneumonia, 50-51
Polyurethane dressings, for pressure ulcers, 67
Positions of bed-bound patients, 64f, 66
Postherpetic neuralgia, 55
Postural hypotension
  falls and, 105-106, 111
  rehabilitation and, 135
Postvoid residual volume, estimate of, 34
PPD test, 22
Prazosin, 40
Pressure-relieving devices, 66
Pressure ulcers, 61-74
  causes, 62
  definitions and stages, 61-62
  epidemiology, 63
  guidelines, for clinical practice, 71
  infected, 53
  multidisciplinary care and other resources, 70-71
  outcomes, 69-70
  prevention, 63-64
    follow-up and reassessment, 67

Pressure ulcers—continued
  identifying patients at risk, 64-65
  measures for, 65-67
  study methods, 61
  treatment, 53
    full-thickness skin loss (stage 3), 68-69
    full-thickness skin loss with extensive destruction
      (stage 4), 69
    newer forms, 69
    nonblanchable erythema (stage 1), 67
    partial-thickness skin loss (stage 2), 68
  trends over time, 71
Prompted voiding protocol, 38-39
Propantheline, 39
Propoxyphene, 95, 134
Propranolol, 162t
Prospective payment system, 4
Prostaglandins, 84
Prostate cancer screening, 22
Prosthetic training for amputees, 136
Protection, 149
  abuse of residents, 150-151
  ethics committees and consultations, 151-152
  psychotropic medication, 150
  resident participation in research, 151
  restraints, 149-150
  risk management, 151
Protein energy undernutrition, 117-120
Proteus, 51
Pseudoephedrine, 39
Pseudomonas aeruginosa, 52, 70
Psychoactive drugs
  antidepressants, 83-84
  in dementia, 159, 161, 162t, 163
    sedation, 81-82
  hypnotics, 82-83
  for protection, 150
  regulations, 10, 80
  side effects, 82t
Pulmonary emboli, 133, 134
Purified protein derivative test, 22
Pyrazolones, 94

Q
Quality improvement, 9-10

R
Readmission evaluation, 19
Records, for incontinence, 32, 33f
Regulation of nursing home care, 3, 9-10, 16-18, 80; *see also*
  Omnibus Budget Reconciliation Act
Rehabilitation, 131-142
  assessment, 132
  challenges in provision of services, 138-140
  long-term services, 136
    ambulation, 136-137
    feeding, bathing, and dressing, 138
    mobility, 137-138
  Medicare reimbursement criteria, 132
  principles, 131
  services, 131-132

  short-term programs, 132
    amputation, 136
    older medical/surgical patients, 136
    orthopedic patients, 132-134
    stroke, 134-136
Reimbursement
  Medicare, for rehabilitation services, 131-132
  of physicians, 10
Relaxation, for pain management, 97
Research
  on drug use, 87-88
  resident participation in, 151
Residency training programs, 12
Resident Assessment Protocols, 9-10, 17-18
  areas covered by, 17t
  for incontinence, 29
Residents of nursing homes
  becoming a resident, 143-144
  characteristics, 4, 5t, 143
  communication with physicians, 8
  types, 15, 16t
Respect , 145
Respiridone, 82
Resting metabolic rate, calculating, 122
Restlessness, 160t
Restraints, 149-150
  falls and, 112-113
Rheumatoid arthritis, stroke rehabilitation and, 135
Rifampin, 54
Risk management, 151

S
Salicylates, 94
Sarcoptes scabies, 53
Scabies, 53
Schizophrenia, 166
Screening
  for delirium, 163-164
  for dementia, 155-156
  in annual review, 22, 23t
Sedation, in dementia, 81-82
Sensory loss, pressure ulcers and, 64, 66
Sepsis, pressure ulcers and, 69-70
Serotinergic agents, 161, 162t
Service utilization patterns, 4-5
Skin infections, 52
Skin loss, 68-69
Sleep
  day-night reversal in, 160t
  hypnotics and, 82, 83
Social Security Act, 3
Sorbitol, 85
Staffing patterns, 5-6
Staphylococcus aureus, 50, 51, 52, 70
  methicillin-resistant, 53-54
State regulation, 10
Stool softeners, 85
Strength training, 126
Streptococci, beta-hemolytic, 52
Streptococcus pneumoniae, 50-51
Stress incontinence, 31t, 39-40

Stress tests in incontinence, 35
Stroke rehabilitation, 134-136
Substituted judgment, 147
Surrogate decision making, 147
Swallowing disorders
  nutrition and, 119
  stroke rehabilitation and, 135
  workup and treatment of dysphagia, 138
Syncope, falls and, 106

T
Tardive dyskinesia, 82
Team approach to care, 7-8, 17t, 18
  for pressure ulcers, 70-71
Terazosin, 40
Tetanus toxoid vaccine, 56-57
Thioridazine, 81
  for dementia, 162t
  side effects, 82t
Thiothixene, side effects, 82t
Thrombophlebitis, deep venous, 133, 134
Tocainide, 96
Toilets, transfer from wheelchairs to, 138
Tooth loss, nutrition and, 119
Toxin assay, 54-55
Training of physicians, 12
Tramadol, 96
Transcutaneous nerve stimulation, 96-97
Transfers, 137-138
Trazodone, 161, 162t
Treatment withdrawal, 148-149
Triazolam, 83
Tricyclic antidepressants, 83-84
Trifluoperazine, side effects, 82t
Trigeminal neuralgia, 96
Tube feedings, 122-124
Tuberculin skin test, 54
Tuberculosis, 22, 54, 85, 120

U
Ulcers
  peptic, from NSAIDs, 94
  pressure; *see* Pressure ulcers
Undergarments for incontinence, 40-41
Urge incontinence, 31t, 40
Urinalysis, in incontinence, 33-34
Urinary incontinence, 29-45

assessment, 32-35
  conditions requiring further evaluation, 34t
  estimate of postvoid residual volume, 34
  history, 33
  physical examination, 33
  urinalysis, 33-34
  urodynamic tests, 35
causes, 30-32
pressure ulcers and, 65
prevalence and morbidity, 29
therapy approaches
  behavioral interventions, 36-39
  catheters and catheter care, 41-42
  drugs, 39-40
  pads and undergarments, 40-41
  reversible factors, 35-36
  surgery, 40
  types, 31-32
Urinary sphincters, artificial, 40
Urinary tract infections, 33-34, 36, 51-52
Urodynamic tests, 35

V
Vaccines, 56-57, 85
Vaginitis, atrophic, 36
Valproate, 96
Vancomycin, 53, 55
Verbal agitation, 161t
Violence, 161t
Vitamin B_{12} deficiency, 124
Vitamin C, 124, 125t
Vitamin D, 86, 125
Vitamins, 117, 124, 125t
Vulnerability, of residents, 144-145

W
Walkers, 137t
Wandering, 160t
Warfarin sodium (Coumadin), 133, 134
Weakness, falls and, 104, 110
Weight loss, nutrition and, 117, 120, 121
Wheelchairs, 137, 138
Wound care, for pressure ulcers, 53, 67-69

Z
Zinc, diabetes mellitus and, 125
Zolpidem, 83